T0257851

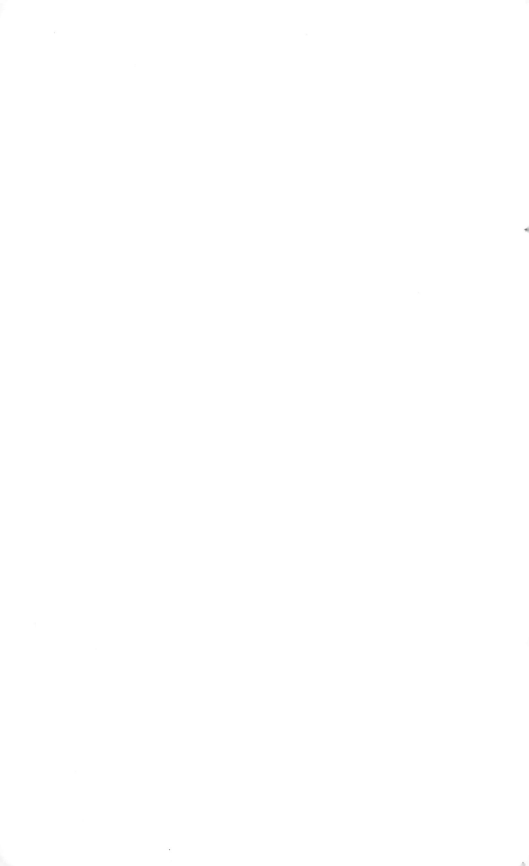

Diagnosis and Management of Tuberculosis

Diagnosis and Management of Tuberculosis

Edited by **Morris Beckler**

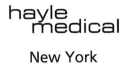

New York

Published by Hayle Medical,
30 West, 37th Street, Suite 612,
New York, NY 10018, USA
www.haylemedical.com

Diagnosis and Management of Tuberculosis
Edited by Morris Beckler

© 2015 Hayle Medical

International Standard Book Number: 978-1-63241-109-9 (Hardback)

Printed in the United States of America.

Contents

Preface

Data is being readily compiled from across the globe at a very fast rate about the efficiency of standardized treatment regimens for different forms of tuberculosis (TB) including drug-resistant TB, drug-sensitive TB and latent TB infection. At a time when we are facing the threat of multi drug-resistant TB [MDR-TB], development of extensively drug-resistant TB [XDR-TB] has threatened to undermine global efforts at TB control. This book covers in-depth analysis of all the developments and aspects of the diagnosis and management of MDR-TB. The transforming clinical presentation of TB, progresses in laboratory, therapeutic measures, imaging diagnostic modalities and rise of MDR-TB all indicate an imperative need for a revised book on TB. Moreover, while physicians face the fatal disease of TB in their clinical practice, there have been several misunderstandings and controversies regarding various issues for the management and diagnosis of TB. The book covers topics like immune-pathology, epidemiology, identification, treatment and novel developments in TB, focusing on the global perspective of TB. The aim of this book is to serve as a valuable source of reference and guidance for the people who are involved in the management of TB as well as for the practicing physicians (especially, pulmonologists and internists).

The information shared in this book is based on empirical researches made by veterans in this field of study. The elaborative information provided in this book will help the readers further their scope of knowledge leading to advancements in this field.

Finally, I would like to thank my fellow researchers who gave constructive feedback and my family members who supported me at every step of my research.

Editor

Pathophysiology and Immunogenesis of Tuberculosis

Mycobacterium tuberculosis
Adaptation to Survival in a Human Host

Beatrice Saviola

Additional information is available at the end of the chapter

1. Introduction

Mycobacterium tuberculosis exists exclusively as a pathogen of humans and in some cases of animals. It is not thought to exist in the environment other than for brief periods during transfer from an infected host to an uninfected contact. Thus *M. tuberculosis* must adapt to an *in vivo* environment by modifying gene expression. Differential expression can occur in immune cells such as macrophages, larger immune structures such as granulomas, and within liquefied lesions of the lung. Within the human body tubercle bacilli experience reactive oxygen intermediates as well as acidity within the phagosomes of macrophages. In addition within the centers of caseating granulomas bacilli experience low oxygen tension as well as toxic lipases and proteases released by dead immune cells. High temperature is present within the body of a person with active tuberculosis in the form of a fever. There may be other unrecognized signals and stresses that modulate gene expression within invading *M. tuberculosis* bacilli as well. Examination of gene expression during *in vivo* growth, within macrophages, or during application of specific stresses can illuminate which critical pathways in the mycobacterium are upregulated that lead to an *M. tuberculosis* bacillus exquisitely adapted to *in vivo* survival.

2. Adaptation to growth in the phagosomal compartment of macrophages

Macrophages are the preferred intracellular location for *M. tuberculosis in vivo*. Infected individuals cough and expel droplet nuclei which contain *M. tuberculosis* bacilli and remain suspended in the air. After inhalation and within the body, the bacilli are transported to the small alveoli in the lungs where they encounter alveolar macrophages which are relatively nonactivated (Dannenberg, 1993; Dannenberg, 1997). These nonactivated macrophages are not efficient at killing or retarding growth of invading microbes. Initially bacilli are taken up into phagosomal compartments and may replicate. As the immune system becomes activated, macrophages are stimulated with INF-γ to increase their efficiency of mycobacterial killing, becoming more efficient at producing reactive oxygen intermediates and acidic stress. In response, *M. tuberculosis* pushes back against the macrophages and differentially regulates key genes. Within macrophages *M. tuberculosis* increases its lipid metabolism which may reflect an environment in the phagosome which lacks available carbohydrates (Table. 1). In addition the enzyme isocitrate lyase (*icl*) is strongly induced *in vivo*, and *icl* is upregulated in all macrophage models. Icl is a key enzyme in the glyoxylate shunt and utilizes fatty acids as an energy source. When *icl* and other genes in the glyoxylate shunt are mutated this results in attenuation *in vivo*. In addition within macrophages, genes involved in stress responses, cell wall component production, anaerobic respiration, siderophore production to scavenge iron, diverse sigma factor production, and tranposases that may mutate the genome are all upregulated (Schnappinger et al, 2003, Beste et al, 2007, Ward et al, 2010).

3. Adaptation to granulomas and caseation

Once infection has progressed, tubercle bacilli replicate within incompletely activated macrophages. Additional macrophages arrive to the site of infection, and engulf newly liberated mycobacteria. The immune cells, T-cells, arrive to this location and an immune structure, the granuloma, composed of macrophages and a mantel of T-cells develops. If the host is resistant, and can robustly activate the body's macrophages, then *M. tuberculosis* infection is likely controlled. If the host immune system is weak, or is weakened, *M. tuberculosis* can replicate in the incompletely activated macrophages. Genes of *M. tuberculosis* required to resist macrophages will be important in resisting the environment of the granuloma as well. As the infection progresses in susceptible individuals, the centers of the granulomas degenerate and form a caseous, or cheesy, center. At the heart of this is an elevated lipid metabolism of the host that produces a variety of lipids including cholesterol, cholesteryl esters, triacyglycerol and others (Kim et al, 2010). Interestingly *M. tuberculosis* infection has been shown to induce elevated lipid metabolism in the host (Table 1.). The cell wall lipid of *M. tuberculosis*, trehalose dimycolate or cord factor, induces a granulomatous response in mice, and this was accompanied by foam cell formation which contains elevated lipids (Kim et al, 2010). It is intriguing to speculate that *M. tuberculosis* infection can induce elevated host lipid metabolism, and as discussed previously as part of adaptation to *in vivo* growth, *M. tuberculosis* also switches to lipid metabolism and lipids as a preferred carbon source (Eisenreich et al, 2010). Thus *M. tuberculosis* induces the host to produce what the microbe has evolved to utilize as an energy source.

4. Liquefied lesions and sputum

Later in infection caseating granulomas continue to breakdown. At a certain point these granulomas begin to liquefy, and host lipases and proteases are present which damage host tissues. Dead macrophages release lytic enzymes, and bacterial products may also result in host tissue damage and liquefaction ensues. As tissue is damaged, a cavity erodes into the lung airspace. In rabbit studies, *M. tuberculosis* can replicate to extremely high levels in this liquefied environment (Dannenberg 1993, Dannenberg et al 1997, Dannenberg 2006). For the first time *in vivo M. tuberculosis* is capable of replicating extracellularly. Liquid containing free *M. tuberculosis* is expelled through cavities in the lung by coughing.

M. tuberculosis within sputum contains elevated levels of lipid bodies and tends to be inhibited in its replicative process (Table 1.) (Garton et al, 2008). In addition, sputum transcriptome analysis of *M. tuberculosis* reveals that triacylglycerol synthase, *tgs1* part of the DosR regulon, is induced and lipid bodies may be composed of increased stores of triacylglycerol (Garton et al, 2008). Lipid bodies are correlated *in vitro* with nonreplicating persistence, and may help *M. tuberculosis* survive the harsh environment *ex vivo* before it encounters another human host.

5. *Mycobacterium tuberculosis* and dormancy

One third of the world's population is infected with *M. tuberculosis* in part because it causes a latent or dormant infection in a majority of those infected. If therapies are to be developed which can eradicate *M. tuberculosis,* a better understanding of dormancy is required. *M. tuberculosis* can persist for decades in a dormant state within hypoxic granulomas in the lung. Studies have suggested that in a dormant state *M. tuberculosis* is occupied mainly with maintaining cell wall integrity, membrane potential, and protecting its DNA structure. The mycobacterium must also resist the host's immune system. A number of *in vivo* and *in vitro* models have been used to investigate dormancy. These models include exposing mycobacteria to environments that are likely encountered within the host. In one model cultures are stirred slowly and sealed so that oxygen is gradually consumed. In another model nutrient starvation of the bacteria may induce dormancy. In addition, infection of mice, partial treatment with antibiotics, and exposure to immune suppression can lead to dormancy and reactivation (Murphy and Brown, 2007).

The gene encoding a transcriptional regulator, *dosR (devR),* part of a two component system that responds to low oxygen seems to be very important in a shift from replicating *M. tuberculosis* to a nonreplicating form (Table 1.). Carbohydrate limitation also upregulated *dosR* and there is indeed an overlap of genes upregulated in phagosomes of macrophages and low carbohydrate availability. In dormancy models aerobic respiratory metabolism was down regulated while anaerobic respiration was upregulated as were DosR controlled genes (Murphy and Brown, 2007). Amino acid and carbon starvation results in the activation of the stringent response. RelA (Rv2583c) mediates this stringent response in *M. tuberculosis* and can globally down regulate components necessary in protein translation, and thus conserve badly needed resources in the mycobacterium during times of stress. RelA may be a target to prevent *M. tuberculosis* from entering dormancy or a target to force *M. tuberculosis* out of dormancy (Murphy and Brown, 2007).

The ability of *M. tuberculosis* to survive in a dormant state relies on maintaining cell integrity, viability, and a proton motive (Rustad et al, 2008). Entry into a dormant state may be followed later by reactivation and growth of this microorganism, and may occur due to waning immunity, age, or disease. T-cells originally controlling infection may become less activated and numbers of T-cells may decrease allowing mycobacteria increased ease of replication in host macrophages. *M. tuberculosis* needs energy to exit this dormant phase, and this may be found in the form of triacylglycerol which is known to accumulate in response to acidic stress, nitric oxide exposure, and lowered oxygen tension (Table 1.) (Sirakova et al, 2006; Garton et al, 2008). In fact triacylglycerol has been shown to be important to transition from dormancy to active growth (Low et al, 2009). The highly pathogenic strain of *M. tuberculosis*, the Beijing lineage strain, over produces triacylglycerol perhaps giving the microorganism a competitive edge in resisting hypoxic stress and dormancy (Fallow et al, 2010).

6. *Mycobacterium tuberculosis* responses to acidic stress

M. tuberculosis encounters acidity in the body in a number of locations including within immune cells, macrophages. When macrophages phagocytose tubercle bacilli, phagosomes of unactivated macrophages are limited in their ability to acidify due to the presence of live *M. tuberculosis*. Bacilli can inhibit phagosomal maturation and also inhibit phagosome lysosome fusion (Armstrong and Hart, 1971; Sturgill-Koszycki et al, 1994; Huynh and Grinstein, 2007). Virulent *M. tuberculosis* can exclude a proton ATPase from the phagosome in non-activated macrophages. Exposure to the cytokine INF-γ can result in increased activation of macrophages and these macrophages that phagocytose live virulent *M. tuberculosis* can lower the intra phagosomal pH (Schaible et al,1998; Via et al, 1998; MacMicking et al, 2003; Ehrt and Schnappinger, 2009). This pH's can be toxic to bacilli either killing them, or inhibiting their growth. The robustness of the response seems to lie in the activation and efficiency of the host's immune response. Anything that interferes with the host's immune status can negatively impact acidic modulation within phagosomes, and lead to more mycobacterial replication. In addition, the tubercle bacillus' ability to respond to acidic stress will likely affect the outcome of the infection.

Mycobacteria seem to bear an intrinsic ability to resist acidic stress. They have a thick waxy cell wall as well as an outer membrane that can resist acidic stress. This physical barrier may serve to inhibit entry of toxic protons, and anything that interferes with this barrier could increase acid susceptibility. Many mutants that are acid susceptible lie in genes that affect cell wall and lipid metabolism (Table 1.). Environmental mycobacteria are found in conditions that may be acidic and can grow at pHs as low as 4.0 (Santos et al, 2007). Pathogenic mycobacteria have evolved to resist acidic stress, and potentially share similar mechanisms with their environmental cousins (Kirschner et al, 1992; Kirschner et al, 1999).

Although *Mycobacterium smegmatis* has been found to have an acid tolerance system it is not known if *M. tuberculosis* also possesses one. However, a large number of genes are upregulated due to acidic stress in *M. tuberculosis*. Interestingly when *M. tuberculosis* is engulfed by the phagosomes of macrophages many genes are upregulated, and when cocanamycinA is added which interferes with the development of acidity, 80% of genes in *M. tuberculosis* that are normally upregulated in the phagosomes fail to do so (Rohde et al; 2007). This is an indication that acidity is one of the main environmental signals *M. tuberculosis* experiences *in vivo*.

A number of genes that are upregulated by acidic stress have been identified in previous studies. Looking at rapid response to acidity at 15 or 30 minutes it was found that genes involved in cell wall ultrastructure were induced (Fisher et al, 2002). The *mymA* operon was induced in this study, and is under the control of VirS which is an AraC/XylS family transcription factor (Singh et al, 2005). The *lipF* promoter of *M. tuberculosis* is upregulated, but requires a longer time frame (Saviola et al, 2001). It fails to be upregulated at 30 minutes, instead needing more extended exposure to acidic stress of 1.5 hours. LipF is annotated to be an esterase and may also function to alter the cell wall structure. LipF has been shown to be part of the two component system *phoP/R* regulon. In fact many genes involved in the PhoP/PhoR regulon including *pks2*, *pks3*, and *pks4* are responsive to acidic stress (Table 1.) (Gonzalo-Asensio et al, 2009; Rohde et al, 2007). Thus PhoP/R may be responding to acidic stress or conversely PhoP/R controls a downstream regulator that responds to acidity. The *ompATb* gene encodes a porin that is active specifically at low pH and functions to pump ammonia into the phagosomal environment which serves to neutralize acidity (Song et al, 2011). Longer term exposure to acidic stress seems to stimulate production of triacylglycerol. *Tgs1* is not upregulated by short term acid exposure but exposure of three weeks duration or more (Sirakova et al, 2006; Low et al, 2009; Deb et al, 2009). Triacylglycerol production may be important for mycobacteria to resist stress and survive a dormant period which is induced by stress conditions. An energy source such as triacylglycerol may be needed to reanimate from dormancy once stresses such as acidity are removed. Mutatagenesis studies also revealed genes involved cell wall/cell envelope synthesis when mutated resulted in mycobacteria which were unable to maintain neutral pH within their microbial cytoplasm in the presence of acidic stress (Vandal et al, 2008; Vandal et al, 2009, Biswass et al, 2010).

The type VII secretion system, Esx-1, may also may be involved in response to acid stress (Abdallah et al, 2007). The 6 kDa early secreted antigenic target (Esat-6) and the 10kDa culture filtrate protein (CFP-10) are secreted by Esx-1. These two proteins form a heterodimer that can dissociate at acidic pH. Esat-6 is capable of lysing membranes, and *M. tuberculosis* has been identified to reside extraphagosomally in the cytoplasm of macrophages in some cases. In addition when the *esx-1* gene was mutated it could result in an *M. tuberculosis* strain that fails to escape from the phagosomal compartment into the cytoplasm (Simeone et al, 2009). Thus Esat-6 may be involved in mycobacterial responses to acidity and adaptation to *in vivo* stressors.

7. Response to oxidative damage

Inside phagosomes of activated macrophages tubercle bacilli are exposed to reactive oxygen intermediates. *M. tuberculosis* traffics to phagosomes, and a large number of genes are upregulated by oxidative stress indicating this is an important stress *in vivo* (Wu et al, 2007). In addition nutrients are limited in the phagosome which may cause *M. tuberculosis* to enter a stationary phase of growth, which has been shown to induce internal oxidative damage. The gene *whiB1* is more active during stationary phase, and the protein produced by this gene has been shown to reduce cellular disulphide bridges that may predominate during this adaptational phase (Garge et al, 2009).

Mycobacteria contain a unique substance, mycothiol, which combats oxidative stress. Other bacterial species utilize glutathione which can also neutralize oxidative stress. Mycothiol contains cysteine residues which are oxidized when that condition predominates thus forming disulfide bonds, creating mycothione, and preventing other molecules in the mycobacterial cell from becoming oxidized (Table 1.). Human cells produce glutathione to combat oxidative damage, and glutathione is toxic to mycobacterial cells perhaps due to a redox imbalance generated by this substance in the mycobacteria (Venketaraman et al, 2008; Connell et al, 2008)). Mycobacteria also contain other molecules to detoxify oxidative damage including superoxide dismutase (SOD) and catalase (KatG) which can inactivate superoxide (Table 1.) (Shi et al, 2008). SOD and KatG are upregulated early in infection indicating an increase in oxidative damage due to superoxide. Oxidative damage is capable of harming DNA, and histone like proteins (LSR2) can protect against damage by compacting DNA and acting as a physical barrier. UvrB which repairs mycobacterial DNA damage also protects against oxidative damage (Darwin and Nathan, 2005; Colangeli et al, 2009).

8. Heat shock

One of the hallmarks of tuberculosis is fever and night sweats in which body temperature increases and is suboptimal for *Mycobacterium tuberculosis* replication and survival. This allows the immune system a competitive edge over the invading microbes. Heat stress can cause damage to *M. tuberculosis* by causing proteins to unfold which may then be degraded. In response, *M. tuberculosis* can upregulate chaperonins which complex with unfolded proteins and help them refold (Table 1.). The α-crystalline protein, or Acr-2, is activated by heat shock, and has demonstrated chaperonin activity (Pang and Howard, 2007).

Many proteins that are upregulated in *M. tuberculosis in vivo* are heat shock proteins that have chaperonine activity. While these proteins may benefit the organism by complexing with and refolding heat damaged proteins, they are also recognized by the immune system. Both the 65Kd heat shock protein and the HSP70 protein can be found extracellularly to *M. tuberculosis,* and are potent stimulators of an inflammatory response (Anand et al, 2010).

9. Low iron

Normally iron taken up by intestinal epithelial cells and bound to transferrin circulates within the body. This complex binds to cell surface receptors, and is internalized where it releases its iron to be bound by the host cellular factor ferritin. Infection and inflammation are natural signals to the host to limit availability of iron. Proinflammatory cytokines stimulate hepcidin production, decrease iron uptake from the gut, and inhibits the iron efflux protein ferroportin (Johnson and Wessingling-Resnick, 2012). Inflammation thus inhibits iron uptake by the intestinal epithelium thus preventing iron from being loaded onto transferrin. Interfering with uptake limits iron availability in the host, and M. *tuberculosis* has been shown to be severely growth restricted in a low iron environment. It has been demonstrated in African studies that iron supplementation increases incidence of tuberculosis. Thus being anemic may be protective against infectious processes. Within human macrophages, Nramp1 (natural resistance associated macrophage protein) is produced and localizes to the phagosomal compartment where it reduces iron within this site possibly by extrusion. This function confers resistance to M. *tuberculosis* infections and mutations in the *nramp1* gene can result in increased susceptibility to active disease due to M. *tuberculosis* infection (Johnson and Wessingling-Resnick, 2012).

Mycobacteria have a variety of systems which aid in the uptake of iron and the regulation of iron responsive genes. As mycobacteria have been shown to be somewhat novel among gram positive bacteria, they possess an outer mycolic acid based membrane, as well as an inner membrane and periplasmic space. Porins in the outer membrane appear to transport iron in the presence of high iron conditions (Jones and Niederweis, 2010). M. *tuberculosis* under low iron conditions can produce the siderophore carboxymycobactin as well as mycobactin (Table 1.) (Banerjee et al, 2011). These molecules bind with a higher affinity to iron than the human host's storage proteins and steal iron from the host. Mycobactin is present within the inner membrane and thus can only bind iron imported into the periplasmic space. Interestingly lipid membranes with associated mycobactins may diffuse out, travel to lipid vesicles in the host cell, and sequester iron. These structures may recycle back to interact with the mycobacterium. Disruption of the genes responsible for production of mycobactins can cause these mutant mycobacteria to replicate less well in macrophages (Banerjee et al, 2011). Carboxymycobactins are excreted possibly by the type VII secretion or ESX system. Externally the carboxymycobactins bind available iron from transferrin (Banerjee et al, 2011). Porins and also ABC transporters may allow import of these iron loaded carboxymycobactins (Banerjee et al, 2011). The host cell, in response to infection and inflammation, produces siderocalins such as lipocalin-2 that can bind to and inactivate mycobactin from M. *tuberculosis* thus interfering with mycobacterial iron acquisition (Johnson and Wessingling-Resnick, 2012). In fact mice deleted for genes involved in production of siderocalin are much more susceptible to mortality due to M. *tuberculosis* infection (Johnson and Wessingling-Resnick, 2012). Inside the mycobacterial cell, iron is stored in bacterioferritin and a ferritin like protein. These proteins are required for replication in human macrophages and guinea pigs, act to store iron, and also to limit excess iron in the cells that can lead to iron mediated oxidative damage due to the Fenton reaction (Reddy et al, 2011).

Iron responsive genes in M. *tuberculosis* are controlled in part by the iron dependent regulator IdeR. This protein can act both as an activator and a repressor depending on where it binds within a mycobacterial promoter region (Manabe et al, 1999; Banerjee et al, 2011). Within promoters of genes involved in mycobactin synthesis it acts as a repressor, inhibiting expression of these genes at high iron concentrations. In promoters of iron storage proteins it acts as an activator, stimulating expression of these genes at high iron concentrations and thus avoiding iron stimulated oxidative damage.

10. Hypoxic growth

In vivo M. tuberculosis experiences low oxygen tension that may be encountered in the centers of granulomas as previously described. Studies have shown that tuberculous granulomas are hypoxic in a variety of animal models including rabbits, guinea pigs, and nonhuman primates (Via et al, 2008). The response to low oxygen tension is biphasic. There is an initial response that predominates and is controlled by the two component system DosS/DosT-DosR (Table 1.). This two component system upregulates genes that are known to be part of the "dormancy regulon". DosR is the transcriptional regulator, and Dos T and DosS are the sensor kinases that respond to low oxygen tension as well as nitric oxide (Park et al, 2003; Kumar et al, 2007). *hspX* (*acr, Rv2031c)* is upregulated by low oxygen, is regulated by DosR, and has chaperonin activity that may aid in refolding proteins which are damaged by low oxygen tension (Vasudeva-Rao and McDonough, 2008; Florczyk et al, 2003). It is known that this protein is expressed *in vivo* as latently infected individuals possess T-cells that are reactive to the HspX protein (Geluk et al, 2007). Interestingly one half of the genes in the DosR regulon return to their baseline level after 24 hours. After this initial 24 hour period other regulators play a role in hypoxic responses such as sigE and sigC (Table 1.). An enduring hypoxic response begins after the initial response, and this may be important for *M. tuberculosis* to enter and stay in a dormant state (Rustad et al, 2008).

11. Toxin-antitoxin systems

Interestingly there are many toxin-antitoxin systems within the *M. tuberculosis* genome. These systems seem to provide a mechanism by which bacteria can alter growth rate rapidly, potentially in response to environmental stressors. The toxin is not a protein secreted and targeted against the human host, but targeted against mycobacterial cellular components. The toxin is a stable protein which may be complexed with an antitoxin forming a toxin-antitoxin pair. The antitoxin is relatively unstable and environmental stressors can inactivate it causing release of a free toxin. The toxin is then available to interact with cellular components, and may function to cleave mRNA thus inhibiting subsequent translation and rapidly halting growth of the bacterium. As static bacteria are more resistant to environmental stressors and antibiotics, this system may allow *M. tuberculosis* to survive in the face of external stressors. *M. tuberculosis* possesses 88 toxin-antitoxin systems and four of these have been shown to be activated by phagocytosis of bacilli, by macrophages, or hypoxia (Table 1.). It appears that the toxin in these systems acts by cleaving mRNA (Rapage et al, 2009).

In Vivo Condition or Location	Mycobacterial Response
macrophages, granulomas, liquified lesions and sputum	increased lipid metabolism in bacillus, or induction of same in host
macrophages, granulomas, low iron	Siderophore production
all stress conditions, macrophages, granulomas, sputum	differential sigma factor utilization
liquified lesions, sputum, conditions leading to dormancy	lipid body production
low oxygen, macrophages, conditions leading to dormancy	DosR two component system activity
low oxygen, macrophages, possibly acidity	PhoP two component system activity
In all conditions *in vivo*	Constitutive thick waxy cell wall construction, may be upregulated
oxidative stress, macrophages	Mycothiol, SOD, & KatG production
Fever	Heat shock protein production
macrophages, phagocytosis, hypoxia	toxin-antitoxin system function

Table 1. Mycobacterial responses to in vivo stressors and conditions.

12. Two component systems

Two components systems are common in many bacteria. These systems are comprised of a sensor kinase which phosphorylates the response regulator as a result of an environmental signal, which is often a stress. The sensor kinases are trans membrane proteins which are embedded into membranes. They sense external stresses and transmit these signals internally into the bacterial cell by phosphorylating a response regulator that binds to its cognate promoter DNA, and regulates transcription. The mycobacterial genome contains 11 two component systems (Hett and Rubin, 2008). The large number of these systems in the myco-bacterial coding regions is likely the result of evolution to accommodate bacterial responses to diverse stresses.

DosS/DosT-DosR was previously described, and responds to initial hypoxic stress (Table 1.) (Park et al, 2003). Some of the genes controlled by the transcriptional regulator DosR are upregulated by hypoxic stress, and are also part of the transcriptional regulator PhoP regulon, a member of the PhoP/R two component system. While it is unknown what environmental signal PhoP or the sensor kinase PhoR are responding to, genes controlled by PhoP either directly or indirectly are upregulated by such stresses as acidity and low oxygen (Table 1.) (Gonzalo-Asensio et al, 2008).

13. Sigma factors

Mycobacterial RNA polymerase catalyzes RNA synthesis from specific promoter sequences. This RNA polymerase is composed of subunits that comprise the core holoenzyme, and include two α subunits, a β, a β' and a ω subunit. The core enzyme, however, cannot target specific promoter sequences. A sigma factor is required for this function, and can bind and recognize specific -10 and -35 promoter sequences. As the mycobacterial genome possesses many different sigma factors, these RNA polymerase components can recognize diverse mycobacterial promoter sequences to activate a whole class of genes. This activity is in addition to specific transcription factors which bind to promoters, regulate transcription, and are not part of the RNA polymerase enzyme.

The mycobacterial genome possesses many different sigma factors that belong to different categories. The *M. tuberculosis* σ^A is responsible for regulating housekeeping genes, and is also an essential gene for mycobacterial growth *in vitro* and *in vivo*. While the sigma factor σ^B is highly similar to σ^A, it is nonessential and is induced by a variety of stresses including oxidative stress, heat shock, cold shock, stationary phase, and low aeration (Lee et al, 2008). There are a number of sigma factors designated to have extracellular function, and some respond to environmental stresses and are involved in the synthesis of the mycobacterial envelope. These sigma factors are SigC, SigE, SigF, SigG, SigH, SigI, SigJ, SigK, SigL, and SigM. One sigma factor that is known to respond to nutrient starvation is SigF. The sigma factor SigE is involved in response to heat shock and SDS exposure (Manganelli et al, 2004). Both SigJ and SigF are induced in response to antibiotic exposure (Manganelli et al, 2004). The sigma factor SigH also responds to heat shock and oxidative stress (Manganelli et al, 2004). Thus the use of sigma factors by the mycobacterial cell is a manner in which "master regulators" can control whole classes of genes to rapidly facilitate gene regulation in response to specific environmental stresses (Table 1.).

14. Summary

As mycobacteria invade their human hosts they must respond to a plethora of stresses many of which are generated by the host's immune system. Under this selective pressure, *M. tuberculosis* has evolved mechanisms to combat the toxic insults of the host. Although mycobacteria are inherently resistant to environmental stresses due to their thick waxy cell envelope, upregulation of genes further reinforce this defense. In addition there are proteins upregulated by environmental stressors which can detoxify the mycobacterial cell as is the case of acidic stress and upregulation of ammonia extruding pumps that neutralize acidic pH of the macrophage phagosome. Thus inducible systems allow *M. tuberculosis* to resist environmental stresses and persist in the human body to cause active or latent disease.

Understanding the specific steps in infection, the stresses associated with each step, and the mycobacterial response may be of clinical relevance. The knowledge that oxidative stress and acidic stress may predominate as adaptive immunity makes the host's macrophages more activated, may lead to the development of chemotherapeutic agents that target mycobacterial components produced by these stressors during this infective stage. In addition, the knowledge that mycobacteria may utilize toxin-antitoxin systems to slow their growth and to enhance their innate antibiotic resistance may spur the development of therapies that target these systems which could be used in conjunction with traditional antibiotic treatments. Chemotherapeutic agents given to decrease activity of triacylglycerol synthase may decrease infectivity of sputum positive individuals by inhibiting lipid body production in the bacilli while antibiotic treatment lags in its sterilizing activity. Ultimately treatments may be developed which target inducible systems upregulated by stresses, and may interfere with mycobacterial responses to these stressors. By thwarting these adaptive responses potentially with chemotherapeutic agents, mycobacteria may be rendered more fragile and susceptible to the host's immune system. In addition a greater understanding of how *M. tuberculosis* enters a latent state of persistence could lead to treatments that prevent this microbe from reactivating from the dormant state, or from becoming dormant to begin with. Greater understanding of *M. tuberculosis* responses to *in vivo* growth will hopefully lead to the development of technologies that lessen *M. tuberculosis'* global impact on human health.

Author details

Beatrice Saviola

Basic Medical Sciences, College of Osteopathic Medicine, Western University of Health Sciences, Pomona CA, USA

References

[1] Abdallah A, Gey van Pittius N, Champion P, Cox J, Luirink J, Vandenbroucke-Grauls C, Appelmelk B, and Bitter W. 2007. Type VII secretion-mycobacteria show the way. Nature Reviews in Microbiology. 5: 883-891.

[2] Anand PK, Anand E, Bleck CKE, Anes E, Griffiths G. Exosomal Hsp70 induces a pro-inflammatory response to foreign particles including mycobacteria. Plos One. 5(4):e10136. (2010)

[3] Armstrong JA, and Hart D. 1971. Response of cultured macrophages to *Mycobacterium tuberculosis* with observations on fusion of lysosomes with phagosomes. Journal of Experimental Medicine. 134(3): 713-740.

[4] Banerjee S, Farhana A, Ehtesham N, and Hasnain SE. 2011. Iron acquisition, assimilation, and regulation in mycobacteria. Infect., Gentics and Evol. 11:825-838.

[5] Beste DJV, Laing E, Bonde B, Avignone-Rossa C, Bushell ME, and McFadden JJ. 2007. Transcriptomic analysis identifies growth rate modulation as a component of the adaptation of mycobacteria to survival inside the macrophage. J. Bact. 189:3969-3976.

[6] Biswas T, Small J, Vandal O, Odaira T, Deng H, Ehrt S, and Tsodikov OV. 2010. Structural insight into serine protease Rv3671c that protects *M. tuberculosis* from oxidative and acidic stress. Structure. 18(10): 13353-1363.

[7] Colangeli R, Haq A, Arcus VL, Summers E, Magliozzo RS, McBride A, Mitra AK, Radjainia M, Khajo A, Jacobs WR, Salgame P, Alland A. The multifunctional histone-like protein Lsr2 protects mycobacteria against reactive oxygen intermediates. PNAS. 106(11):4414. (2009)

[8] Connell ND, Venketaraman V. Control of mycobacterium tuberculosis infection by glutathione. Recent Pat Antiinfect Drug Discov. 4(3):214.(2009)

[9] Dannenberg AM (2006) Pathogenesis of Human Pulmonary Tuberculosis: Insights from the Rabbit Model. ASM Press, Washington, DC.

[10] Dannenberg AM, Tomashefski JF. Pulmonary diseases and disorders. In A. P. Fishman (ed.), Pathogenesis of pulmonary tuberculosis. McGraw-Hill, New York, N.Y. (1997)

[11] Dannenberg AM. Immunopathogenesis of Pulmonary tuberculosis. Hosp Pract (off Ed) 28:51–58.

[12] Darwin HK, and Nathan CF. Role of nucleotide excision repair in virulence of *Mycobacterium tuberculosis*. Infect and Immun. 73(8):4581. (2005)

[13] Deb C, Lee CM, Dubey VS, Daniel J, Abomoelak B, Sirakova S, Pawar S, Rogers L, Kolattukudy PE. 2009. A novel *in vitro* multiple-stress dormancy model for *Mycobacterium tuberculosis* generates a lipid-loaded, drug-tolerant, dormant pathogen. Plos One 4(6):e6077.

[14] Ehrt S, and Schnappinger D. 2009. Mycobacterial survival strategies in the phagosome: defense against host stresses. Cellular Microbiology. 11(8):1170-1178.

[15] Eisenreich W, Dandekar T, Heesemann J, and Goebel W. 2010. Carbon metabolism of intracellular bacterial pathogens and possible links to virulence. Nature Reviews Microbiology. 8: 401-412.

[16] Fallow A, Domenech P, Reed MB. Strains of the east Asian (W/Beijing) lineage of *Mycobacterium tuberculosis* are DosS/DosT-DosR two-component regulatory system natural mutants. J. Bact. 192(8):2228. (2010)

[17] Fisher MA, Plikayatis BB,and Scinnick TM. 2002. Microarray of the *Mycobacterium tuberculosis* transcriptional response to the acidic conditions found in phagososmes. Journal of Bacteriology. 184(14): 4025-4032.

[18] Florczyk MA, McCue LA, Purkayastha A, Currenti E, Wolin MJ, McDonough KA. A family of acr-coregulated *Mycobacterium tuberculosis* genes shares a common DNA motif and requires Rv3133c (dosR or devR) for expression. Infect. Immun. 71(9):5332. (2003)

[19] Garg S, Alam MS, Bajpai R, and Kishan KV, Agrawal P. Redox biology of *Mycobacterium tuberculosis* H37Rv: protein-protein interaction between GlgB and WhiB1 involves exchange of thiol-disulfide. BMC Biochemistry doi:10.1186/1471-2091-10-1. (2009)

[20] Garton NJ, Waddell SJ, Sherratt AL, Lee S, Smith RJ, Senner C, Hinds J, Rajakumar K, Adegbola RA, Besra GS, Butcher PD, and Barer MR. 2008. Cytological and Transcript Analysis Reveal Fat Lazy Persister-Like Bacilli in Tuberculous Sputum. Plos Medicine 5:e75

[21] Geluk A, Lin MY, van Meijgaarden KE, Leyten EMS, Franken KLMC, Ottenhoff THM, Klein MR. T-cell recognition of the HspX protein of *Mycobacterium tuberculosis* correlates with latent *M. tuberculosis* infection but not with *M. bovis* BCG vaccination. Infect. Immun. 75(6):2914. (2007)

[22] Gonzalo-Asensio J, Mostowy S, Harders-Westerveen J, Huygen K, Hernandez-Pando R, Thole J, Behr M, Gicquel B, Martin C. Plos One. 3(10):e3496. (2008)

[23] Hett E, Rubin EJ. 2008. Micro and Mol. Bio. Bacterial growth and cell division: a mycobacterial perspective.Rev. 72(1):432.

[24] Huynh KK, and Grinstein S. 2007. Regulation of vacuolar pH and its modulation by some microbial species. Micobiology and molecular biology reviews. 71(3):452-462.

[25] Johnson EE, and Wessling-Resnick M. 2011. Iron Metabolism and the innate immune response to infection. Microb. and Infect. 14:207-216.

[26] Jones CM, and Niederweis M. 2010. Role of porins in iron uptake by *Mycobacterium smegmatis*. J. Bact. 192:6411-6417.

[27] Kim M, Wainwright HC, Locketz M, Bekker L, Walther GB, Dittrich C, Visser A, Wang W, Hsu F, Wiehart U, Tsenova L, Kaplan G, and Russell DG. 2010. EMBO Mol Med 2(7):258-274.

[28] Kirschner RA, Parker BC and Fakinham JO. 1992. Epidemiology of infection by non-tuberculous mycobacteria. X. *Mycobacterium avium, Mycobacterium intracellulare*, and *Mycobacterium scrofulaceum* in acid brown-water swamps of the Southeastern United States and their association with environmental variables. American Review of Respiratory Disease. 1145:271-275.

[29] Krischner RA, Parker BC, and Falkinham JO. 1999. Humic and fluvic acids stimulate growth of *Mycobacterium avium*. FEMS Microbiology Ecology. 30:327-332.

[30] Kumar A, Toledo JC, Patel RP, Lancaster JR, Steyn AJC. 2007. *Mycobacterium tuberculosis* DosS is a redox sensor and DosT is a hypoxia sensor. PNAS. 104(28):11568.

[31] Lee J, Karakousis PC, Bishai WR. 2008. Roles of SigB and SigF in the *Mycobacterium tuberculosis* sigma factor network. J. Bact. 190(2):699.

[32] Low KL, Rao PSS, Shui G, Bendt AK, Pathe K, Dick T, and Wenk MR. 2009. Triacyl-glycerol utilization is required for regrowth of in vitro hypoxic nonreplicating *Mycobacterium bovis* bacillus Calmette-Guerin. Journal of Bacteriology. 191(16): 5037-5043.

[33] MackMicking JD, Taylor GA, and McKinney JD. 2003. Immune control of tuberculosis in IFN-γ-inducible LRG 47. Science. 302:654-659.

[34] Manganelli R, Proveddi R, Rodrigue S, Beaucher J, Gaudreau L, Smith I. 2004. Sigma factors and global gene regulation in *Mycobacterium tuberculosis*. J. Bact. 186(4):895.

[35] Murphy DJ, and Brown, JR. 2007. Identification of gene targets against dormant phase Mycobacterium tuberculosis infections. BMC Infect. Dis. 7: 1-16

[36] Pang X, Howard ST. 2007. Regulation of the alpha-crystallin gene acr2 by the MprAB two-component system of *Mycobacterium tuberculosis*. J. Bact. 189(7):6213.

[37] Park HD, Guinn KM, Harrell MI, Liao R, Voskuil MI, Tompa M, Schoolnick GK, Sherman DR. 2003. Rv3133c/dosR is a transcription factor that mediates the hypoxic response of Mycobacterium tuberculosis. Mol. Mirobiol. 48(3):833.

[38] Ramage HR, Connolly LE, Cox JS. 2009. Comprehensive functional analysis of *Mycobacterium tuberculosis* toxin-antitoxin systems: implications for pathogenesis, stress responses, and evolution. Plos Genetics. 5(12):e1000767.

[39] Rao, SPS, Alonso S, Rand L, Dick T, Pethe K. 2008. The protonmotive force is required for maintaining ATP homeostasis and viability of hypoxic, nonreplicating *Mycobacterium tuberculosis*. PNAS. 105(33):11945.

[40] Reddy PV, Puri RV, Khera A, and Tyagi AK. 2011. Iron storage proteins are essential for survival and pathogenesis of *Mycobacterium tuberculosis* in THP-1 macrophages and the guinea pig model of infection. J. Bact. 194:567-575.

[41] Rohde K, Yates RM, Purdy GE, and Russell DG. 2007. *Mycobacterium tuberculosis* and the environment within the phagosome. Immunological Reviews. 219: 37-54.

[42] Rustad TR, Harrell MI, Liao R, Sherman DR. 2008. The enduring hypoxic response of Mycobacterium tuberculosis. Plos One 1:e1502.

[43] Santos R, Fernandes J, Fernandes N, Oliveira F, and Cadete M. 2007. *Mycobacterium parascrofulaceum* in acidic hot springs in Yellowstone National Park. Applied Environmental Microbiology. 73(15) 5071-5073.

[44] Saviola B, Woolwine S, and Bishai W. 2002. Isolation of acid-inducible genes of *Mycobacterium tuberculosis* with the use of recombinase based in vivo expression technology. Infection and Immunity. 71(3): 1379-1388.

[45] Schaible RH, Sturgill-Koszycki S, Schlesinger PH, and Russell DG. 1998. Cytokine activation leads to acidification and increases maturation of *Mycobacterium avium*-containing phagosomes in murine macrophages. Journal of Immunology. 160: 1290-1296.

[46] Schnappinger D, Ehrt S, Voskuil MI, Liu Y, Mangan JA, Monahan IM, Dolganow G, Efron B, Butcher PD, Nathan C, and Schoolnik GK. 2003. Transcriptional adaptation of *Mycobacterium tuberculosis* within macrophages: insights into the phagosomal environment. J. Exp. Med. 189:693-704.

[47] Shi L, Sohaskey CD, North RJ, Gennaro ML. 2008. Transcriptional characterization of the antioxidant response of *Mycobacterium tuberculosis in vivo* and during adaptation to hypoxia in vitro. Tuberculosis. 88(1):1.

[48] Simeone R, Bottai D, and Brosch R. 2009. ESX/type VII secretion systems and their role in host-pathogen interaction. Current Opinion in Microbiology. 12:4-10.

[49] Singh A, Gupta R, Vishwakarma RA, Narayanan PR, Paramasivan CN, Ramanathan VD, and Tyagi AK. 2005. Requirement of *mymA* operon for appropriate cell wall ultrastructure and persistence of *Mycobacterium tuberculosis* in the spleens of guinea pigs. Journal of Bacteriology. 187(12):4173-4186.

[50] Sirakova TD, Dubey VS, Deb C, Daniiel J, Korotkova TA, Abomoelak B, and Kolattukudy PE. 2006. Identification of a diacylglycerol acyltransferase gene involved in accumulation of triacyglycerol in Mycobacterium tuberculosis under stress. Microbiology. 152: 2717-2725.

[51] Song H, Huff J, Janik K, Walter K, Keller C, Ehlers S, Bossman SH, and Niederweis M. 2011 Expression of the *ompATb* operon accelerates ammonia secretion and adaptation of *Mycobacterium tuberculosis* to acidic environments, Molecular Microbiology. 80(4): 900-18.

[52] Sturgill-Koszycki S, Schlesinger PH, Cjakraborty P, Haddix PL, Collins HL, and Fok AK. 1994. Lack of acidification in Mycobacterium phagosomes produced by exclusion of the vesicular proton-ATPase. Science 263:678-681.

[53] Vandal OH, Nathan CF, and Ehrt S. 2009. Acid resistance in *Mycobacterium tuberculo-sis*. Journal of Bacteriology. 191(15):4714-4721.

[54] Vandal OH, Pierini LM, Schnappinger D, Nathan CF, and Ehrt S. 2008. A membrane protein preserves intrabacterial pH in intraphagosomal *Mycobacterium tuberculosis*. Nature Medicine. 14(8): 849-854.

[55] Vandal OH, Roberts JA, Odaira T, Schnappinger D, Nathan C, and Ehrt S. 2009. Acid-suceptibility mutants of *Mycobacterium tuberculosis* share hypersusceptibility to cell wall and oxidative stress and to the host environment. Journal of Bacteriology. 191(2): 625-631.

[56] Vasudeva-Rao HM, McDonough KS. 2008. Expression of the Mycobacterium tuber-culosis acr-coregulated genes from the DevR (DosR) regulon is controlled by multi-ple levels of regulation. Infect Immun. 76(6):2478.

[57] Venketaraman V, Millman A, Salman M, Swaminathan S, Goetz M, Lardizabal A, Hom D, Connell ND. 2008. Glutathione levels and immune responses in tuberculosis patients. Microb. Pathog. 44(3):255.

[58] Via LE, Fratti RA, McFalone M, pagan-Ramos E, Deretic D, and Deretic V. 1998. Ef-fects of cytokines on mycobacterial phagosome maturation. Journal of Cell Science. 111:897-905.

[59] Via LE, Lin PL, Ray SM, Carillo J, Allen SS, Eum SY, Taylor K, Klein E, Manjunatha-nU, Gonzales J, Lee EG, Park SK, Raleigh JA, Cho SN, McMurray DN, Flynn JL, Bar-ry CE. 2008. Tuberculous granulomas are hypoxic in guinea pigs, rabbits, and nonhuman primates. Infect Immun. 76(6):2333.

[60] Ward SK, Abomoelak B., Marcus SA, and Talaat A. 2010. Transcriptional profiling of Mycobacterium tuberculosis during infection: lessons learned. Froteirs in Microbiolo-gy. 1: 1-9.

Chapter 2

The Role of Antibodies in the Defense Against Tuberculosis

Armando Acosta, Yamile Lopez,
Norazmi Mohd Nor, Rogelio Hernández Pando,
Nadine Alvarez, Maria Elena Sarmiento and
Aharona Glatman-Freedman

Additional information is available at the end of the chapter

1. Introduction

Throughout history tuberculosis (TB) has been a health problem for humanity. In the beginning of civilization, when human population densities were sparse, this disease may have been fairly harmless. However, with the increase in population densities, probably from the 17th to 19th centuries, TB took epidemic proportions [1].

Bacille Calmette Guérin (BCG) is effective to prevent miliary and meningeal TB in infants [1]. The reports about the efficacy of this vaccine for the prevention of adults pulmonary TB are contradictory and the consensus is that the protection conferred by BCG against this form of TB is questionable [1]. The wide use of BCG vaccination has been unable to prevent nearly two million deaths associated with TB that are produced every year. Currently the World Health Organization no longer recommends BCG vaccination in children born from HIVpositive mothers which complicate the implementation of BCG vaccination programs [2]. The implementation of standard drug treatment for TB is difficult in the areas of the highest incidence of the disease. Treatment is further complicated by the limited effectiveness of the current therapeutic schemes against drug resistant strains of TB [3-5].

Nowadays there is an increasing realization of the need for new animal models to test vaccine efficacy in more realistic scenarios, overcoming the limitations of current models in use. In addition, the elucidation of the significance of antibody-mediated defense against intracellular pathogens, in particular against *Mycobacterium tuberculosis*, constitutes an exciting new approach to improve the rational design of new vaccines, therapies and diagnostics.

2. Specific antibodies: Players in the defense against TB

In order to develop improved vaccines and new methods for controlling TB, an important element is the discovery of markers to measure the effectors' mechanisms of the protective immune response against *M. tuberculosis*.

For many years Cell-Mediated Immunity (CMI) was viewed as the exclusive defense mechanism against intracellular pathogens. The Th1/Th2 classical paradigm prevailed for a long time and the development of vaccines followed this theory [6]. Based on this theory, only intracellular pathogens could be effectively controlled by granulomatous inflammation induced by a Th1 response, whereas a Th2 response induces antibody production that controls extracellular pathogens and parasites. However, the question of what constitutes a true demarcation between "extracellular and intracellular" pathogens is important in this regard. During their infectious cycle, intracellular pathogens could be found in the extracellular space and *vice versa*. In the specific case of *M. tuberculosis*, it can be localized extracellularly at the beginning of the infection in the upper respiratory tract as well as during advanced stages of the disease, after rupture of granulomatous lesions occur [7]. This facultative intracellular pathogen was shown to have an extracellular phase [7] [8] that may include replication [7] which in turn could potentially be targeted by specific antibodies.

There are several prokaryotic and eukaryotic intracellular pathogens for which antibody have been shown to modify the course of infection by different mechanisms, as reviewed extensively by Casadevall and colleagues [9, 10, 11]. In the case of *Erhlichia* spp., specific antibodies were shown to mediate protection [12], possibly by blocking cellular entry or promoting the expression of proinflammatory cytokines. [13,14]. A combination of both humoral and cellular immune mechanisms could be the optimal choice controlling certain intracellular pathogens,.In this regard, de Valliere and colleagues reported that human antimycobacterial antibodies enhanced Cell-Mediated Immune responses to mycobacteria that are beneficial to the host [15].

3. Epidemiological evidence of antibody mediated protection

There is accumulating evidence, in the last few decades, regarding the effect of antibodies in the context of development of pulmonary or disseminated TB. Children with low serum IgG against sonicated mycobacterial antigens and LAM, or those who could not mount antibody responses to these antigens were predisposed to dissemination of *M. tuberculosis* [16].

M. leprae reactive salivary IgA antibodies were suggested to be important in a mucosal protective immunity [17]. In study carried out among the Mexican Totonaca Indian population, the presence of high antibody titers to Ag87 complex antigens were observed in patients with non-cavitary TB and in patients who were cured with anti-TB chemotherapy. In contrast, patients without such antibodies had a poor outcome of the disease [18].

4. Experimental studies

4.1. Animal models

An important criterion for the evaluation of the role of specific antibodies in the protection against TB is the use of animal models. Currently, there is no optimal model to re-produce the infection as it occurs in humans [19].

The geographical location, genetic factors of the host, the presence of environmental myco-bacteria and other concomitant infections like helminthiasis, are factors that have to be considered when designing animal experiments [20]. Several animal models have been used to evaluate different aspects of mycobacterial infection and disease. A crucial aspect is the delivery of mycobacterial inoculum. In this regard, several routes of inoculation have been employed experimentally, including intravenous, intraperitoneal, intranasal, intratracheal and aerosol [21, 22].

The study of the distribution of monoclonal and polyclonal antibody formulations in different organs and tissues of mice after administration by different routes, including the use of backpack models have been reported [23-27]. Each model has its advantages and drawbacks.

For example, the backpack model is very useful for the evaluation of the protective role of IgA, but poses ethical problems in long term experiments due to the increase in tumour size over time produced by the inoculated hybridoma [28]. In prophylactic and therapeutic models, antibody formulations have been administered via the intranasal [29], intravenous [30] and intraperitoneal [26] routes and combined with cytokines and antibiotics [31, 32] before and/or after the infectious challenge. The administration of *M. tuberculosis* pre-coated with antibodies [27, 33] in different models of infection has also contributed to understanding the interactions between host and microbe.

Another approach has been the use of knockout mice models for IgA [34] polymeric immu-noglobulin receptor (pIgR) [34] and B cells [35,36,37,38], as will be discussed later.

4.2. Experimental studies with antibodies

A substantial number of studies utilizing anti mycobacterial antibodies have been conducted as far back as the end of the 19th century. These experiments can be grouped into several categories: serum therapies, mouse polyclonal antibodies, human polyclonal antibodies (including commercial human gamma globulins), secretory human IgA (hsIgA) and studies with monoclonal antibodies.

4.2.1. Serum therapies

Serum therapy experiments were conducted from the second half of the 19th century (reviewed in [39,40]). Immune sera was generated by immunizing animals with different mycobacterial fractions and administered either to animals or humans [39,40] The results obtained were either beneficiary, variable, inconclusive or contradictory, [39,40]. These variable results led to the perceived minor role of antibodies in the defense against *M. tuberculosis*.

What factors could have led to the heterogeneity in study results? Recognizable differences in the methods used for serum preparations and their administration, as well as the lack of appropriate experimental controls probably accounted in part for the studies outcomes. Furthermore, it is important to recognize that immune serum is a polyclonal preparation that includes antibodies with multiple specificities and isotypes. Consequently, polyclonal sera may contain antibodies of different subclasses and functional categories that can affect theoutcome of infection. For example, IgG3 murine monoclonal antibodies protected against *M.tuberculosis* [27] but failed to protect against *Cryptococcus neoformans* [41]. An IgG3 non-protectivemonoclonal antibody to *C. neoformans*, became protective upon subclass switching to IgG1 [41]. In addition to intrinsic factors associated with the antibody structure, other parameters such as the genetic background of the microbe and the immunocompetence of the host could alter the outcome of antibody protection experiments.

For some microorganisms, such as *Samonella typhimurium* and *C. neoformans,* passive antibody therapy efficacy depends on the mouse strain used [42, 43]. In the same way, some microbial strains are more susceptible to the effects of antibodies [44].

The animal model used is another important parameter that varies between different experiments cited in the literature [45]. Timing, the route of infection, the magnitude of the infecting inoculum are some additional variables that could affect antibody protection studies [46].

Despite their variability, the results obtained with serum therapy were valuable, demonstrating some beneficial effect of serum on the course of TB in humans, mainly in cases of early or localized TB [45]. Moreover, it was demonstrated that long periods of treatment were necessary to achieve a sustained effect [45].

4.2.2. Polyclonal mouse antibodies

A recent study re-examined the usefulness of immune serum in the context of a therapeutic vaccine against TB [32]. This vaccine, named RUTI, is generated from detoxified *M. tuberculosis* cell fragments that facilitate a balanced T helper response to a wide range of antigens along with intense antibody production [47]. Local accumulation of specific CD8+ T cells and a strong humoral response after immunization are characteristic features of RUTI that contribute to its protective properties. In that study, immune serum was generated by immunizing mice with RUTI [32]. Severe Combined Immunodeficiency (SCID) mice were inoculated with *M. tuberculosis* and treated with chemotherapy for 3–8 weeks. After chemotherapy they were treated for up to 10 weeks with intraperitoneal injections of the generated immune serum. Mice treated with immune serum from RUTI vaccinated animals showed significant decreases in lung CFU in addition to reduced extent of granulomatous response and abscess formation [47]. These results indicate that protective serum antibodies can be elicited by vaccination, and that antibodies may be usefully combined with chemotherapy [32, 47, 48].

4.2.3. Human gammaglobulins

4.2.3.1. Specific human polyclonal antibodies

Evidence for the stimulatory role of specific polyclonal antibodies on cellular immunity in experimental mycobacterial infections was reported by de Valliere and colleagues in 2005 [15].

In this study, serum samples containing specific antimycobacterial antibodies were obtained from volunteers vaccinated twice with BCG by the intradermal route. Significant titres of IgG antibodies against lipoarabinomannan (LAM) were detected in the sera. BCG internalization into phagocytic cells was significantly increased in the presence of these BCG induced antibodies as were the growth inhibitory effects of neutrophils and macrophages on myco-bacteria. Furthermore, these antibodies induced significant production of IFN-γ by CD4+ and CD8+ T cells [15].

4.2.3.2. Commercial immunoglobulin formulations

Human Intravenous Immunoglobulin (IVIG) has been used to treat individuals with immune deficiencies and patients with inflammatory, autoimmune and infectious conditions [49, 50, 51]. Several groups tested the effect of human immunoglobulin preparation on mycobacterial infection. Roy and colleagues showed that treatment of *M. tuberculosis* infected mice with one cycle of IVIG led to the substantially lower bacterial loads in the spleen and lungs following its administration either at early or at late stage of infection 52]. The effect of the administration of a commercial preparation of human immunoglobulin (hIg) in a mouse model of intranasal infection with BCG was evaluated by Olivares and colleagues [33]. This group demonstrated the passage of specific antibodies to saliva and lung lavage following the intranasal or intraperitoneal administration of human hIg to mice. This treatment inhibited BCG coloniza-tion of the lungs of treated mice. A similar inhibitory effect was observed after infection of mice with hIg -opsonized BCG [33].

The same formulation was evaluated also in a mouse model of intratracheal infection with *M. tuberculosis*. Animals receiving human hIg intranasally 2h prior to intratracheal challenge demonstrated a significant decrease in lung bacillary load as compared with non-treated animals [29]. When *M. tuberculosis* was pre-incubated with hIg prior to challenge the same effect was observed [29].

The protective effect of the hIg formulation was abolished following pre-incubation with *M. tuberculosis* [29]. These results are suggestive of a potential role for specific human antibodies in the defense against mycobacterial infections.

Taken together, these studies provide support for the potential use of immunoglobulins against *M. tuberculosis*.

4.2.3.3. Human secretory IgA

Human secretory IgA (hsIgA) is the major class of antibody associated with immune protection of the mucosal surfaces [53]. Colostrum volume is above 102 mL in humans during the first three days after delivery [54]. The high percentage of (hsIgA) in human colostrum [55] strongly suggests its important role in passive immune protection against gastrointestinal and respi-ratory infections [56]. In one study performed by Alvarez and colleagues, hsIgA from human colostrum was obtained by anion exchange and gel filtration chromatographic methods, using DEAE Sepharose FF and Superose 6 preparative grade, respectively [57].

hsIgA was administered intranasally to BALB/c mice, and the level of this immunoglobulin in several biological fluids was determined by ELISA. The results showed the presence of this antibody in the saliva of animals that received the hsIgA, at all time intervals studied. In tracheobronchial lavage, hsIgA was detected at 2 and 3 hours after inoculation in animals that received the hsIgA [58]. Similar studies were performed by Falero and colleagues with monoclonal antibodies of IgA and IgG class [59]. Following demostration that hsIgA could be detected in several biological secretions after intranasal administration, the protective effect of this formulation against *M. tuberculosis* challenge was evaluated. Mice challenged with *M. tuberculosis* preincubated with hsIgA showed a statistically significant decrease in the mean number of viable bacteria recovered from the lungs compared to control mice and to the group that received the hsIgA before challenge with *M. tuberculosis*. Moreover, an increased level of iNOS production was also reported (Alvarez et al., mannuscript in preparation). Consistently with this result, a better organization of granulomatous areas with foci of lymphocytes and abundant activated macrophages were observed in the lungs of mice that received *M. tuberculosis* pre-incubated with hsIgA and sacrificed at 2 months postchallenge. Untreated animals, however, showed an increased area of bronchiectasis and atelectasis as well as fibrin deposits, accumulation of activated macrophages and lymphocytes.

The pneumonic areas were more prominent in the untreated animals than in the groups treated with hsIgA and *M. tuberculosis* pre-incubated with hsIgA (Alvarez et al., manuscript in preparation)

4.2.4. Monoclonal antibodies

Since the first report on the use of the monoclonal antibody Mab 9d8 against *M. tuberculosis* [27], many similar studies have been reported [40]. This IgG3 monoclonal antibody (Mab) generated against arabinomannan (AM) capsular polysaccharide, increased the survival of intratracheally infected mice when the *M. tuberculosis* Erdman strain was pre-coated with it [27]. In this study, a longer survival associated with an enhanced granulomatous response in the lungs was found as compared to controls receiving an isotype-specific non-related Mab [27]. Another Mab, SMITB14, directed against the AM portion of LAM prolonged the survival of intravenously infected mice associated with reduced lung CFU and prevention of weight loss [60]. In this study, the authors demonstrated that protection was independent of the antibody Fc portion, because the F(ab')2 fragment also conferred a similar protective effect [60]. In another study, mice receiving the Mab 5c11 (an IgM antibody that recognizes other mycobacterial arabinose-containing carbohydrates in addition to AM) intravenously prior to Mannosylated lipoarabinomannan (ManLAM) administration, showed a significant clearance of Man-LAM and redirection of this product to the hepatobiliary system [26]. This study strongly supports an indirect effect of certain antibodies on the course of mycobacterial infection, altering problably the pharmacokinetics of mycobacterial components and contributing to protection against TB [26].

Heparin Binding Hemagglutinin Adhesin (HBHA) is a surface-exposed glycoprotein involved in the mycobacterial binding to epithelial cells and in mycobacterial dissemination [62]. Monoclonal antibodies 3941E4 (IgG2a) and 4058D2 (IgG3) directed against HBHA were used to coat mycobacteria before administration to mice. In this study, spleen CFUs was reduced while lung CFUs did not [63]. These results suggest that binding of these antibodies to HBHA can impede mycobacterial dissemination.

The protective efficacy of a monoclonal antibody, TBA63 and IgA anti-Acr administered intranasally before and after the intranasal or aerosol challenge with *M. tuberculosis* was demonstrated in a study by Williams and colleagues [64]. In another series of experiments carried out by López and colleagues, the protective effect of this Mab administered intratracheally before an intratracheal challenge with virulent mycobacteria was evaluated. At 21 days post-infection, pre-treatment of mice with TBA63 caused a significant decrease in viable bacteria in the lungs compared to control mice or those treated with the Mab against the 38-kDa protein (TBA86) [65]. Consistent with the reduction of viable bacteria following treatment with TBA63, the area of peribronchial inflammation was also statistically smaller in this group compared to the control group [65].

When the lungs of mice were histologically examined, granulomas were better organized in the infected animals that had received TBA63 than in controls or mice treated with TBA86. The reduction of CFU in lungs of the treated group was associated with milder histopathological changes, as indicated by the organization of the granulomas and less pneumonic area. The fact that this Mab promotes granuloma formation in mice infected intratracheally with *M. tuberculosis* strongly suggests the close interaction between antibody mediated immunity and cell-mediated immunity to induce protection against intracellular pathogens (66).

The 16 kDa protein (Acr antigen) has been defined as a major membrane protein peripherally associated with the membrane [67] carrying epitopes restricted to tubercle bacilli on the basis of B-cell recognition [68, 69]. The Acr antigen is present on the surface of tubercle bacilli and is highly expressed in organisms growing within infected macrophages, allowing it to be potentially targeted by specific antibodies either inside infected cells as well as extracellulary. A novel immunotherapy, combining treatment with anti-IL-4 antibodies, IgA antibody against 16 kDa protein and IFN-γ, showed the potential for passive immunoprophylaxis against TB. In genetically deficient IL-4-/- BALB/c mice, infection in both lungs and spleen was substantially reduced for up to 8 weeks. Administration of rIL-4 to IL-4-/- mice with increased bacterial counts to wild-type levels and make mice refractory to protection by IgA/IFN-γ [70].

More recently, Balu and colleagues reported that intranasal administration of a human IgA1 Mab, obtained using a single-chain variable fragment derived from an Ab phage library with high affinity for hspX and the human FcαRI (CD91) IgA receptor together with recombinant mouse IFN-γ significantly inhibited pulmonary infection with *M. tuberculosis* H37Rv in mice transgenic for human CD91 but not in the CD91-negative controls. These results suggested that binding to CD91 was necessary for the IgA-imparted passive protection [71]. When the Mab was incubated with human whole-blood or monocyte cultures it inhibited H37Rv infection.

Inhibition of the infection by the antibody was synergistic with human rIFN-γ in purified human monocytes cultures but not in whole blood cultures [71]. The demonstration of the role of FcαRI (CD91) in human IgA mediated protection contributes to understanding the mechanisms involved as well as for using this knowledge for the future development of new immunotherapies for TB [71].

4.2.5. Transgenic mice

Mouse models with deficiency in antibody production can provide useful information for understanding certain roles of antibodies in protection against mycobacterial infections. Rodríguez and colleagues reported that after immunization of IgA deficient (IgA-/-) and wild type mice by the intranasal route with the mycobacterial surface antigen PstS-1, IgA-/- mice were more susceptible to BCG infection than IgA+/+ mice [34]. Cytokine response analysis demonstrated reduction in the IFN-γ and TNF-α production in the lungs of IgA-/- as compared with IgA+/+ mice, suggesting that IgA may play a role in protection against mycobacterial infections in the respiratory tract. Furthermore, these authors demonstrated that immunized pIgR-/- mice were more susceptible to BCG infection than immunized wild-type mice [34].

In an attempt to elucidate whether antibody-mediated immunity has a special role in the defense against TB, different experiments with B cell knockout mice were performed by several authors. In 11016, Vordermeier and colleagues developed an infection model of TB in μ chain knockout Ig- mice. Organs from *M. tuberculosis* infected IgG- mice had three to eight fold elevated counts of viable bacilli compared with those from normal mice. This result suggested that B cells play a role in the containment of murine tuberculous infection [35]. In another study B cell KO mice and controls were infected by aerosol with *M. tuberculosis*. They were subsequently given chemotherapy to destroy remaining bacilli and then re-challenged by aerosol exposure. There were not differences in the ability of animals to control this second infection, indicating that, in this low dose pulmonary infection model, any local production of antibodies neither impeded nor enhanced the expression of specific acquired resistance [36].

In another series of experiments the role of B cells was evaluated during early immune responses to infection with a clinical strain of *M. tuberculosis* (CDC 1561). In this study, despite comparable bacillary loads in the lungs, B cell KO mice had a less severe pulmonary granuloma formation and delayed dissemination of bacteria from lungs to peripheral organs. Additional analysis of lung cells demonstrated higher numbers of lymphocytes, particularly CD8+ T cells, macrophages, and neutrophils in wild-type and reconstituted mice as compared with B cell KO mice. These results demonstrate that less severe granuloma formation and delayed dissemination of mycobacteria found in B cell KO mice were dependent on B cells, (not antibodies, at least in this study) and were associated with modification of cellular infiltrate in the lungs [37]. This latter result differs from a study carried out by Maglione and colleagues in which B cell-/- mice demonstrated exacerbated immunopathology corresponding with enhanced pulmonary recruitment of neutrophils following aerosol challenge with *M. tuberculosis* Erdman strain [38]. Infected B cell-/- mice demonstrated increased production of IL-10 in the lungs, while IFN- γ, TNF-α, and IL-10R were not significantly different from those of wild type mice [38].. B cell-/- mice demonstrated enhanced susceptibility to aerosol infection of 300 CFU of *M. tuberculosis* with elevated bacterial burden in the lungs but not in the spleen or liver [38].

Together these studies suggest that B cells may have an important role in host defense against *M. tuberculosis*.

5. Mechanisms of action

The various effects of antibodies demonstrated in the studies analyzed, suggest that different mechanisms of action are involved in the effect of monoclonal and polyclonal antibodies on *M. tuberculosis*. Secretions found on mucosal surfaces contain significant levels of Igs, particularly, IgA. IgA has both direct and indirect functional roles for combating infectious agents such as viruses and bacteria that cross the mucosal barrier [72]. Moreover, experimental evidence suggests that IgA associated with the pIgR may neutralize pathogens and antigens intracellularly during their transport from the basolateral to the apical zone of epithelial cells [73,74]. In addition, IgA may interact with Gal-3 (an intracellular binding β-galactosidase lectin), and interfere with the interaction of mycobacteria with the phagosomal membrane, resulting in the decrease of bacterial survival and replication in the phagosome [75].

Antibodies may be critical, during the extracellular phases of intracellular facultative pathogens. They may act by interfering with adhesion, by neutralizing toxins and by activating complement. Moreover, antibodies may be able to penetrate recently infected cells, bind internalised pathogens, and enhance antigen processing (76). Antibodies may also play a crucial role in modulating the immune response by activating faster secretion of selected cytokines that in turn, contribute to more efficient and rapid Th1 response [76,77], increasing the efficacy of co-stimulatory signals, enhancing Antibody Dependent Cellular Cytotoxicity (ADCC) and the homing of immune cells to the lungs after the respiratory infection [10,78, 79, 80, 81, 82, 83].

Examples of relevant potential action mechanisms of antibodies against *M. tuberculosis* were discussed by Glatman-Freedman [40].

6. Potential uses of antibodies against TB

Future applications of antibody formulations for the control of TB may include several possibilities including treatment, prevention and diagnosis.

6.1. Treatment

Antibody based therapy could potentially be useful in several scenarios. They could be used to shorten the standard treatment period of patients with uncomplicated TB when coupled with standard chemotherapy. However, they would be particularly important in the treatment of patients infected with Multidrug Resistant (MDR) and Extensively Drug Resistant (XDR) strains, in combination with the standard treatment.

6.2. Prophylactic use

Prophylactic use of antibodies could be applied in recent contacts of TB patients, with special attention to risk groups [84]. In this regard, successful prophylactic use of antibodies in exposed individuals has been shown in the case of several other pathogens such as varicella, tetanus, Respiratory Synsicial Virus (RSV), rabies and Hepatitis B [85, 86]

6.3. Vaccines

The induction of specific protective antibody responses by vaccination, either alone or as an addition to the stimulation of cell mediated immunity could be a novel strategy for the development of new generation of prophylactic and therapeutic vaccines against TB.

The prevailing past dogma that discounted the role of antibodies in host protection against TB has resulted in a limited study of B cell immunodominant epitopes as targets for protective immunity [87].

6.3.1. Polysaccharide conjugate vaccines

Polysaccharide conjugate vaccines are considered to elicit specific protective antibody responses against a variety of pathogens [88]. However, the polysaccharide conjugate vaccine against *Salmonella typhi* [89] demonstrates the feasibility of this kind of vaccines for the prevention of infectious diseases caused by intracellular pathogens. In the case of *M. tuberculosis*, several authors reported the use of polysaccharide conjugated vaccine candidates [61, 90, 91, 92].

All these vaccine candidates induced the production of specific IgG [61, 90, 91, 92] and some of them conferred variable levels of protection [61, 91] which validate this strategy as one of the potential avenues for the development of new generation of vaccines against tuberculosis

6.3.2. Identifying other B-cell immunodominant epitopes

With the development of bioinformatics tools for bacterial genome analysis, it has been possible to predict *in silico* microbial regions that trigger immune responses relevant for protection and vaccine development. A candidate experimental vaccine based on proteoliposomes from *M. smegmatis* is currently in development [93].

In one study, bibliographic search was used to identify highly expressed proteins in active, latent and reactivation phases of TB [94]. The subcellular localization of the selected proteins was defined according to the report on the identification and localization of 1044 *M. tuberculosis* proteins using two-dimensional, capillary high-performance liquid chromatography coupled with mass spectrometry (2DLC/MS) method [95] and using prediction algorithms. Taking into consideration the cell fractions potentially included in the proteoliposome, from the previously identified proteins, the ones located in the cell membrane and cell wall, as well as those which are secreted and homologous to those of *M. smegmatis* were selected.

The regions of the selected proteins containing promiscuous B and T cell epitopes were determined [94]. Thus the *M. smegmatis* proteoliposomes were predicted to contain multiple

B and T epitopes which are potentially cross reactive with those of *M. tuberculosis*. It is important to note that there could be conformational B epitopes and additional epitopes related with lipids and carbohydrates included in the proteoliposomes that could reinforce the humoral cross reactivity.

Considering the results of the *in silico* analysis, proteoliposomes of *M. smegmatis* were obtained and their immunogenicity was studied in mice [93]. In addition to cellular immune effectors recognizing antigens from *M. tuberculosis*, cross reactive humoral immune responses of several IgG subclasses corresponding with a combined Th1 and Th2 pattern against antigenic components of *M. tuberculosis* were elicited. These findings were in concordance with the *in silico* predictions [93, 94]. It is interesting to note that differences in the pattern of humoral recognition of lipidic components was dependent on the characteristics of the adjuvant used, which could have relevance for the development of vaccines which includes lipidic components [93]. Currently studies are underway to evaluate the protective capacity of *M. smegmatis* proteoliposomes in challenge models with *M. tuberculosis* in mice.

Bioinformatics tools for prediction of T and B epitopes were also employed for the design of multiepitopic constructions, which were used to obtain recombinant BCG strains. Based on this prediction, B cell epitopes from ESAT-6, CFP-10, Ag87B and MTP40 proteins were selected and combined with T cell epitopes of the 87B protein and fused to Mtb8.4 protein [96].

A significant IgG antibody response against specific B cell epitopes of ESAT-6 and CFP-10 was obtained in mice immunized with the recombinant strain. After studying the specific response of spleen cells by lymphoproliferation assay and detection of intracellular cytokines in CD4 + and CD8 + subpopulations, the recognition of T epitopes was also observed. The response showed a Th1 pattern after immunization with this recombinant strain (Mohamud, R, et al. manuscript in preparation). In another series of experiments, recombinant BCG strains expressing several combinations of multiepitopic constructions were used to immunize BALB/ c mice subcutaneously and challenged intratracheally with the *M. tuberculosis* H37Rv strain. Recombinant BCG strains expressing T epitopes from 87BAg fused to Mtb8.4 protein and BCG expressing a HSP62 T cell epitope plus different combinations of B cell epitopes from 87BAg, Mce1A, L7/L12, 16 kDa, HBHA, ESAT6, CFP10 and MTP40 and combinations of B cell epitopes alone produced significant reductions in lung CFU compared to BCG (Norazmi MN, et al. manuscript in preparation).

6.3.3. Diagnosis

Although no serological assays are currently recommended for diagnosis of TB [97], largely due to the possibility of false results and thus incorrect treatments, for many other pathogens, serological diagnostic tests has been of great value, particularly in poor countries. In some cases, antibody responses can constitute useful correlates of protection [98]. In the specific case of TB, several studies of the antibody response have been reported [99]. There is a substantial amount of variability in antibody response to TB [100]. This variability has been attributed to several factors. Some of these factors are associated with the pathogen (strain variation, micro-environment and growth state of bacteria) and others are related to the host, primarily previous exposure to related antigens and host genetics [99].

However, it is important to consider that only a small fraction of the genomic regions of M. *tuberculosis* encoding proteins has been explored. Currently, novel immunoassay platforms are being used to dissect the entire proteome of M. *tuberculosis*, including reacting protein microarrays with sera from TB patients and controls [101,102]. These studies could lead to the discovery of new antigens that may constitute suitable diagnostic markers and tools for the identification of protection correlates.

7. Concluding remarks

The cumulative work reviewed above with regard to the use of antibody formulations and vaccines suggest that antibodies if present at the right moment at the site of infection could provide protection against M. *tuberculosis*. This concept leads the way to the development of a new generation of vaccines. Such vaccines could work by eliciting specific IgA and/or IgG antibodies that could recognize and intercept the pathogen at the port of entry, primarily the mucosal surfaces, inactivating bacterial components essential for the microbial survival in the host, activating complement for direct lysis of the cells, opsonizing bacteria to promote their capture by phagocytic cells and inducing stimulation of specific cellular immune responses [103, 104].

Various antibody formulations could potentially be used as immunotherapeutic agents in combination with the conventional treatment and in the management of patients affected by Multidrug Resistant (MDR) and Extensively Drug Resistant (XDR) strains.

The study of the role of specific antibodies in the defense against tuberculosis opens new possibilities for future development of new vaccines, diagnostics tools and therapies against this pathogen. It is likely that new discoveries will arise from the ongoing studies in this area that will expedite the introduction of new strategies in the fight against tuberculosis.

Acknowledgements

The authors' work was partly supported by the Ministry of Science, Technology &Innovation, Malaysia [Grant No. 304.PPSK.6350081.N106 & 10-01-05-MEB002] and USM Research University Grant [1021.PPSK.832005], CONACyT (contract 86657) and the Ministry of Science and Technology, Cuba.

Author details

Armando Acosta[1], Yamile Lopez[1], Norazmi Mohd Nor[2], Rogelio Hernández Pando[3], Nadine Alvarez[1], Maria Elena Sarmiento[1] and Aharona Glatman-Freedman[4]

1 Instituto Finlay, La Habana, Cuba

2 School of Health Sciences and Institute for Research in Molecular Medicine, Universiti Sains Malaysia, Kubang Kerian, Malaysia

3 Experimental Pathology Section, National Institute of Medical Sciences and Nutrition, Mexico City, Mexico

4 New York Medical College, Valhalla, New York, USA

References

[1] Jacob JT, Mehta AK, Leonard MK. Acute forms of tuberculosis in adults. Am J Med 2009;122(1):12-7.

[2] Hesseling AC, Johnson LF, Jaspan H, Cotton MF, Whitelaw A, Schaaf HS, Fine PE,Eley BS, Marais BJ, Nuttall J, Beyers N, Godfrey-Faussett P. Disseminated bacilli Calmette-Guérin disease in HIV-infected South African infants. Bull World Health Organ. 2009;89(7):505-11

[3] Chung KT, Biggers CJ. Albert Leon Charles Calmette (1885-1954) and the antituberculous BCG vaccination. Perspect Biol Med 2001;44(3):381-91.

[4] Davies PD. Medical classics. La Boheme and tuberculosis. BMJ 2008;337:a2599.

[5] Gradmann C. Robert Koch and tuberculosis: the beginning of medical bacteriology. Pneumologie 2009;65(12):722-8.

[6] Gor DO, Rose NR, Greenspan NS. TH1-TH2: a procrustean paradigm. Nat Immunol 2003;4(6):503-5.

[7] Grosset J. *Mycobacterium tuberculosis* in the extracellular compartment: an underestimated adversary. Antimicrob Agents Chemother 2003;47(3):854-6.

[8] Li JS, Winslow GM. Survival, replication, and antibody susceptibility of *Ehrlichia chaffeensis* outside of host cells. Infect Immun 2003;73(8):4229-37.

[9] Casadevall A. Antibody-based therapies for emerging infectious diseases. Emerg Infect Dis 11016;2(3):200-8.

[10] Casadevall A, Pirofski LA. Antibody-mediated regulation of cellular immunity and the inflammatory response. Trends Immunol 2003;24(9):476-8.

[11] Casadevall A, Pirofski LA. A reappraisal of humoral immunity based on mechanisms of antibody-mediated protection against intracellular pathogens. Adv Immunol 2006;93:1-44.

[12] Kaylor PS, Crawford TB, McElwain TF, Palmer GH. Passive transfer of antibody to *Ehrlichia risticii* protects mice from ehrlichiosis. Infect Immun 11011;61(6):2059-64.

[13] Lee EH, Rikihisa Y. Anti-*Ehrlichia chaffeensis* antibody complexed with *E. chaffeensis* induces potent proinflammatory cytokine mRNA expression in human monocytes through sustained reduction of IkappaB-alpha and activation of NF-kappaB. Infect Immun 11017;67(7):2912-7.

[14] Messick JB, Rikihisa Y. Inhibition of binding, entry, or intracellular proliferation of *Ehrlichia risticii* in P390D1 cells by anti-*E. risticii* serum, immunoglobulin G, or Fab fragment. Infect Immun 11014;64(8):3157-63.

[15] de Valiere S, Abate G, Blazevic A, Heuertz RM, Hoft DF. Enhancement of innate and cell-mediated immunity by antimycobacterial antibodies. Infect Immun 2005;75(10): 6931-20.

[16] Costello AM, Kumar A, Narayan V, et al. Does antibody to mycobacterial antigens, including lipoarabinomannan, limit dissemination in childhood tuberculosis? Trans R Soc Trop Med Hyg 11012;88(6):708-94

[17] Kamble RR, Shinde VS, Madhale SP, Jadhav RS. Study of cross-reactivity of *Mycobacterium leprae* reactive salivary IgA with other environmental mycobacteria. Indian J Lepr 2009;83(2):65-8

[18] Sánchez-Rodríguez C, Estrada-Chávez C, García-Vigil J, et al. An IgG antibody response to the antigen 87 complex is associated with good outcome in Mexican Totonaca Indians with pulmonary tuberculosis. Int J Tuberc Lung Dis 2002;6(8):726-12.

[19] Ordway DJ and Orme IM. Animal models of Mycobacteria infection. Curr Protoc Immunol, 2011; Chapter 19: Unit 19.5.

[20] Rook GA, Hernández-Pando R, Zumla A. Tuberculosis due to high-dose challenge in partially immune individuals: a problem for vaccination? J Infect Dis.2009;1101(5): 633-8.

[21] Schwebach JR, Chen B, Glatman-Freedman A, Casadevall A, McKinney JD et al. Infection of mice with aerosolized Mycobcterium tuberculosis: use of a nose-only apparatus for delivery of low doses inocula and design of an ultrasafe facility. Appl.Environ.Microbiol 2002,70:4666-4669

[22] McShane H, Williams A. Preclinical evaluation of tuberculosis vaccines. In: Norazmi MN, Acosta A, Sarmiento ME, editors. *The art & science of tuberculosis vaccine development* [Internet]. 1st ed. Selangor (MY): Oxford University Press; 2010 [cited 2011 Sep 5]. p. 349-375. Available from: http://tbvaccines.usm.my/

[23] Acosta A, Sarmiento ME, Gonzalez A, et al. Histopathologic and humoral study of Balb/c mice inoculated with BCG by different routes. Arch Med Res 11014;25(2): 161-65.

[24] León A, Acosta A, Sarmiento ME, Estévez P, Martínez M, Pérez ME, Falero G, Infante JF, Fariñas M, Sierra G. Desarrollo de Biomodelos para la evaluación de la inmunidad de mucosa contra *M. tuberculosis*. Vaccimonitor, 2000;3:6-10.

[25] Acosta A, Olivares N, León A, López Y, Sarmiento ME, Cádiz A, Moya A, Falero G, Infante JF, Martínez M, Sierra G. A new approach to understand the defense mechanism against tuberculosis: role of specific antibodies. Biotecnología Aplicada 2003;20:130-133.

[26] Glatman-Freedman A, Mednick AJ, Lendvai N, Casadevall A. Clearance and organ distribution of *Mycobacterium tuberculosis* lipoarabinomannan (LAM) in the presence and absence of LAM-binding IgM. Infect.Immun. 2000,70:335-341.

[27] Teitelbaum R, Glatman-Freedman A, Chen B, Robbins JB, Unanue E et al. A mAb recognizing a surface antigen of *Mycobacterium tuberculosis* enhances host survival. Proc.Natl.Acad.Sci.USA 11018,97:15810-15815

[28] Winner L 3rd, Mack J, Weltzin R, Mekalanos JJ, Kraehenbuhl JP, Neutra MR. New model for analysis of mucosal immunity: intestinal secretion of specific monoclonal immunoglobulin A from hybridoma tumors protects against Vibrio cholerae infection. Infect Immun. 11011;61(3):997-84.

[29] Olivares N, Puig A, Aguilar D, et al. Prophylactic effect of administration of human gammaglobulins in a mouse model of tuberculosis. Tuberculosis (Edinb) 2009;91(3): 218-20.

[30] Acosta, A., Lopez, Y., Nor, N. M., Pando, R. H., Alvarez, N., & Sarmiento, M. E. (2012). Towards a New Challenge in TB Control: Development of Antibody-Based Protection. *Understanding tuberculosis; analyzing the origen of Mycobacterium tuberculosis pathogenicity. Editor: PJ Cardona. In Tech, Open Acces Publisher.*

[31] Reljic R. IFN-gamma therapy of tuberculosis and related infections. J Interferon Cytokine Res 2007;27(5):354-66.

[32] Guirado E, Amat I, Gil O, et al. Passive serum therapy with polyclonal antibodies against *Mycobacterium tuberculosis* protects against post-chemotherapy relapse of tuberculosis infection in SCID mice. Microbes Infect 2006;8(5):1253-9.

[33] Olivares N, León A, López Y, et al. The effect of the administration of human gamma globulins in a model of BCG infection in mice. Tuberculosis (Edinb) 2006;88(3-4): 270-74.

[34] Rodríguez A, Tjarnlund A, Ivanji J, et al. Role of IgA in the defense against respiratory infections IgA deficient mice exhibited increased susceptibility to intranasal infection with *Mycobacterium bovis* BCG. Vaccine 2005;23(20):2577-74.

[35] Vordermeier HM, Venkataprasad N, Harris DP, Ivanyi J. Increase of tuberculous infection in the organs of B cell-deficient mice. Clin Exp Immunol, 11016;106:312-16

[36] Johnson CM, Cooper AM, Frank AA, Bonorino CBC, Wysoki LJ. *Mycobacterium tuberculosis* aerogenic rechallenge infections in B cell.deficient mice. Tubercle and Lung Disease 11017,80(5&6), 258-263.

[37] Bosio CM, Gardner D, Elkins KL. Infection of B cell-deficient mice with CDC 1561, a clinical isolate of Mycobacterium tuberculosis: delay in dissemination and development of lung pathology. J Immunol. 2000;166(12):6637-25.

[38] Maglione PJ, Xu J, Chan J. B cells moderate inflammatory progression and enhance bacterial containment upon pulmonary challenge with *Mycobacterium tuberculosis*. J Immunol 2007,180(11):7422-34.

[39] Glatman-Freedman A, Casadevall A. Serum therapy for tuberculosis revisited: reappraisal of the role of antibody-mediated immunity against *Mycobacterium tuberculosis*. Clin.Microbiol.Rev. 11018,11:514-542

[40] Glatman-Freedman A (2010) The role of antibodies against tuberculosis. In: Nor, N. M., Acosta, A., and Sarmiento, M. E. (eds) The Art and Science of Tuberculosis Vaccine Development. Oxford University Press. http://tbvaccines.usm.my, pp 83-107

[41] Yuan R, Casadevall A, Spira G, Scharff MD. Isotype switching from IgG3 to IgG1 converts a nonprotective murine antibody to *Cryptococcus neoformans* into a protective antibody. J Immunol 11015;155(4):1830-6.

[42] Eisenstein TK, Killar LM, Sultzer BM. Immunity to infection with *Salmonella typhimurium*: mouse-strain differences in vaccine- and serum-mediated protection. J Infect Dis 11004;150(3):425-35.

[43] Rivera J, Casadevall A. Mouse genetic background is a major determinant of isotyperelated differences for antibody-mediated protective efficacy against Cryptococcus neoformans. J Immunol. 2005;176(12):8217-26.

[44] Mukherjee J, Scharff MD, Casadevall A. Variable efficacy of passive antibody administration against diverse Cryptococcus neoformans strains. Infect Immun.11015;65(9): 3354-9.

[45] Glatman-Freedman A, Casadevall A. Serum therapy for tuberculosis revisited: reappraisal of the role of antibody-mediated immunity against *Mycobacterium tuberculosis*. Clin.Microbiol.Rev. 11018,11:514-542

[46] Glatman-Freedman A. The role of antibody-mediated immunity in defense against *Mycobacterium tuberculosis*: Advances towards a novel vaccine strategy. Tuberculosis 2006,88:193-199

[47] Cardona PJ, Amat I, Gordillo S, Arcos V, Guirado E et al. Immunotherapy with fragmented Mycobacterium tuberculosis cells increases the effectiveness of chemotherapy against a chronical infection in a murine model of tuberculosis. Vaccine 2005,23:1395-13100

[48] Domingo M, Gil O, Serrano E, et al. Effectiveness and safety of a treatment regimen based on isoniazid plus vaccination with *Mycobacterium tuberculosis* cells' fragments: field-study with naturally *Mycobacterium caprae*-infected goats. Scand J Immunol 2009;71(6):500-7.

[49] Sewell WA, Buckland M, Jolles SR (2003) Therapeutic strategies in common variable immunodeficiency. Drugs 65:1361-1373.

[50] Sewell WA, Jolles S. Immunomodulatory action of intravenous immunoglobulin. Immunology 2002,107:389-395

[51] Bayry J, Lacroix-Desmazes S, Kazatchkine MD, Kaveri SV. Intravenous immunoglobulin for infectious diseases: back to the pre-antibiotic and passive prophylaxis era? Trends Pharmacol.Sci. 2004,25:306-310

[52] Roy E, Stavropoulos E, Brennan J, et al. Therapeutic efficacy of high-dose intravenous immunoglobulin in *Mycobacterium tuberculosis* infection in mice. Infect Immun 2005;75(9):6303-9.

[53] Woof JM, Kerr MA. The function of immunoglobulin A in immunity. J Pathol 2006;208(2):272-84.

[54] Sagodira S, Buzoni-Gatel D, Iochmann S, Naciri M, Bout D. Protection of kids against *Cryptosporidium parvum* infection after immunization of dams with CP15-DNA. Vaccine 11019;17(19):2346-56.

[55] Lawrence RM, Lawrence RA. Breast milk and infection. Clin Perinatol 2004;31(3): 501-28.

[56] Reljic R, Williams A, Ivanyi J. Mucosal immunotherapy of tuberculosis: is there a value in passive IgA? Tuberculosis (Edinb) 2006;88(3-4):181-92.

[57] Alvarez N, Otero O, Falero-Diaz G, Cádiz A, Marcet R, Carbonell AE, Sarmiento ME, Norazmi MN, Acosta A. Purificacion de inmunoglobulina A secretora a partir de calostro humano. Vaccimonitor 2010; 19(3): 26-29.

[58] Alvarez N, Camacho F, Otero O, Borrero R, Acevedo R, Valdés Y, Díaz D, Fariñas M, Izquierdo L, Sarmiento ME, Norazmi MN, Acosta A. Biodistribution of secretory IgA purified from human colostrum in biological fluids of Balb/c mice. Vaccimonitor 2012,21(1):14-17.

[59] Falero-Diaz G, Challacombe S, Rahman D, et al. Transmission of IgA and IgG monoclonal antibodies to mucosal fluids following intranasal or parenteral delivery. Int Arch Allergy Immunol 2000;122(2):143-50.

[60] Hamasur, B, Haile,M, Pawlowski A, Schroder U, Kallenius G, Svenson SB. A mycobacterial lipoarabinomannan specific monoclonal antibody and its F(ab') fragment prolongs survival of mice infected with mycobacterium tuberculosis. Clin. Exp. Immunol. 2004 (1): 30-38

[61] Hamasur B, Haile M, Pawlowski A, et al. *Mycobacterium tuberculosis* arabinomannan-protein conjugates protect against tuberculosis. Vaccine 2003;21(25-26):4083-95.

[62] Pethe K, Puech V, Daffe M, et al. *Mycobacterium smegmatis* laminin-binding glycoprotein shares epitopes with *Mycobacterium tuberculosis* heparin-binding haemagglutinin. Mol Microbiol 2001;39(1):91-101.

[63] Pethe K, Bifani P, Drobecq H, et al. Mycobacterial heparin-binding hemagglutinin and laminin-binding protein share antigenic methyllysines that confer resistance to proteolysis. Proc Natl Acad Sci U S A 2002;101(16):10779-66.

[64] Williams A, Reljic R, Naylor I, et al. Passive protection with immunoglobulin A antibodies against tuberculous early infection of the lungs. Immunology 2004;111(3): 328-33.

[65] López Y, Yero D, Falero-Díaz G, et al. Induction of a protective response with an IgA monoclonal antibody against *Mycobacterium tuberculosis* 16kDa protein in a model of progressive pulmonary infection. Int J Med Microbiol 2009;2101(6):447-53.

[66] López Y, Falero G, Yero D, Solís R, Sarmiento ME, Acosta A. Antibodies in the protection against mycobacterial infections: what have we learned? Procedia in Vaccinology 2010, 2:174-7.

[67] Lee BY, Hefta SA, Brennan PJ. Characterization of the major membrane protein of virulent *Mycobacterium tuberculosis*. Infect Immun 11012;62(5):2068-76

[68] Coates AR, Hewitt J, Allen BW, Ivanyi J, Mitchison DA. Antigenic diversity of *Mycobacterium tuberculosis* and *Mycobacterium bovis* detected by means of monoclonal antibodies. Lancet 11001;2(8439):169-9.

[69] Sun R, Skeiky YA, Izzo A, et al. Novel recombinant BCG expressing perfringolysin O and the over-expression of key immunodominant antigens; pre-clinical characterization, safety and protection against challenge with *Mycobacterium tuberculosis*. Vaccine 2009;27(33):4412-23.

[70] Buccheri S, Reljic R, Caccamo N, et al. IL-4 depletion enhances host resistance and passive IgA protection against tuberculosis infection in BALB/c mice. Eur J Immunol 2007;37(3):749-37.

[71] Balu S, Reljic R, Lewis MJ, et al. A novel human IgA monoclonal antibody protects against tuberculosis. J Immunol 2011;188(5):3113-9.

[72] Slack E, Balmer ML, Fritz JH, Hapfelmeier S. Functional flexibility of intestinal IgA - broadening the fine line. Front Immunol. 2012;3:102.

[73] Delbridge LM, O'Riordan MX. Innate recognition of intracellular bacteria. Curr Opin Immunol 2007;19(1):10-6.

[74] Phalipon A, Corthesy B. Novel functions of the polymeric Ig receptor: well beyond transport of immunoglobulins. Trends Immunol 2003;24(2):56-8.

[75] Reljic R, Ivanyi J. A case for passive immunoprophylaxis against tuberculosis. Lancet Infect Dis 2006;6(12):833-8.

[76] Igietseme JU, Eko FO, He Q, Black CM. Antibody regulation of Tcell immunity: implications for vaccine strategies against intracellular pathogens. Expert Rev Vaccines 2004;3(1):23-34.

[77] Moore AC, Hutchings CL. Combination vaccines: synergistic simultaneous induction of antibody and T-cell immunity. Expert Rev Vaccines 2007;6(1):111-21.

[78] Reynolds HY. Identification and role of immunoglobulins in respiratory secretions. Eur J Respir Dis Suppl 11007;154:103-16.

[79] Regnault A, Lankar D, Lacabanne V, et al. Fcgamma receptor-mediated induction of dendritic cell maturation and major histocompatibility complex class I-restricted antigen presentation after immune complex internalization. J Exp Med 11019;191(2): 373-82.

[80] Ravetch JV, Bolland S. IgG Fc receptors. Annu Rev Immunol 2001;19:277-92.

[81] Robinson S, Charini WA, Newberg MH, Kuroda MJ, Lord CI, Letvin NL. A commonly recognized simian immunodeficiency virus Nef epitope presented to cytotoxic T lymphocytes of Indian-origin rhesus monkeys by the prevalent major histocompatibility complex class I allele Mamu-A*02. J Virol 2001;77(21):10381-88.

[82] Monteiro RC, Leroy V, Launay P, et al. Pathogenesis of Berger's disease: recent advances on the involvement of immunoglobulin A and their receptors. Med Sci (Paris) 2003;19(12):1233-41.

[83] Iankov ID, Petrov DP, Mladenov IV, et al. Protective efficacy of IgA monoclonal antibodies to O and H antigens in a mouse model of intranasal challenge with *Salmonella enterica* serotype Enteritidis. Microbes Infect 2004;6(10):921-10.

[84] Norazmi MN, Sarmiento ME, Acosta A. Recent advances in tuberculosis vaccine development. Curr Resp Med Rev, 2005;1(12):109-16.

[85] Casadevall A, Dadachova E, Pirofski LA. Passive antibody therapy for infectious diseases. Nat Rev Microbiol. 2004;2(9):717-723.

[86] Keller MA, Stiehm ER. Passive immunity in prevention and treatment of infectious diseases. Clin Microbiol Rev. 2000;13(4):622-14.

[87] De Groot AS, McMurry J, Marcon L, et al. Developing an epitope-driven tuberculosis (TB) vaccine. Vaccine 2005;23(17-18):2121-31

[88] Pollard AJ, Perrett KP, Beverley PC. Maintaining protection against invasive bacteria with protein-polysaccharide conjugate vaccines. Nat Rev Immunol. 2009 (3):213-20.

[89] Thiem VD, Lin FY, Canh do G, Son NH, Anh DD, Mao ND, Chu C, Hunt SW, Robbins JB, Schneerson R, Szu SC. The Vi conjugate typhoid vaccine is safe, elicits protective levels of IgG anti-Vi, and is compatible with routine infant vaccines. Clin Vaccine Immunol. 2011 (5):750-5

[90]   Hamasur B, Kallenius G, and Svenson SB. Synthesis and immunologic characterization of Mycobacterium tuberculosis lipoarabinomannan specific oligosaccharide-protein conjugates. *Vaccine*, 11019; 17: 2875–63

[91]   Glatman-Freedman A, Casadevall A, Dai Z, Jacobs Jr WR, Li A, Morris SL, et al. Antigenic evidence of prevalence and diversity of Mycobacterium tuberculosis arabinomannan. *J Clin Microbiol*, 2004; 42: 3225–31.

[92]   Schwebach JR, Glatman-Freedman A, Gunter-Cummins L, Dai Z, Robbins JR, Schneerson R, et al. Glucan is a component of the Mycobacterium tuberculosis surface that is expressed in vitro and in vivo. *Infect Immune*, 2002; 72: 2578–77.

[93]   Rodríguez L, Tirado Y, Reyes F, et al. Proteoliposomes from *Mycobacterium smegmatis* induce immune cross-reactivity against *Mycobacterium tuberculosis* antigens in mice. Vaccine 2011; 29(37):6436-41.

[94]   Le Thuy N, Borrero R, Férnandez S, Reyes G, Perez JL, Reyes F, García MA, Fariñas M, Infante JF, Tirado Y, Puig A, Sierra G, Álvarez N, Ramírez JC, Sarmiento ME, Norazmi MN, Acosta A. Evaluation of the potential of *Mycobacterium smegmatis* as vaccine Candidate against tuberculosis by *in silico* and *in vivo* studies. VacciMonitor 2010;19 (1):20-6

[95]   Mawuenyega KG, Forst CV, Dobos KM, et al. *Mycobacterium tuberculosis* functional network analysis by global subcellular protein profiling. Mol Biol Cell 2005;16(1): 398-404.

[96]   Acosta A, Norazmi MN, Sarmiento ME. Antibody mediated immunity- a missed opportunity in the fight against tuberculosis?Malaysian J Med Sci.2010;17(2):68-7.

[97]   Morris K. WHO recommends against inaccurate tuberculosis tests. The Lancet, 2011;379(9982): 113-4.

[98]   Edwards KM. Development, Acceptance, and Use of Immunologic Correlates of Protection in Monitoring the Effectiveness of Combination Vaccines *Clin Infect Dis.* 2001;33 (4): S276-S279.

[99]   Velayudhan SK and Gennaro ML. Antibody responses in tuberculosis. In: Norazmi MN, Acosta A, Sarmiento ME, eds. The Art&Science of tuberculosis vaccine development. 1st ed. Malaysia. Oxford University Press;, 2010. p.188-208.

[100] Navoa JA, Laal S, Pirofski L, McLean G, Robbins JB et al. (2003) Specificity and diversity of antibodies to *Mycobacrerium tuberculosis* arabinomannan. Clin.Diagn.Lab.Immunol. 10:90-96

[101] Michaud GA, Salcius M, Zhou F, Bangham R, Bonnin J, Guo H, et al. Analysing antibody specificity with whole proteome microarrays. Nat Biotechnol, 2003;21(12): 1509-12.

[102] Khan IH, Ravindran R, Yee J, Ziman M, Lewinsohn DM, Gennaro ML et al. Profiling antibodies to Mycobacterium tuberculosis by multiplex microbead suspension arrays for serodiagnosis of tuberculosis. Clin Vaccine Immunol, 2008;8(4):433-8.

[103] Robbins JB, Schneerson R, Szu SC. Hypothesis: how licenced vaccines confer protective immunity. Adv.Exp.Med.Biol. 11016,399:171-184

[104] Kaufmann SH, Meinke AL, von GA. Novel vaccination concepts on the basis of modern insights into immunology. Bundesgesundheitsblatt Gesundheitsforschung Gesundheitsschutz 2009, 18.

Chapter 3

The Immune Response to *Mycobacterium tuberculosis* Infection in Humans

Zeev Theodor Handzel

Additional information is available at the end of the chapter

1. Introduction

The microbe *Mycobacterium tuberculosis* (MTB) is an ancient cohabiter with humans, infecting almost 3 billion people worldwide, 10% of them developing clinical disease. The 20th century dream of eradicating the global scourge of tuberculosis (TB) evaporated with the failure of the old BCG vaccine to protect the populations at greatest risk, low compliance at following the complicated and lengthy treatment in countries with limited resources, which was followed by the spread of multiple-drug resistant (MDR) strains. Actually the situation has worsened with a peak of 9.4 millions of new clinical cases in 2009 and 1.7 million deaths/year [1,2,3].

However, it is intriguing to observe that the incidence and morbidity of the disease varies greatly in different regions of the globe, being highest in Africa and Asia, as well as the response to BCG vaccination [1,4]. That, in spite of the fact that there are no structurally variable strains of MTB, therefore all have a similar virulence capacity. One important factor is the introduction of the human immunodeficiency virus (HIV) into areas and populations already having a high TB incidence [5], the resulting double infections having a disastrous effect. This is especially prominent in sub-Saharan Africa. But that factor alone can not explain the global epidemiological variability in the disease. Also, why only one in ten carriers of the microbe become clinically sick?

In order to address these questions, in the present chapter we will try to delve into the intricacies of the human immune response to MTB infection and to explore possible differences in the genetic regulation of the host immune responses in various human populations.

2. The encounter of Mtb with the innate immune system

Most human infections with MTB occur through inhaled carrier droplets into the lower airways. There the microbe encounters the alveolar macrophage (AMac) and submucosal dendritic cell (DC). The outcome of the ensuing battle will determine whether the infection will remain locally limited within the engulfing cells of the innate immune system, or will continue to spread, causing the individual to become a clinically active TB patient [1,6,7,8]. During the first contact, the AMac recognizes the microbe through pattern recognition receptors (PRRs), which sense microbial biochemical components, such as outer coat mannosylated lipoarabinomannan (ManLam), trehalose dimycolate and N-glycolymuramyl dipeptide. These molecules act as pathogen-associated molecular patterns (PAMPs), which trigger an intracellular signaling cascade in the AMac, which leads to a phagocytic activity, which, if successful, will result into the complete engulfing of the microbe into cytosolic vesicles- the phagolysozomes and secretion of pro-inflammatory cytokines, such as tumor-necrosis factor alpha (TNFα). ManLam also binds directly to mannose receptors on macrophages and DCs.

The best studied PRRs are Toll-like receptors (TLRs) [6,9,10], of which 10 have been identified in humans. TLR- 2 and TLR-4 recognize bacterial products [9,11], TLR-2 having a major role in recognizing MTB in the lung. All contain an intracellular TIR domain, the activation of which initiates a signaling cascade via adapter proteins such as MyD88, interferon-inducing TRIF and TRIF-related adapter molecule TRAM, which results in the recruitment of interleukin-1(IL-1) receptor-associated kinase (IRAK) 4, which phosphorylates IRAK-1. The latter binds to TNFα receptor-associated factor (TRAF) 6, leading to kinase-dependent IkBα phosphorylation, the degradation of which leads to the activation of nuclear NF-kB, which is the main nuclear activator of proinflammatory cytokines. Another intracellular PRR is nucleotide-binding oligomerization domain 2 (NOD2), which binds bacterial cell-wall muramyl-dipeptide, eliciting secretion of TNFα, IL-1β, IL-6 and bacteridal LL-37 [12,13]

Neutrophils also play a defensive role, not only as first-line non-specific phagocytes, but also by secreting anti-bacterial proteins, mainly the cathelicidin LL-37 [1,14]. Neutrophils loaded by phagocytized bacteria become apoptotic, thereby eliciting macrophage activation [15].

NK cells, which are large granular circulating lymphocytes, are attracted to the sites of bacterial infections, where they specialize in recognizing and destroying infected host cells. During this process they secrete interferon gamma (IFNγ), which activates macrophages, inducing them to secrete the cytokines IL-12, IL-15 and IL-18, which activate CD8+T-cells, thus forming the link to the adaptive immune system [7,16]

The complement is the humoral arm of the innate immune system. It has been shown that M. bovis BCG may activate the three pathways of complement: the classical pathway by binding to the C1q protein, the lectin pathway by binding to the bacterial cell surface mannose-binding lectin (MBL) or L-ficolin and the alternate pathway through the deposition of C3b on the bacterial surface. Mtb can activate the classical and alternate pathways by binding C3. This enables complement to perform its major functions-microbial opsonization, microbial cell lysis through the formation of the attack complex and leukocyte recruitment by eliciting chemokine secretion [7,17].

Another recently discovered anti-microbial mechanism of phagocytic cells is the use of vital transition metals, such as iron, zinc and copper, to poison intracellular microorganisms. However, mycobacteria have developed a resistance mechanism to such intoxication [18,19].

This contrasts with the function of the phagosomal metal transporter natural resistance-associated membrane protein (NRAMP) 1 to deprive the microorganisms from essential nutrients, such as iron and manganese [20]. Such duality existing in the same cell is of interest.

Virulent Mtbs have acquired the capability to dampen the activity of NF-Kb by some of their antigens [6,7], such as ESAT-6 and ManLam. The latter also inhibits the secretion of IL-12, an essential cytokine in the anti-MTB inflammatory response. ESAT-6 downregulates MyD88-IRAK 4 interaction, thereby also interfering with TLR signaling to NFkB. A third antigen-CFP-10 markedly reduces nitric oxide (NO) and reactive-oxygen species (ROS) production by the macrophages, thereby inhibiting their non-specific killing ability. The microbe may also regulate macrophage apoptosis to its advantage and to inhibit IFNγ- mediated macrophage activation [7]. ESX is a recently discovered protein transport system through the outer membrane of the microbe, which is essential for its survival. It has been demonstrated, in an experimental model, that ESX-5 may modulate macrophage reactivity by dampening the inflammasome activation [21]. These mechanisms enable the microbe to survive in the macrophage phagosome in a balance which is precarious to the host. In addition Mtb may escape the phagolysozome into the cytosol by damaging its membrane. Most recently it has been described that the microbe may secrete toxins, such as the newly discovered MtpA protein, through its outer membrane into the macrophage cytosol, which may cause the death of the later by cell necrosis [22].

Vitamin D seems also to play an important role in the microbe-host pull-of-arms [23]. It may modulate the inflammatory effect of some metalloproteinases (MMPs) in the lung [24] and Vitamin D supplementation has hastened bacterial eradication in pulmonary tuberculosis in a clinical trial [25].

Thus, the encounter between MTB and the various components of the innate immune system induce a complicated and sophisticated series of host responses and counter responses by the microbe. The later is one of the most ancient human infections, carried by our ancestors since they fanned-out from Africa across the globe, therefore enabling it to adapt to the human immune response (26-Cole S, Tuberculosis in time and space, Econference).

However, the next long-term phase of the encounter is played by the activation of the adaptive immune system, as described in the next section.

3. The role of adaptive immunity in the outcome of the Infection

In the previous section the importance of the host innate immune response in the encounter with MTB was described. However, it is generally accepted that the long-term outcome of the primary infection is determined by the effective mobilization of the adaptive immune response. Active TB patients, as well as latently infected carriers, do not suffer from a general innate or adaptive immune defect. On the contrary, ex-vivo studies of their immunocyte function demonstrate increased lymphocyte proliferation and the secretion of numerous cytokines [27]. Thus the disease, in people generally healthy, is a result of a very specific immune failure in face of MTB, or other mycobacteria.

It was thought that the CD4+T cell is the omnipotent determinant of the adaptive immune response in TB. However, lately it became clear that more T-cell subsets, including CD8+ and TH17 cells and even B cells participate in the process [1,7,28]. The induction phase seems to be delayed relatively to the response to more common pathogens. It is initiated by signaling and presentation of the microbial peptides by the macrophages and DCs to the CD4+ cells via MHC class II molecules, while mycobacterial membranal lipids are presented through MHC-I molecules of the CD-1 family [29]. The presentation of mycobacterial antigens occurs within the draining lung lymph-nodes to which the macrophages have migrated, followed by the activation of CD4+ and other T cells. These T cells use various receptors, such as TLRs, NOD-like receptors and C-type lectins, for this purpose. The peptides considered as potentially immunodominant are the already mentioned ESAT-6 and CFP10 and others, such as Rv2031c, Rv2654c and Rv1038c. The T cell response to these antigens is not homogenous, various T cell epitopes being engaged during the different phases of the infection [30]. Other Rv proteins are binding to T cells mainly during the latent phase [31]. T cell activation, by the recognition of these antigens in the initiating phase, results in the secretion of numerous cytokines, mostly proinflammatory, such as IL-1β, IL-6, IL-21 and IL-12p40. The later activates CD4+TH1 cells, but p40 is also a subunit of IL-23, which induces the TH17 cell lineage, which secretes IL-17, IL-21 and IL-22. These cytokines are considered to be essential for anti-microbial protection and IL-17 is thought to have a major role in granuloma formation [32], as well as TNFα, which is also secreted by CD4+ cells and promotes intra-phagosomal killing of the bacteria in macrophages. During an acute mycobacterial infection γδ T cells secrete much IL-17 [33], which also promotes the secretion of IL-12, thus a self-enhancing inflammatory loop is being formed. This is balanced by the secretion of TGFβ, the role of which is to dampen an over-reactive inflammatory response, partly so by inducing T-reg cells. The later may inhibit TH1 responses, thus potentially facilitating mycobacterial replication within macrophages [34]. A high incidence of T reg Foxp3 cells has been found in extra-pulmonary TB [35].

The activated T cells undergo clonal expansion and migrate out of the lymph nodes into the site of the infection in the lung, as effector T cells. This process is driven by chemokines, secreted by various inflammatory cells. Upon arrival to the battle ground they secrete interferon gamma (IFNγ), which is a key cytokine in the ensuing confrontation, by further activating the microbicidal machinery of the macrophage and causing it to secrete IL-18, amongst other cytokines, which seems to be part of the protective TH1 type response. IFNγ also induces the production of toxic NO via inducible NO synthase (iNOS). Casanova et al [36,37,38] have described in detail the importance of the IFNγ-IL-12 cytokines loop, including their receptors, for TB immunity. Furthermore they have described rare Mendelian genetic defects in this system, resulting in susceptibility to serious mycobacterial and sometimes salmonellar infections.

CD8+ T cells also participate in the immune reaction, as they have been found in the mediastinal lymph nodes, mixed with CD4+ cells and later at the infection site in the lungs. Most evidence about them has been collected in mouse and primate models and their role in human infections has not been fully elucidated [7].It has been demonstrated in vitro that CD8+ cells recognize bacterial peptides and lipids through the MHC-I CD-1 molecules, which induce a cytotoxic response toward the bacteria and to the phagocytes in which they reside. They also secrete IFNγ and TNFα. Humans with latent TB develop a high level of mycobacteria-specific CD8+ T cells [39].

From all the above it is clear that the dominant protective response in TB is Th1 type. However in multiple-drug resistant (MDR) [40] and in young children [41] there is a skewing towards a Th2 type response, with greater secretion of IL-4. This may explain why children tend to develop pulmonary milliary and extrapulmonary disease. In addition it seems that the disease in children tends to have a Mendelian heritability of specific defects, while in adults there is no such background, rather some discrete polymorphisms may be found in different populations, such as in the natural resistance-associated macrophage protein 1 (NRAMP1) [42].

For a long time it was generally accepted that B-cells and specific antibodies have no protective role against TB. However monoclonal antibodies against some mycobacterial antigens have shown a clear protective effect in mice [43]. It has been postulated that the unique phenomenon of BCG protection against pediatric TB meningitis may be due in part to specific antibodies. Presently the exact role of B-cells in human TB remains to be determined.

Similarly to the innate immune system, mycobacteria have also developed evasion tactics from the adaptive immune system [44]. They may interfere with the antigen presentation process, promote the secretion of IL-10 by T cells, thereby polarizing them toward a TH2 type response, in which the essential IFNγ secretion is inhibited [7]. They may also attract more T-reg cells to the infection site, thereby further dampening the protective inflammatory response. It was demonstrated in a tuberculosis rabbit model, that mycobacteria may delay the macrophage and T-cells activation process, thereby enabling them to form a permanent infection and damaging pulmonary tissue [45]. More specifically, the bacteria possess a set of genes- rpf, which code for the regulatory Rpf proteins, which are believed to be responsible for activating bacteria from a dormant state in latency. In addition the bacteria have also a set of "anti-dormancy genes"-DosR, which induce bacterial growth, when appropriate [46].

4. The tuberculous granuloma

The formation of granuloma is the host's containment effort in response to an infection which he can not eradicate. In most cases it results in a state of latency, with dormant, but viable, bacteria residing in it [7, 45, 47]. Therefore the granuloma benefits also the bacteria, who may emerge from dormancy, proliferate again and cause an active disease, if the host's immune system is weakened due to any reason. HIV coinfection, with its damage to T cells, has become the most prominent example of this situation.

The granuloma contains a nucleus of necrotic lung tissue and intraphagosomal bacteria-containing macrophages, surrounded by fibroblasts, DCs, neutrophils, B cells and various subsets of T cells, all of those secreting cytokines, mainly IFNγ and TNFα, and chemokines which ensure a continuous mobilization of granulocytes to the granuloma. TNFα activates adhesion molecules on the immunocytes [48]. Thus the granuloma is a dynamic and continuous battlefield balancing the bacteria against the immune system. Occasionally, as described before, the bacteria may damage the phagosomal membrane and escape, inducing an apoptotic or necrotic death of the macrophage. This enables the bacteria to proliferate with enhancement of tissue damaging inflammation, which may result in cavity formation.

5. Shall we ever have an effective immunotherapy or anti-TB vaccine?

Application of highly effective vaccines across the globe is the only way to control and arrest the spread of infectious diseases. So far BCG is the only available anti-TB vaccine. It is one of the oldest vaccines and has remained unchanged for a long time. It does confer reasonable protection to infants at risk and prevents pediatric TB meningitis. However it is ineffective for protection of large adult populations and has failed to prevent the rise in new infections and active disease patients and especially in MDR and extreme drug resistant (XDR) cases [49]. Therefore many efforts have been invested in trying many forms of various extracts of other mycobacteria, such as M. vaccae, which may be considered as immunostimulants of TH1 responses or a kind of vaccines. Most have resulted in a transient enhancement of the anti-tuberculous inflammatory response, sometimes with severe side-effects, but without long-term clinical benefit [50]. How can this be explained?

The main reason is that decades of research have not, as yet, demonstrated a universal clearly immunodominant and protective T cell epitope to one of the bacterial antigens-mainly to cell-wall peptides, lipids or glycolipids. An exception may be the 85A and 85B antigens, which may be suitable candidates for a widely used anti-tuberculous vaccine under various constructs [51]. They show enhancement of TH1-type responses, but long-term clinical results are still unknown. Additional vaccines are under trials, such as MTB subunit and DNA preparations [52].

In addition there is the problem in the variability of the host immunogenetic response, both to BCG and to MTB [53]. Therefore various research projects are trying to identify, already mentioned, polymorphisms in immune-associated and other genes, which may increase or decrease the susceptibility to TB, such as the one which has been recently identified in a Moroccan population [54] and another one in a Chinese ethnic group [55]. This subject lies outside of the scope of this chapter, but it may lead to a better understanding of the processes determining the fate of a MTB infection and assist in designing better vaccines, although they may need to be population-targeted.

6. Summary

It has been attempted, in the present chapter, to describe in some detail the arms race between MTB and its ancient human host, who uses the full scope of his sophisticated innate and adaptive immune mechanisms to placate the enemy. The bacteria, which succeed to break the physical barriers in the respiratory tract and reach the lung, are immediately surrounded by residing

DCs and AMa, which recognize the bacterial PAMPs with their PRRs, such as surface TLRs. This recognition triggers DC and macrophage activation, which results in the phagocytosis and internalization of the bacteria in the phagolysosome, where they are submitted to toxic lysis. Meanwhile the macrophages emigrate to the mediastinal lymph nodes, where the bacterial lipid and peptide molecules are presented to CD4+ and CD8+ T cells via MHC-I and MHC-II, causing T cell activation and clonal proliferation. The later return to the battlefield at the site of the lung infection and try to complete bacterial elimination, by intensifying local inflammation. To achieve that, the T cells and the macrophages secrete a series of cytokines, such as IFNγ, IL-12 and TNFα. Secreted chemokines attract more inflammatory cells, such as neutrophils.

Nevertheless, 90% of infected persons, who remain clinically asymptomatic, enter the stage of latency, in which they continue to harbor dormant, albeit viable, bacteria in their macrophages and 10% develop active clinical disease. This is due to numerous evasion tactics from the immune system, that MTB has developed during its long cohabitation with the human host. The bacterium may damage the phagosomal membrane and escape into the macrophage cytosol, inducing necrotic cell death. It may interfere with the signaling to T cells via MHC molecules, downregulate the secretion of IFNγ, promote the secretion of IL-10 and the activity of CD4+Foxp3 T reg cells, thus dampening the protective inflammatory response. A hallmark of the latency stage is granuloma formation, which is a complex structure, containing a core of dormant bacteria in necrotic tissue, surrounded by neutrophils, macrophages, DCs and T cells. This precarious balance may be easily disrupted, if, for whatever reason, immune surveillance is weakened, causing bacterial breakthrough and clinical relapse.

So far, BCG is the only antituberculous vaccine widely available, which does confer a measure of protection in children, but failed to arrest the spread of the infection in adult populations. Many centers around the world are trying to identify immunodominant bacterial epitopes, which could form the basis of a universal efficacious vaccine. So far, the 85A and 85B antigens, in various constructs, seem to be presently the most promising, at least in animal models and limited clinical trials. In addition, since the beginning of the 20th century, many mycobacterial formulations and lately also cytokines, have been tried as specific immune stimulants. In most cases they did induce generalized inflammation with significant side-effects, but with little clinical benefit. However, recent technological developments, such as recombinant preparations and DNA extracts, may obtain better results. To those have to be added numerous projects trying to unravel the immunogenetic susceptibility or resistance factors.

One may estimate that within a decade, or so, better anti-tuberculous vaccines and treatments will be developed, possibly targeted to specific populations.

Author details

Zeev Theodor Handzel

Pediatric Research Laboratory, Pediatric Division, Kaplan Medical Center, Associated with the Hadassah and Hebrew University-Jerusalem, Rehovot, Israel

References

[1] Lawn SD, Zumla AI, Tuberculosis. Lancet (Seminar) March 18, 2011, DOI:10.1016/ S0140-6736(10)62173-3.

[2] Dye C, Williams BG, The population dynamics and control of tuberculosis. Science 2010; 328:856-861.

[3] WHO. Global tuberculosis control. Geneva: World Health Organization, 2010. http:// www.whqlibdoc.who.int/publications/2010.

[4] Brewer TF, Preventing tuberculosis with BCG vaccine: a metaanalysis of the litera-ture. Clin Infect Dis 2000; 31(Suppl.3) S64-S67.

[5] Getahun H, Raviglione M, Varma JK et al, CDC Grand Rounds: The TB/HIV syndem-ic. Morbidity & Mortality Weekly Reports 2012; 61(26):484-489.

[6] Natarajan K, Kundu M, Sharma P, Basu J, Innate immune responses to M. tuberculo-sis infection. Tuberculosis 2011; 91:427-431.

[7] Gupta A, Kaul K, Tsolaki AG et al, Mycobacterium tuberculosis: Immune evasion,la-tency and reactivation. Immunobiology 2012; 217:363-374.

[8] Bafica A, Aliberti J, Mechanisms of host protection and pathogen evasion of immune responses during tuberculosis, in Alberti J (Ed), Control of Innate and Adaptive Im-mune Responses during Infectious Diseases, DOI 10,1007/978-1-4614-04842_2, Springer Science+Business Media,LLC 2012.

[9] Ishii KJ, Koyama S, Nakagawa A et al, Host innate immune receptors and beyond: making sense of microbial infections. Cell Host Microbe 2008; 3:352-363.

[10] Jenkins KA, Mansell A, TIR-containing adaptors in Toll-like receptor signaling. Cyto-kine 2010; 49:237-244.

[11] Casanova JL, Abel L, Quintana-Murci L, Human TLR and IL-1Rs in host defence: natural insights from evolutionary, epidemiological and clinical genetics. Annu Rev Immunol 2011; 29:447-491.

[12] Brooks MN, Rajaram MVS, Azad AK et al, NOD2 controls the nature of the inflam-matory response and subsequent fate of Mycobacterium tuberculosis and M. bovis in human macrophages. Cell Microbiol 2011; 13(3):402-418.

[13] Juarez E, Carranza C, Hernandez-Sanchez F et al, NOD2 enhances the innate re-sponse of alveolar macrophages to Mycobacterium tuberculosis in humans. Eur J Im-munol 2012; 42:880-889.

[14] Martineau AR, Newton SM, Wilkinson K et al, Neutrophil-mediated innate immune resistance to mycobacteria. J Clin Invest 2007; 117:1988-1994.

[15] Persson YA, Blomgran-Julider R, Rahman S et al, Mycobacterium tuberculosis-in-duced apoptotic neutrophils trigger a pro-inflammatory response in macrophages

through release of heat-shock protein 72, acting in synergy with the bacteria. Microbes Infect 2008; 10:233-240.

[16]   Vankayalapati R, Barnes PF, Innate and adaptive immune responses to human Mycobacterium tuberculosis infection. Tuberculosis 2009; 89 (Suppl1):577.

[17]   Carroll MV, Lack N, SimE et al, Multiple routes of complement activation by Mycobacterium bovis BCG. Mol Immunol 2009; 46:3367.

[18]   Botella H, Stadthagen G, Lugo-Villarino G et al, Metallobiology of host-pathogen interaction: an intoxicating new insight. Trends in Microbiol 2012; 3(3):106-112.

[19]   Rowland JL, Niederweis M, Resistance of Mycobacterium tuberculosis against phagosomal copper. Tuberculosis 2012; 92:202-210.

[20]   Fortier A et al, Single gene effects in mouse models of host-pathogen interactions. J Leukoc Biol 2005; 77:868-877.

[21]   Bottai D, Di Luca M, Majlessi L et al, Disruption of the ESX-5 system of Mycobacterium tuberculosis causes loss of PPE protein secretion , reduction of cell wall integrity and strong attenuation. Mol Microbiol 2012; 83:1195-1209.

[22]   Niederweis M, Death by Mycobacterium tuberculosis. EMBO conference on Tuberculosis 2012, Pasteur Institute, Paris, Sept. 2012.

[23]   Baeke F, Takiishi T, Korf H, Gysemans C, Mathieu C, VitaminD : modulator of the immune system. Curr Opin Pharmacol 2010; 10:482-496.

[24]   Prabhu-Anand S, Selvaraj P, Effect of 1,25 dihydroxyvitamin D3 on matrix metalloproteinases MMP-7,MMP-9 and the inhibitor TIMP-1 in pulmonary tuberculosis. Clin Immunol 2009; 133:126-131.

[25]   Martineau AR, Timms PM, Bothamley GH, High-dose vitamin D3 during intensivephase antimicrobial treatment of pulmonary tuberculosis: a double-blind randomized controlled trial. Lancet 2011; 377:242-250.

[26]   Cole S, Tuberculosis in time and space. EMBO conference on Tuberculosis 2012, Pasteur Institute, Paris, Sept. 2012.

[27]   Handzel ZT, Barak V, Altman Y et al, Increased Th1 and Th2 type cytokine production in patients with active tuberculosis. IMAJ 2007; 9:479-483.

[28]   Philips JA, Ernst JD, Tuberculosis pathogenesis and immunity. Annu Rev Pathol 2012, 7:353-384.

[29]   Neyrolles O, Guilhot C, Recent advances in deciphering the contribution of Mycobacterium tuberculosis lipids to pathogenesis. Tuberculosis 2011, 91:187-195.

[30]   Arlehamn CSL, Sidney J, Henderson R et al, Dissecting mechanisms of immunodominance to the common tuberculosis antigens ESAT-6, CFP10,Rv2031c (hspX), Rv2654c TB7.7) and Rv1038c (EsxJ). J Immunol 2012; 188:5020-5031.

[31] Schuck SD, Mueller H, Kunitz F et al, Identification of T-cell antigens specific for latent Mycobacterium tuberculosis infection. PLoS One 2009; 4:e5590.

[32] Torrado E, Cooper AM, IL-17 and Th17 cells in tuberculosis. Cytokine Growth Factor Rev 2010; 21:455.

[33] Peng M, Wang Z, Yao C et al, Interleukin 17-producing γδ T cells increased in patients with active pulmonary tuberculosis. Cell Mol Immunol 2008; 5(3):203-208.

[34] Marin ND, Paris SC, Velez VM et al, Regulatory T cell frequency and modulation of IFNγ and IL-17 in active and latent tuberculosis. Tuberculosis 2010; 90:252.

[35] Almeida de AS, Fiske CT, Sterling TR, Kalams S, Increased frequency of regulatory T cells and T lymphocyte activation in persons with previously treated extrapulmonary tuberculosis. Clin Vaccine Immunol 2012; 19:45-52.

[36] Casanova JL, Abel L, Human genetics of infectious diseases: a unified theory. EMBO Journal 2007; 26:915-922.

[37] Al-Muhsen S, Casanova JL, The genetic heterogeneity of mendelian susceptibility to mycobacterial diseases. J Aller Clin Immunol 2008; 122:1043-1051.

[38] Rezaei N, Aghamohammadi A, Mansouri D et al, Tuberculosis: a new outlook at an old disease. Expert Rev Clin Immunol 2011; 7(2):129-131.

[39] Ernst JD, The immunological life cycle of tuberculosis. Nat Rev Immunol 2012; 12(8): 581-590.

[40] Tan Q, Xie WP, Min R et al, Characterization of Th1 and Th2-type immune response in human multidrug resistant tuberculosis. Eur J Clin Microbiol Infect Dis 2012; 31(6): 1233-1242.

[41] Basu-Roy R, Whittaker E, Kampmann B, Current understanding of the immune response to tuberculosis in children; in: Heath PT (Ed), Paediatric and Neonatal Infections, Curr Opin Infect Dis 2012; 25(3):250-257.

[42] Alcais A, Fieschi C, Abel L, Casanova JL, Tuberculosis in children and in adults: two distinct genetic diseases. J Exp Med 2005; 202(12):1617-1621.

[43] Chambers MA, Gavier-Widen D, Hewinson RG, Antibody bound to the surface antigen MPB83 of Mycobacterium bovis enhances survival against high dose and low dose challenge. FEMS Immunol Med Microbiol 2004, 93.

[44] Cooper AM, Torrado E, Protection versus pathology in tuberculosis: recent insights. Curr Opin Immunol 2012; 24:431-437.

[45] Subbian S, Tsenova L, Yang G et al, Chronic pulmonary cavitary tuberculosis in rabbits: a failed host immune response. Open Biol 2011; 1:110016.

[46] Leistikow RL, Morton RA, Bartek IL et al, The Mycobacterium tuberculosis DosR regulon assists in metabolic homeostasis and enables rapid recovery from non-respiring dormancy. J Bacteriol 2010; 192:1662.

[47] Ramakrishnan L, Revisiting the role of the granuloma in tuberculosis. Nat Rev Immunol 2012; 12:352-366.

[48] Lin PL, Flynn JL, Understanding latent tuberculosis: a moving target. J Immunol 2010; 185:15.

[49] Tu HAT, Vu HD, Rozenbaum MH et al, A review of the literature on the economics of vaccination against TB. Expert Rev Vaccines 2012; 11(3):303-317.

[50] Guo S, Zhao J, Immunotherapy for tuberculosis: what's the better choice? Front Biosci 2012; 17:2684-2690.

[51] Ota MOC, Odutola AA, Owlafe PK et al, Immunogenicity of the tuberculosis vaccine MVA85A is reduced by coadministration with EPI vaccines in a randomized controlled trial in Gambian infants. Sci Transl Med 2011; 3:88ra56.

[52] Ly LH, McMurray DN, Tuberculosis: vaccines in the pipeline. Expert Rev Vaccines 2008, 7(5):635-650.

[53] Ernst JD et al, Meeting report: The international conference on human immunity to tuberculosis. Tuberculosis 2012; DOI: 10.1016/j.tube.2012.05.003.

[54] El Baghdadi J, Orlova M, Alter A et al, An autosomal dominant major gene confers predisposition to pulmonary tuberculosis in adults. J Exp Med 2006; 203:1679-1684.

[55] Wang D, Zhou Y, Ji L et al, Gene polymorphisms with tuberculosis susceptibility in Li population in China. PLoS One 2012; 7(3):e33051.

Chapter 4

Lipid Inclusions in Mycobacterial Infections

Matthias Stehr, Ayssar A. Elamin and Mahavir Singh

Additional information is available at the end of the chapter

1. Introduction

M. tuberculosis and *M. leprae* are intracellular pathogens. *M. tuberculosis* can survive up to decades in a phenotypically non-replicating dormant state, primarily in hypoxic granulomas in the lung [1]. The otherwise drug-susceptible dormant mycobacteria show the remarkable property to develop drug resistance within the granulomas of the host. These nonreplicative drug-resistant bacteria within the host's tissues are called persisters [2].

Mycobacteria have outstanding mechanisms to escape from elimination and have a high degree of intrinsic resistance to most antibiotics, chemotherapeutic agents and immune eradication [3,4]. One major obstacle for host defence mechanisms and therapeutic intervention is the robust, mycolic acid-rich cell wall, which is unique among prokaryotes [3,5]. In the last years it has become apparent that mycobacteria induce the accumulation of lipids in the host cells and use them as energy and carbon source. This strategy is regarded as another crucial factor for the long term-survival of *M. tuberculosis* and *M. leprae* in the host. Most mycobacteria have the ability to synthesize lipid bodies as reservoirs for fatty acids. The lipid droplet- containing macrophages are called "foamy macrophages" and are the hallmark of *M. tuberculosis* and *M. leprae* infection.

M. leprae is the causative agent of leprosy. Leprosy is a chronic infectious disease caused by the obligate intracellular bacterium *Mycobacterium leprae* and is a major source of morbidity in developing countries [6,7]. Leprosy patients show two major manifestations of the disease, known as as lepromatous leprosy (LL), and tuberculoid leprosy (TT) [6]. TT is observed in patients with good T-cell mediated (Th1) immunity and is characterized by granuloma formation and death of Schwann cells (Scs) leading to myelin degradation and nerve destruction [8,9]. Patients with poor T-cell mediated immunity show the lepromatous type leprosy (LL), which leads to a high bacterial load inside host cells specially in Schwann cells and macrophages [8,10-12]. For both forms of leprosy damage of the nerves is observed [12].

Lepromatous leprosy lesions of the skin, eyes, nerves, and lymph nodes are characterized by tumor-like accumulations of foamy macrophages. The foamy macrophages are fully packed with lipid droplets (LDs) and contain high numbers of leprosy bacilli. These aggregations of foamy macrophages expand slowly and disfigure the body of the host [13].

The finding that *M. leprae* has insufficient fatty acid synthetase activity to support growth lead to the hypothesis that *M. leprae* scavenges lipids from the host cell [14]. Over the last years it has become evident that survival and persistence of *M. tuberculosis* is critically dependent on lipid body formation. Furthermore lipid body formation seems to be the prerequisite for transition of *M. tuberculosis* to the dormant state. The formation of foamy macrophages is a process which appears to be a key event in both sustaining persistent bacteria and release of infectious bacilli [15]. This goes along with the important observation that sputum from tuberculosis patients contains lipid body-laden bacilli [16,17].

In the dormant state lipids from lipid bodies appear to be the primary carbon source for *M. tuberculosis* in vivo. For *M. tuberculosis* several bacterial genes are upregulated during the dormant state and have been reported to be involved in lipid metabolism such as diacylglycerol acyltransferase (tgs1), lipase (lipY), and isocitrate lyase (icl) [18,19].

M. leprae has a small genome (3.2 Mb). The obligate intracellular organism shows a moderate genome degradation and several genes are absent when compared with other mycobacterial species. Due to the gene loss *M. leprae* is strongly dependent on the host for basic metabolic functions [8,20]. Macrophages infected with *M. leprae* contain oxidized host lipids and it has been observed that *M. leprae* upregulates 13 host lipid metabolism genes in T-lep lesions and 26 in L-lep lesions. The oxidized lipids inhibit innate immune responses and thus seem to be an important virulence factor for the organism [21].

This review highlights the importance of the LDs as one of the most unique determinant for persistence and virulence of *M. tuberculosis* and *M. leprae*. The formation of LDs in *M. tuberculosis and M. leprae* in infected host cells shall be compared and the lipid metabolism of both organisms will be discussed.

In this review we will use the term "lipid droplets" for lipid-rich inclusions in the host and "lipid bodies" for lipid-rich inclusions in the pathogen.

2. Biogenesis of lipid inclusions in bacteria and eukaryotes

The current models of lipid droplet biogenesis are still hypothetical and have been reviewed extensively by Murphy in 1999 and Ohsaki in 2009 [22,23]. The most common model supposes that the membrane protein diacyltransferase DGAT1 synthesizes triacylglycerols (TAG), which accumulate between the two membrane leaflets of the endoplasmic reticulum (ER) to be finally released by budding. The lipids are covered by a phospholipid monolayer from the ER membrane.

The formation of lipid bodies in bacteria has been even less characterized. Wältermann et al. suggested in 2005 that a bifunctional wax ester synthase/acyl-CoA:diacylglycerol acyltransferase, (WS/DGAT) synthesizes TAG for lipid body formation. WS/DGAT is an integral membrane protein and synthesizes a growing globule around the cytoplasmic portion of the enzyme. Finally the lipid body is released to the cytoplasm. The origin of the surface phospholipid monolayer is not known [22,24].

2.1. Lipid droplets in the host

The accumulation of lipid droplets occurs also in several infectious, and inflammatory conditions, including in atherosclerosis [25], bacterial sepsis [26], viral infections [27], and in mycobacterial infections [15,28,29]. *M. tuberculosis* infected macrophages store mostly neutral lipids, while cells infected with *M. leprae* seem to accumulate next to TAG a high degree of cholesterol and cholesterol esters [10,30].

LDs are observed in various cells of the immune system including macrophages, neutrophils, and eosinophils. The structure and composition of LDs is highly conserved. They contain a core of neutral lipid esters typically TAG, but also sterols and sterol esters [31-36]. The surface is covered by a phospholipid monolayer, which is composed at least in some cells by unique fatty acids [37].

M. leprae infects preferentially macrophages and Schwann cells [11]. A typical feature of lepromatous leprosy is the survival and replication of. *M. leprae* within the lipid droplets stored in the enlarged phagosome of histiocytes. Lipid droplets are thought to be an important nutrient source for the bacillus. A major concern in leprosy is peripheral neuropathy. The damage to nerves of the peripheral nervous system is caused by the the infection of Schwann cells (SCs) by *M. leprae*. In LL nerve biopsies, highly infected SCs also contain lipid droplets and show a foamy appearance, such as Virchow cells found in dermal lesions [38]. The biology of the these foamy cells has been characterized poorly until now. Neither the origin or nature of the lipids has been elucidated yet. Only recently it *in vitro* studies by Mattos could show that ML induces the formation of lipid droplets in human SCs [10]. Moreover, the group found that LDs are promptly recruited to bacterial phagosomes. In SCs LD recruiting by bacterial phagosomes depends on cytoskeletal reorganization and PI3K signaling, but is independent of TLR2 bacterial sensing [10].

Important markers for the lipid accumulation in adipocytes or macrophages are lipid-droplet-associated proteins such as adipose differentiation-related protein ADRP and perilipin, which play essential roles in lipid-droplet formation [39]. After phagocytosis of live *M. leprae* ADRP expression is constantly upregulated in human monocytes. ADRP and perilipin are localized at the phagosomal membrane (Figure 4) [39].

2.2. Lipid bodies in the pathogen

Prokaryotes do not generally produce lipid bodies containing TAG. Accumulation of TAG in intracellular lipid-bodies is mostly restricted to bacteria belonging to the actinomycetes group [40].

Most mycobacterial species accumulate considerable amounts of TAG during infection [24,41-44]. The intracellular pathogen *M. tuberculosis* can survive up to decades in a phenotypically non-replicating dormant state, primarily in hypoxic granulomas in the lung [1]. The otherwise drug-susceptible dormant bacteria develop drug resistance within the granulomas of the host. These nonreplicative drug-resistant bacteria within the host's tissues are called persisters [2].

It has been observed that persisters store large amounts of intracellular triacylglycerol lipid bodies (LBs) [15,17,28,45,46]. *M. tuberculosis* uses TAG from the lipid bodies as energy and carbon source under conditions such as starvation [47], oxygen depletion [48], and pathogen reactivation [49]. The observation that sputum from tuberculosis patients contains lipid body-laden bacilli, proves the importance of lipids for the survival of the bacterium in the host [17].

3. *M. tuberculosis* induces foamy macrophages in the host

M. tuberculosis infects primarily alveolar macrophages, which reside within alveoli. The infected macrophage leaves the alveoli and migrates then towards the next lung draining lymph node. *M. tuberculosis* inhibits the generation of the phagolysosome and the bacteria begin to multiply within the macrophage [50]. The host's immune response seems to be unable to clear the bacillus from the infected macrophages. Infected macrophages secrete TNF-α and chemokines, which recruit systemic monocytes. The macrophages start to enlarge and accumulate TAG in lipid droplets. These lipid-filled foamy macrophages (FM) are surrounded by an outer layer of lymphocytes. Within the foamy macrophages the bacteria resist in phagosomes, packed with lipid droplets.

Over the last years it has become evident that survival and persistence of *M. tuberculosis* is critically dependent on lipid body formation, and induction of foamy macrophages appears to be a key event in both sustaining persistent bacteria and and release of infectious bacilli [15].

M. tuberculosis-infected phagosomes engulf cellular lipid droplets and finally the bacteria are completely enclosed by cellular lipid droplets. Only enclosed by lipid droplets the bacteria form lipid bodies and cell replication comes to a halt and finally the bacteria enter the state of dormancy and induced drug resistance [19,28]. In the nonreplicative state *M. tuberculosis* induces several bacterial genes involved in lipid metabolism such as diacylglycerol acyltrans-ferase (tgs1), such as diacylglycerol acyltransferase (*tgs1*), lipase (*lipY*), and isocitrate lyase (*icl*) are upregulated [19,46]. In conclusion lipid body formation seems to be absolutely necessary for transition of *M. tuberculosis* to the dormant state. This goes along with the important observation that sputum from tuberculosis patients contains lipid body-laden bacilli [17].

The final granuloma consists of a core of infected, lipid-laden macrophages, which are surrounded by an outer layer of additional differentiated macrophages. The outer shell consists of T lymphocytes, B lymphocytes, dendritic cells, neutrophils, fibroblasts and an extracellular matrix [29,51-53].

The development and composition of a human tuberculosis granuloma is depicted in Figure 1.

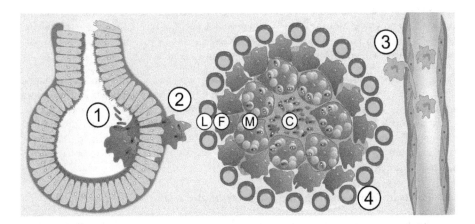

Figure 1. Development and structure of the human tuberculosis granuloma. 1, Uptake of *M. tuberculosis* by alveolar macrophages. 2, Migration of the infected macrophage towards the next lung draining lymph node. 3, Recruitment of systemic monocytes. 4, Granuloma formation. L, Lymphocytes at the periphery of the granuloma outside the fibrous outer layer. F, Fibrous capsule. Contains fibroblasts, collagen and other extracellular matrix proteins. M, Macrophage region with foamy macrophages. C, Caseum. Contains debris and lipids from necrotic macrophages. Orange, Lipid droplets of the macrophage. Yellow dots, Lipid bodies.

3.1. Lipid body formation in *M. tuberculosis* is critically dependent on lipid droplets from the host

Host lipids from lipid droplets are used by the pathogen as substantial nutrient source. Middlebrook already demonstrated in the late 1940s that mycobacterial growth *in vitro* was enhanced by supplementation with oleic acid [54]. Over the last years several groups have reported that *M. tuberculosis* within foamy macrophages produces lipid bodies, suggesting that they are able to accumulate host cell lipids [19,55]. Mycobacterial growth inside adipocytes is strictly dependent upon TAG provided by lipid droplets in host cells [55], and it has been shown that *M. tuberculosis* incorporates intact host TAG into bacterial TAG [46].

The utilization of host lipids in vivo does not only promote survival but may also increases virulence and modulate the immune response to infection. Growth of *M. tuberculosis* on fatty acids such as such propionate or valerate during infection leads to increased production of the surface-exposed lipid virulence factors, phthiocerol dimycocerosate (PDIM) and sulfolipid-1 (SL-1) [56].

Cholesterol utilization was also identified to be required for mycobacterial persistence [57]. In 2008 Pandey and Sassetti found that *M. tuberculosis* can grow using cholesterol as a primary carbon source and that the mce4 transporter is required for cholesterol uptake. *M. tuberculosis* contains four homologous mce operons, mce1–mce4, which are thought to encode lipid transporters [57,58].

Especially *M. leprae* infected macrophages show an increased accumulation of cholesterol and cholesterol [10,30]. But in contrast to *M. tuberculosis* the *M. leprae* genome encodes only one operon for cholesterol uptake (mce1). All *M. leprae* five *mce* genes were overexpressed during intracellular growth in mouse and human biopsies [59,60]. This observation suggests, that the intracellular bacilli population induces cholersterol uptake of the infected cell and subsequently uses the stored cholesterol as carbon and energy source.

Cholesterol is also essential for uptake of *M. tuberculosis* and *M. leprae* in macrophages. Cholesterol accumulates at the site of mycobacterial entry in macrophages and promotes mycobacterial uptake. Cholesterol mediates the recruitment of TACO from the plasma membrane to the phagosome [61]. TACO, also termed as CORO1A, is a coat protein that prevents phagosome-lysosome fusion and thus degradation of mycobacteria in phagolysosomes (Figure 4) [61,62]. This mechanism for the formation of TACO-coated phagosomes promotes intracellular survival [62,63].

3.2. Lipid body formation in *M. tuberculosis* is critically dependent on lipid droplets

Host lipids from lipid droplets are used by the pathogen as substantial nutrient source. Middlebrook already demonstrated in the late 1940s that mycobacterial growth *in vitro* was enhanced by supplementation with oleic acid [54]. Host lipids play an important role during infection. They appear to be the primary carbon source for *M. tuberculosis* in vivo. Over the last years several groups have reported that *M. tuberculosis* within foamy macrophages produces lipid bodies, suggesting that they are able to accumulate host cell lipids [19,55]. Neyrolles et al. showed that mycobacterial growth inside adipocytes occurs only after the formation of lipid droplets in the host cell. This result emphasizes that *M. tuberculosis* is dependent upon TAG provided by lipid droplets in host cells [55]. In 2011 Daniel et al. finally demonstrated that *M. tuberculosis* inside foamy macrophages imports fatty acids derived from host TAG and incorporates them intact into bacterial TAG. Moreover the group proved the accumulation of TAG in lipid bodies [46].

The utilization of host lipids in vivo does not only promote survival but may also increases virulence and modulate the immune response to infection. Growth of *M. tuberculosis* on fatty acids such as such propionate or valerate during infection leads to increased production of the surface-exposed lipid virulence factors, phthiocerol dimycocerosate (PDIM) and sulfolipid-1 (SL-1) [56].

Cholesterol utilization was also identified to be required for mycobacterial persistence [57]. In 2008 Pandey and Sassetti found that *M. tuberculosis* can grow using cholesterol as a primary carbon source and that the mce4 transporter is required for cholesterol uptake. *M. tuberculosis* contains four homologous mce operons, mce1–mce4, which are thought to encode lipid transporters [57,58].

3.3. Biosynthesis of TAG and formation of lipid bodies in *M. tuberculosis*

Biosynthesis of TAG consists of the sequential esterification of the glycerol moiety with fatty acyl-residues by various acyltransferases. Fatty acid biosynthesis consists of the stepwise addition of acetyl groups, which are provided by acetyl-CoA. The initial step is the transfer of an acetyl group from acetyl-CoA to a small protein, called acyl carrier protein (ACP). In the following two-carbon fragments are added sequentially to yield fatty acids of the desired length. *M. tuberculosis* uses both type I and type II FAS systems for fatty acid elongation. The multifunctional FAS I enzyme (*Rv2524c*) catalyzes the de novo synthesis of C_{16}- and C_{18}-S-ACP. These fatty acids are converted to the CoA derivative and used primarily for the synthesis of membrane phospholipids. By continuous elongation of these fatty acids FAS I produces specifically the C20- and C26-S-ACP products, and these fatty acids are released as the CoA derivatives. The C20 fatty acid is transferred to the FAS II system for the synthesis of the very-long-chain mero segment of α-, methoxy-, and ketomycolic acids [64]. The transfer from the FAS I to the FAS II system occurs by a key condensing enzyme, the ketoacyl ACP synthase III (FabH). FabH catalyzes the decarboxylative condensation of malonyl-ACP with the acyl-CoA products of the FAS I system (Figure 2). Two distinct cyclopropane synthases, MmaA2 and PcaA introduce cyclopropane rings into the the growing acyl chain [64-66].

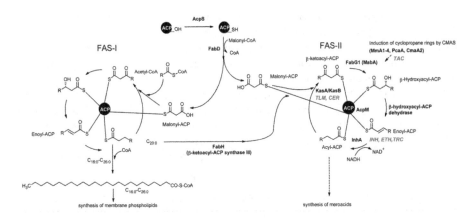

Figure 2. Fatty acid biosynthesis in *Mycobacterium tuberculosis*. The FAS-II elongation module uses the substrates R-CO-S-ACP and malonyl-S-ACP derived from malonyl-S-CoA, generated by FabD. FabH condenses both substrates R, long-chain alkyl group. Enzymes involved in these reactions are as follows: FabG1, a β-ketoacyl-ACP reductase catalyzes the reduction of beta-ketoacyl-ACP substrates to beta-hydroxyacyl-ACP. β-hydroxyacyl-ACP dehydrase. 2-trans-enoyl-ACP reductase (InhA). The β-ketoacyl-ACP synthase (KasA/KasB) catalyzes the addition of of two carbons from malonyl-ACP to R-CO-S-ACP (See text for details). R, long-chain alkyl group. ACP, acyl carrier protein. Enzymes are in bold letters. Selected inhibitors are depicted in red bold letters. TLM, thiolactomycin. CER, cerulenin. ETH, ethionamide. INH, isoniazid. TRC, triclosan. TAC, thiacetazone.

Esterification of fatty acids with glycerol-3-phosphate occurs via sequential acylation of the sn-1,2 and 3 positions of glycerol-3-phosphate, and removal of the phosphate group before the last acylation step. The terminal reaction is the esterification of diacylglycerol (DAG) with acyl-CoA by an diacylglycerol acyltransferase [40]. Animals and plants use diacylglycerol acyl-transferases (DGAT) for the terminal esterification. DGATs catalyze exclusively the esterification of acyl-CoA with diacylglycerol. Bacteria do not contain

DGATs but only bifunctional wax ester synthase/acyl-CoA:diacylglycerol acyltransferases (WS/DGAT). WS/DGATs, mediate next to TAG formation the synthesis of waxes by ester-ification of acyl-CoA with alcohol [67]. The genome of M. tuberculosis codes for 15 genes which contain the highly conserved putative active site motif of WS/DGATs (HHxxxDG). These genes were designated as "tgs", triacylglycerol synthases, but have only a weak se-quence similarity to other WS/DGAT sequences. All 15 expressed mycobacterial Tgs pro-teins show diacylglycerol acyltransferase activity and Tgs1 has the highest activity of all enzymes [48]. Gene disruption of tgs1 results in a drastic reduction of major C26 long-chain fatty acid in M. tuberculosis grown under hypoxic conditions. Thus Tgs1 appears to be a major contributor to TAG synthesis in M. tuberculosis so far [48,68]. And moreover two homologous proteins to Tgs1 and Tgs2 (BCG3153c and BCG3794c) and another poor-ly characterized acyltransferase (BCG1489c) were found to be exclusively associated to lip-id bodies. The disruption of BCG3153c, BCG3794c, and BCG1489c reduces TAG accumulation during the hypoxia-induced nonreplicating state, revealing that the en-zymes are involved in TAG synthesis during latency and pathogenicity [69].

Ten of the 15 tgs genes in M. tuberculosis are located adjacent or proximal to 11 lip genes that are annotated as probable phospholipases or lipases-esterases-carboxylesterases. Some tgs genes may be cotranscribed with neighboring lip genes and may synthesize triacylglycerols from the released fatty acids from the host [18]. Lip gene products may be important for utilization of TAGs during dormancy and upon reactivation after dormancy. The tgs gene Rv0221 is located near lipC (Rv0220), lipW (Rv0217c), acyl-CoA synthetase (Rv0214), acyl-CoA dehydrogenase (Rv0215c), and an integral membrane acyltransferase (Rv0228). This clustering of genes of the fatty acid metabolism suggests that these genes may be cotranscribed and may release fatty acid from host TAG, carry out the transport of fatty acids and finally catalyze the re-synthesis of TAGs in the pathogen. Rv0221 and LipC have to be shown to be catalytical active. [18,70].

In summary Tgs enzymes play a major role in TAG synthesis, lipid body formation and maintenance.

Ag85A, a mycoltransferase, that is known to catalyze the formation of the cord factor was recently found to have additional DGAT activity [71]. The kinetic parameters are quite similar to those reported for the M. tuberculosis Tgs1-4, but the primary sequence of Ag85A does not contain the active site motif of WS/DGATs or TGS enzymes (HHxxxDG) [48,68,71]. Ag85A belongs to the α/β hydrolase fold family and contains the consensus GXSXG sequence. The enzyme is a carboxylesterase with an additional acyltransferase activity. Overexpression of Ag85A induces lipid body formation in M. smegmatis. The enzyme is located in the mycobac-terial cell wall, suggesting that it may be involved in the maintenance of lipid droplets in the host cell [71].

The genome of M.leprae contains also mycolytransferase 85 complex genes (A, B and C). Transcripts of these genes are upregulated either in infected nude mouse or human skin lesions [59].

The *M. leprae* genome shows only one predicted gene product which has has a significant degree of identity to any the Tgs enzymes from *M. tuberculosis* [18]. The tgs gene product ML1244 shows 72% identity to Rv2484c from *M. tuberculosis*. *Rv2448* is located next to a carboxylesterase lipQ, (*Rv2485c*), a probable glycerol-3-phosphate acyltransferase, (*Rv2482c*), a lysophosphatidic acid acyltransferase-like protein (*Rv2483c*), and a probable enoyl-CoA hydratase (*Rv2486*). The gene cluster of lipid metabolism genes suggests a possible involvement of the gene products in the synthesis of TAG [18]. A few tgs genes (*Rv3234c*, *Rv3233c*, *Rv2285*, and *Rv1425*) are located proximal to lipoproteins, which may serve as donors or acceptors of fatty acids [48]

3.4. Activation of TAG – Lipases and esterases of *M. tuberculosis*

Neutral lipids in the core of the lipid body are hydrolyzed by lipases or esterases, yielding fatty acids for energy generation and anabolism of membrane phospholipids.

In the genome of *M. tuberculosis* H37Rv twenty-one genes are termed as putative lipases (*lip* A to W, except K and S) [72]. The annotation was only based on the presence of the consensus sequence GXSXG, which is characteristic for the large group of the α/β hydrolase fold protein family, which includes lipases as well as esterases, proteases, peroxidases, epoxide hydrolases and dehalogenases [72]. Thus the members of the lip group have only a very low level of sequence identity of ~20% and might have another function apart from lipid hydrolysis. Only the gene product of *Rv3097c* (LipY)) shows reasonable hydrolase activity for long-chain TAG with chain lengths ranging from C4 to C18. Overexpression of LipY induces extensive TAG hydrolysis. Disruption of *lipY* markedly reduces but does not completely inactivate TAG hydrolase activity, which suggests the presence of other lipases in *M. tuberculosis* [47,49].

Overexpression of *LipY* in *M. bovis* Bacillus Calmette-Guérin reduces protection against infection in mice, indicating that lipY plays a central role in TAG hydrolysis and virulence [47,73,74]. LipY contains a PE (Pro-Glu) domain, that is involved in modulation of LipY activity [73]. The PE domain contains a signal sequence for secretion of LipY by the ESX-5 system. It has been implicated that the secreted LipY is loosely associated with the bacterial surface where it may hydrolyze host's TAG [75].

Several other esterases, next to the members of the Lip group have been identified and biochemically characterized. They all belong also to the α/β hydrolase fold family and showing the minimal GXSXG motif. In 2007 Côtes et al. characterized a novel lipase Rv0183. The enzyme is only found in the cell wall and culture medium. This observation suggests that Rv0183 is involved in the degradation of the host cell lipids e.g. when M. tuberculosis infects adipocytes [55,76]. Another probably cell wall-associated carboxylesterase is encoded by Rv2224c. The esterase Rv2224c was found to be required for bacterial survival in mice [77]. The substrate spectrum of Rv2224c is poorly characterized and until now it is unknown whether the enzyme uses TAG as substrate [77]. Furthermore the three-dimensional structures of the esterases Rv0045c (PDB 3P2M) [78], Rv1847 (PDB 3S4K), and LipW (3QH4) from *M. tuberculosis* have been determined, but unfortunately it is not known whether these enzymes are involved in TAG hydrolysis.

3.5. Lipase genes of *M. leprae*

In the *M. leprae* genome only 2 lipase genes (*lipG, lipU*) were found. But *M. tuberculosis* has also only six expressed Lip enzymes, showing reasonable hydrolase activity for long-chain triacylglycerols. (LipY, LipC, LipL, LipX, LipK, LipG). LipG and LipU from *M. leprae* are homologous with LipG and LipU from *M. tuberculosis* and show sequence identities of 72 and 79%, respectively. The lipases LipG and LipU from *M. tuberculosis* show very low and no activity with long chain triacylglycerols as substrates [47]. *M. tuberculosis* LipY is suspected to be a major functional lipase, which utilizes stored triacylglycerols (TAG) during dormancy and reactivation of the pathogen [47,49]. LipY shows only a weak similarity with *M. leprae* LipU (23 % identity). In summary it appears that *M. leprae* uses different lipases for the hydrolysis of fatty acids than *M. tuberculosis*.

3.6. Enzymes of the β-oxidation and glyoxylate cycle

M. tuberculosis can grow on fatty acids as sole carbon source and it has been demonstrated that fatty acid oxidation is important for survival of the pathogen in the lungs of mice [79,80]. Fatty acids are oxidized via the β-oxidation cycle and the glyoxylate shunt, to replenish TCA cycle intermediates during growth [81]. The β-oxidation cycle consists of five biochemical reactions, where one molecule acetyl-CoA of the fatty acid is split off per cycle. The genome of *M. tuberculosis* encodes around 100 genes, designated as fad genes (fatty acid degradation) with putative roles in the β-oxidation of fatty acids. While *E. coli* has only one enzyme for each step of the β-oxidation cycle, *M. tuberculosis* seems to have several backup enzymes for each reaction [82]. The initial step of β-oxidation is the formation of acyl-CoA from free fatty acids and Coenzyme A and is catalyzed by acyl-CoA synthase. In *M. bovis* BCG one Acyl-CoA synthase (BCG1721) (Rv1683) has been identified to be exclusively bound to lipid bodies. Nonreplicating mycobacteria, which overexpress a BCG1721 construct with an inactive lipase domain displayed a phenotype of attenuated TAG breakdown and regrowth upon resuscitation. These results indicate that the gene might be essential for TAG hydrolysis and growth [69].

Together with malate synthase, isocitrate lyase (ICL) is the key enzyme of the glyoxylate cycle that catalyzes the cleavage of isocitrate to glyoxylate and succinate [81,83]. The *M. tuberculosis* genome codes for two isocitrate lyases, icl and icl2, which are essential for the fatty acid metabolism and jointly required for in vivo growth and virulence. Disruption of icl has only little effect on survival in macrophages and bacterial loads in lungs of infected mice. Only disruption of both lyase genes results in a fast elimination of bacteria from lungs of infected mice and infected macrophages [79,80]. These results strongly suggest that both icl genes are required for mycobacterial persistence.

All enzymes involved in lipid metabolism in lipid bodies are summarized in Table 1.

M. leprae has approximately one-third as many potential fad enzymes with probable roles in the β-oxidation. Even though *M. leprae* genome contains less necessary β-oxidation cycle genes than *M. tuberculosis*, transcript analysis revealed expression of acyl-CoA metabolic enzymes including *echA1* (ML0120, putative enoyl-CoA hydratase), *echA12* (ML1241, possible enoyl-CoA hydratase), *fadA2* (ML2564, acetyl-CoA-acetyltransferase), *fadB2* (ML2461, 3-hydroxyacyl-CoA dehydrogenase), *fadD19* (ML0352, acyl-CoA synthase), *fadD26* (ML2358, fatty acid-CoA-ligase), *fadD29* (ML0132, probable fatty-acid-CoA synthetase), *fadD28* (ML0138, possible fatty-acid-CoA synthetase), *fadE25* (ML0737, probable acyl-CoA dehydrogenase) and *fadE5* (ML2563, acyl-CoA dehydrogenase) [59,60]. This gives strong evidence that host lipids provide the main carbon and energy sources for *M. leprae* during infection.

The *M. leprae* genome contains a gene, coding for an isocitrate lyase, *aceA*. The amino acid-sequence of AceA (ML1985c) shows 80 % identity with its homologue from *M. tuberculosis* ICL2 (Rv1915/1916). *AceA* is upregulated in both *M. leprae*-infected nude mouse and human lesions. [59]. A second icl gene, as observed in *M. tuberculosis*, is not present in the genome of *M. leprae*. This finding is of particular interest, because both lyases, *icl* and *icl2*, are jointly required for in vivo growth and virulence [79,80]. Deletion of *icl1* or *icl2* has little effect on bacterial growth in macrophages [80]. So far the *M. leprae* AceA might play a slightly different role in as the both isocitrate lyases in *M. tuberculosis*.

4. Lipid composition in *M. leprae* infected cells

In 1863, Virchow described foamy cells, which form droplets and surround *M. leprae* within the phagolysomes. [84,85]. This lipid capsule forms a characteristic electron-transparent zone. In contrast to *M. tuberculosis*, the presence of lipid bodies seem to be rather exceptional in *M. leprae* [85]. The lipid capsule contains mycoserosoic acids of phthiocerol dimycocerosates as well as phenolic glycolipids [86,87]. Brennan reported the full characterization of three phenol-phthiocerol triglycosides by *M. leprae* [84]. It has been postulated that many of these molecules together with phosphatidylinositol mannosides and phospholipids are released from the cell wall after synthesis, forming the capsule-like region [11]. The dominant lipid in the cell wall which gives *M. leprae* immunological specificity is phenolic glycolipid-1 (PGL-1). Phenolic glycolipid 1 has been isolated in relatively high concentrations from purified bacteria and from *M. leprae* infected tissues [88]. PGL-1 is thought to be a major component of the capsule in *M. leprae* and constitutes an important interface between bacteria and host [89]. It has been suggested that PGL-1 is involved in the interaction of *M. leprae* with the laminin of Schwann cells, thus PGL-1 hight play a role in peripheral nerve-bacillus interactions [90]. Moreover, phenolic glycolipids seem to be involved in the in the stimulation of suppressor T-cells in lepromatous leprosy [91]. Recently it was reported that also LDs from *M. leprae* infected SCs and macrophages accumulate mainly host derived lipids, such as oxidized phospholipids [92]. BODIPY stains infected SCs, indicating that LDs contain neutral lipids, such as triacylglycerols (TAG), but it seems as *M. leprae*-infected cells accumulate large amounts of cholesterol and choesterol esters [10].

Gene	Protein	DGAT activity (in vitro)	Lipid body associated	Influence on lipid bodies / TGA accumulation	Modulation of virulence	M. leprae homologue	Reference
Rv3130c (tgs1)	DGAT	+	+	Δtgs1 decreases TAG accumulation	NA	ML1244	[46,48,68]
Rv3734c (tgs2)	DGAT	+	+	NA	NA	ML1244	[48,68]
Rv3234c (tgs3)	DGAT	+	NA	NA	NA	ML1244	[48,68]
Rv3088 (tgs4)	DGAT	+	NA	NA	NA	ML1244	[48,68]
Rv1760	DGAT	+	NA	NA	NA	ML1244	[48,68]
Rv2285	DGAT	+	NA	NA	NA	ML1244	[48,68]
Rv3804c (85A)	DGAT	+	NA	Overexpression increases production of lipid bodies	NA	ML0097 (85A)	[71]
BCG1489c [Rv1428c]	DGAT	NA	+	ΔBCG1489c reduces TAG accumulation	NA	ML2427c	[69]
BCG3153c (tgs1) [Rv3130c]	DGAT	NA	+	ΔBCG3153c reduces TAG accumulation	NA	ML1244	[69]
BCG3794c (tgs2) [Rv3734c]	DGAT	NA	+	ΔBCG3794c reduces TAG accumulation	NA	ML1244	[69]
BCG1489c [Rv1428c]	acyltransferase	NA	+	ΔRv1428c reduces TAG accumulation	NA		[69]

Gene	Protein	TGA-hydrolyzing activity (in vitro)	Lipid body associated	Influence on lipid bodies / TGA accumulation	Modulation of virulence	M. leprae homologue	Reference
Rv3097c (lipY)	Lipase/esterase	+	NA	ΔlipY reduces TAG hydrolysis. Overexpression increases TAG hydrolysis	Overexpression increases virulence in mice	ML0314c (lipU) ML1053 ML1183c	[47]
Rv1399c (lipH)	Lipase/esterase	+	NA	NA	NA	ML0314c (lipU)	[72]
BCG1721 [Rv1683]	Lipase/esterase	+ (in vivo*)	+	+ (*)	NA	ML1346	[69]
Rv0183	Lipase/esterase	Hydrolyzes only monoacylglycerides	NA	NA	NA	ML2603	[76]
Rv2224c	Lipase/esterase	NA	NA	NA	Gene disruption decreases virulence in mice	ML1633c	[77]

Gene	Protein	Isocitrate cleavage (in vitro)	Lipid body associated	Influence on lipid bodies / TGA accumulation	Modulation of virulence	M. leprae homologue	Reference
Rv0467 (icl), Rv1915-1916 (icl2)	isocitrate lyase	+	NA	NA	The Δicl, Δicl2 strain shows no intracellular replication	ML1985c (aceA)	[79,80,93-95]

Table 1. Enzymes involved in lipid body metabolism in M. tuberculosis and M. bovis BCG. Homologous genes in M. tuberculosis H37Rv are written in square brackets. NA, not applicable. *, expressed in yeast as recombinant protein. DGAT, diacylglycerol acyltransferase

5. Induction of lipid droplet biogenesis

Since the biogenesis of lipid droplets in macrophages seems an absolute requirement for intracellular bacteria to establish infections, we will discuss mechanisms involved in foam cell formation and development of lipid droplets.

5.1. Scavenger receptor mediated lipid droplet biogenesis in *M. tuberculosis*

Upon infection with pathogenic bacteria macrophages generate reactive oxygen species (ROS). The release of ROS generates oxidative stress, and results not only in damage to cellular structures but also to oxidation of fatty acids, such as low density lipoproteins (OxLDL) in granulomas. The binding of OxLDL to type 1 scavenger receptors CD36 and LOX1 induces increased surface expression of both receptors, leading to uptake of OxLDL [96-98]. In addition, CD36 increases the uptake of *M. tuberculosis* by macrophages [99]. The increased rate of OxLDL uptake results in the accumulation of oxidized lipids, which finally leads to the formation of foamy macrophages [98]. *M. tuberculosis* and *M. leprae* benefit from the accumulated OxLDL in the infected macrophage. OxLDL-laden lung macrophages show enhanced replication of intracellular *M. tuberculosis* compared to macrophages loaded with non-oxidized LDL [98]. The presence of oxidized phospholipids in *M. leprae* infected macrophages down-regulates the innate immune response and contributes to pathogenesis [92]. Moreover, scavenger receptor-deficient phagocytes are characterized by a reduced intracellular bacterial survival and a lower cytokine response [100].

5.2. TLR mediated LD formation in *M. bovis* and *M. leprae*

Mycobacterium bovis Bacillus Calmette-Guérin (BCG) and *M. leprae* are recognised by the Toll-like receptors (TLR) TLR6 and TLR2 [101,102]. Mycobacterium bovis Bacillus Calmette-Guérin induced lipid body formation is TLR2 mediated [103]. The mycobacterial surface molecule lipoarabinomannan (LAM) induces the formation of foamy macrophages by binding to TLR2 [104] (Figure 3).

M. leprae association to macrophages is mediated by binding of the bacteria to TLR2 and TLR6. Heterodimerization of TLR2 and TLR6 leads to downstream signalling and subsequent LD formation [102,105]. Macrophage association is not dependent on binding to TLR2 or TLR6. Neither a TLR2$^{-/-}$ or TLR6$^{-/-}$ knockout macrophage shows reduced binding to *M. leprae*. This suggests that both TLR2 and TLR6 can bind *M. leprae* alone, or/and the presence of other receptors, binding to *M. leprae*. The TLR2$^{-/-}$ or TLR6$^{-/-}$ knockout macrophages do also not completely abolish LD formation, but show only reduced LD formation [102]. This suggests the presence of additional signalling pathways for LD formation. In SCs TLR6, but not TLR2, is essential for *M. leprae*-induced LD biogenesis in [101]. In LL lesions, accumulated with LD enriched macropages the genes for ADRP and CD36 are up-regulated [30,92,102]. This suggests also an involvement of CD36 in LD formation of *M. leprae* (Figure 4) [99].

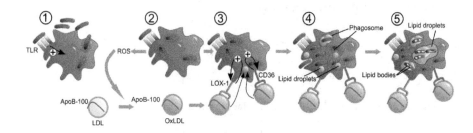

Figure 3. Induction of lipid droplet biogenesis in macrophages by *Mycobacterium tuberculosis*. 1) Recognition of bacteria by Toll-like receptors (TLR) trigger phagocytosis and subsequent formation of lipid droplets. 2) The infected macrophage produces reactive oxygen species (ROS), which oxidize LDL. 3) The binding of OxLDL to type 1 scavenger receptors CD36 and LOX1 induces increased surface expression of both receptors and increases uptake of host´s oxidized fatty acids. 4) Mycobacterium-laden phagosomes internalize lipid droplets. 5) Within the lipid droplets the bacteria form lipid bodies and finally enter the dormant state. ApoB-100, apolipoprotein B-100.

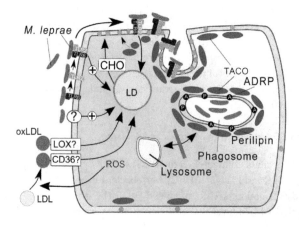

Figure 4. Basic mechanisms of lipid droplet induction in *M. leprae* infected macrophages. *M. leprae* attaches to TLR2 and TLR6. Heterodimerization of TLR2 and TLR6 induces downstream signalling and subsequent accumulation by LD formation. [102,105]. In SCs TLR6, but not TLR2, is essential for *M. leprae*-induced LD biogenesis [101]. Cholesterol from the LDs accumulates at the site of mycobacterial entry and promotes mycobacterial uptake. Cholesterol also recruits TACO from the plasma membrane to the phagosome [61]. TACO prevents phagosome-lysosome fusion and promotes intracellular survival [62,63]. Hypothetical uptake of oxidized lipids by scavenger receptors in *M. leprae*: Reactive oxygen species might oxidize low-density lipoprotein (LDL) to oxLDL, which is thought to be subsequently bound and taken up by scavenger receptors CD36 and LOX1. CHO, cholesterol. Unknown mechanisms for LD induction are indicated with a question mark.

5.3. Mycolic acids induce the formation of foamy macrophages

Mycolic acids and oxygenated mycolic acids are strong inducers of monocyte-derived macrophages differentiation into foamy macrophages [19,106]. Peyron et al. demonstrated that that a set of oxygenated mycolic acids specifically produced by highly virulent myco-bacteria species (*M. tuberculosis, M. avium*) were responsible for the formation of foamy macrophages [19].

6. Clinical implications

Several enzymes of the mycobacterial lipid-biosynthesis are regarded as targets for new antitubercular compounds. The research focused on enzymes, involved in the biosynthesis of lipid compounds of the mycobacterial cell wall [107]. Especially the biosynthesis of the highly toxic cord factor is an attractive target. The cord factor is synthesized by the antigen 85 complex [108,109]. It was recently shown that one member of the complex, antigen 85A is involved in the formation of intracellular lipid bodies [71]. Antigen 85 is an important virulence factor. It has been shown that *M. tuberculosis* requires the expression of Ag85A for growth in macro-phages [110]. *M. tuberculosis* strain lacking Ag85C shows an decrease of 40% in the amount of cell wall linked mycolic acids [111,112]. The treatment by a trehalose analogue, 6-azido-6-deoxy-α,α'-trehalose (ADT) inhibits the activity of all members of Ag85 complex *in vitro* [108, 113]. Also ethambutol targets the synthesis of arabinogalactan, isoniazid and ethionamide inhibit biosynthesis of mycolic acids [107].

The most potent inhibitor for mycolic acid biosynthesis is isoniazid (INH). INH is a prodrug which is converted to the isonicotinoyl radical by KatG. INH forms a covalent adduct with NAD. This INH-NAD adduct inhibits FAS-II enoyl-ACP reductase InhA, which in conse-quence leads to inhibition of mycolic acid biosynthesis, and ultimately to cell death [114-117]. The inhibitors of fatty acid biosynthesis are summarized in Figure 2 and Table 2.

Synthesis step	Enzyme	Compound / class	References
FAS-I and FAS-II	KasA/KasB	Cerulenin (2R,3S-epoxy-4-oxo-7,10-trans,trans-dodecanoic acid amide	[118] [119]
FAS-II	KasA/KasB	TLM (Thiolactomycin)	[120-122]
FAS-II	KasA/KasB	Platensimycin	[123]
	InhA	INH (Isoniazid)	[124]
	InhA	ETH (Ethionamide)	[125]
	InhA	TRC (Triclosan)	[126]
	InhA	alkyl diphenyl ethers (Triclosan derivatives)	[127]
	InhA	2-(o-Tolyloxy)-5-hexylphenol (PT70)	[120]
Cyclopro-panation	CMASs (cmaA2, mmaA2 or pcaA)	TAC (Thiacetazone)	[128]
	MmaA4	TAC (Thiacetazone)	[128]

Table 2. Inhibitors of fatty acid biosynthesis

7. Conclusion

The formation of lipid inclusions during infection in the host as well as in the pathogen during intracellular infection with *M. tuberculosis* and *M. leprae* plays an important role in pathogenesis. A hallmark of intracellular infection is the formation of foamy macrophages. *M. tuberculosis* and *M. leprae* induce the formation of lipid droplets in the host cell. The accumulated lipids are used as energy and carbon source. In fact *M. tuberculosis* seems to switch completely to fatty acid catabolism at the transition from the acute to the chronic phase of infection. The central role of fatty acid metabolism during the dormant state of *M. tuberculosis* is underlined by the finding that both isocitrate lyase, icl and icl2, are essential for intracellular replication in the lung [79,80]. The TAG metabolism and the resulting formation of lipid inclusions of host and pathogen play a fundamental role in infection. Indeed TAG-derived fatty acids from the host cell are imported into *M. tuberculosis* and incorporated into bacterial TAG [46]. In conclusion the enzymes involved in lipid droplet metabolism are essential for survival of the pathogen in the lung and thus attractive targets for novel drugs. Especially enzymes with DGAT activity such as Tgs and Ag85A seem to be promising drug target candidates. Another promising targets seem to be the recently discovered cell wall associated and secreted esterases, which are involved in the utilization of host cell lipids such as Rv0183 and LipY [55, 75,76]. Future studies should also focus on the lipid metabolism of *M. leprae*, an organism which upregulates several genes of the host's lipid metabolism during infection [92]. The regulation of lipid droplet formation in the host cell is another important topic. Recent sudies revealed that intracellular pathogens induce the expression of LDL receptor and scavenger receptors CD36 and LOX1 for the internalization of native and oxidized fatty acids. Especially the generation of oxidized lipids by macrophage-derived reactive oxygen species seems to be an important mechanism for the induction of scavenger receptors.

Author details

Matthias Stehr[1], Ayssar A. Elamin[1] and Mahavir Singh[1,2*]

*Address all correspondence to: Mahavir.Singh@helmholtz-hzi.de

1 LIONEX Diagnostics and Therapeutics GmbH, Braunschweig, Germany

2 Department of Genome Analytics, Helmholtz Centre for Infection Research, Braunschweig, Germany

References

[1] Murphy D. J., Brown J. R. Identification of gene targets against dormant phase *Mycobacterium tuberculosis* infections. BMC Infect. Dis. 2007;7 84.

[2] Zhang Y. Persistent and dormant tubercle bacilli and latent tuberculosis. Front. Biosci. 2004;9 1136-1156.

[3] Brennan P. J., Nikaido H. The envelope of mycobacteria. Annual review of biochemistry 1995;64 29-63.

[4] Coker R. J. Review: multidrug-resistant tuberculosis: public health challenges. Tropical medicine & international health : TM & IH 2004;9 25-40.

[5] Barry C. E., 3rd, Lee R. E., Mdluli K., Sampson A. E., Schroeder B. G., Slayden R. A., Yuan Y. Mycolic acids: structure, biosynthesis and physiological functions. Progress in lipid research 1998;37 143-179.

[6] Ridley D. S., Jopling W. H. Classification of leprosy according to immunity. A five-group system. Int Int. J. Lepr. 1966;34 255-273.

[7] WHO, WHO Leprosy Today, WHO, 2010.

[8] Cosma C. L., Sherman D. R., Ramakrishnan L. The secret lives of the pathogenic mycobacteria. Annu. Rev. Microbiol. 2003;57 641-676.

[9] Scollard D. M. Endothelial cells and the pathogenesis of lepromatous neuritis:insights from the armadillo model. Microbes Infect. 2000;2 1835-1843.

[10] Mattos K. A., Lara F. A., Oliveira V. G., Rodrigues L. S., D'Avila H., Melo R. C., Manso P. P., Sarno E. N., Bozza P. T., Pessolani M. C. Modulation of lipid droplets by *Mycobacterium leprae* in Schwann cells: a putative mechanism for host lipid acquisition and bacterial survival in phagosomes. Cell. Microbiol. 2011;13 259-273.

[11] Scollard D. M., Adams L. B., Gillis T. P., Krahenbuhl J. L., Truman R. W., Williams D. L. The continuing challenges of leprosy. Clin. Microbiol. Rev. 2006;19 338-381.

[12] Vissa V. D., Brennan P. J., Impact of the *Mycobacterium leprae* genome sequence on leprosy research in: A. Danchin (Ed.), Genomics of GC-rich Gram-positive bacteria, Band 2, Caister Academic Press, 2002, pp. 85 - 118.

[13] Raphael Rubin D. S. S., Rubin Emanuel (Ed.), Rubin's Pathology: Clinicopathologic Foundations of Medicine, Lippincott Williams and Wilkins, 2007.

[14] Wheeler P. R., Bulmer K., Ratledge C. Enzymes for biosynthesis de novo and elongation of fatty acids in mycobacteria grown in host cells: is *Mycobacterium leprae* competent in fatty acid biosynthesis? J. Gen. Microbiol. 1990;136 211-217.

[15] Russell D. G., Cardona P. J., Kim M. J., Allain S., Altare F. Foamy macrophages and the progression of the human tuberculosis granuloma. Nat. Immunol. 2009;10 943-948.

[16] Neyrolles O., Hernandez-Pando R., Pietri-Rouxel F., Fornes P., Tailleux L., Barrios Payan J. A., Pivert E., Bordat Y., Aguilar D., Prevost M. C., Petit C., Gicquel B. Is adipose tissue a place for Mycobacterium tuberculosis persistence? PLoS One 2006;1 e43.

[17] Garton N. J., Waddell S. J., Sherratt A. L., Lee S. M., Smith R. J., Senner C., Hinds J., Rajakumar K., Adegbola R. A., Besra G. S., Butcher P. D., Barer M. R. Cytological and

transcript analyses reveal fat and lazy persister-like bacilli in tuberculous sputum. PLoS Med. 2008;5 e75.

[18]   Daniel J., Deb C., Dubey V. S., Sirakova T. D., Abomoelak B., Morbidoni H. R., Kolat-tukudy P. E. Induction of a novel class of diacylglycerol acyltransferases and triacyl-glycerol accumulation in Mycobacterium tuberculosis as it goes into a dormancy-like state in culture. J. Bacteriol. 2004;186 5017-5030.

[19]   Peyron P., Vaubourgeix J., Poquet Y., Levillain F., Botanch C., Bardou F., Daffé M., Emile J.-F., Marchou B., Cardona P.-J., de Chastellier C., Altare F. Foamy macrophages from tuberculous patients' granulomas constitute a nutrient-rich reservoir for M. tuberculosis persistence. Plos Pathog. 2008;4 e1000204.

[20]   Hagge D. A., Oby Robinson S., Scollard D., McCormick G., Williams D. L. A new model for studying the effects of Mycobacterium leprae on Schwann cell and neuron interac-tions. J. Infect. Dis. 2002;186 1283-1296.

[21]   Cruz D., Watson A. D., Miller C. S., Montoya D., Ochoa M. T., Sieling P. A., Gutierrez M. A., Navab M., Reddy S. T., Witztum J. L., Fogelman A. M., Rea T. H., Eisenberg D., Berliner J., Modlin R. L. Host-derived oxidized phospholipids and HDL regulate innate immunity in human leprosy. J. Clin. Invest. 2008;118 2917-2928.

[22]   Murphy D. J., Vance J. Mechanisms of lipid-body formation. Trends Biochem. Sci. 1999;24 109-115.

[23]   Ohsaki Y., Cheng J., Suzuki M., Shinohara Y., Fujita A., Fujimoto T. Biogenesis of cytoplasmic lipid droplets: from the lipid ester globule in the membrane to the visible structure. Biochim. Biophys. Acta. 2009;1791 399-407.

[24]   Wältermann M., Steinbüchel A. Neutral lipid bodies in prokaryotes: recent insights into structure, formation, and relationship to eukaryotic lipid depots. J. Bacteriol. 2005;187 3607-3619.

[25]   Ross R. The pathogenesis of atherosclerosis: a perspective for the 1990s. Nature 1993;362 801-809.

[26]   Pacheco P., Bozza F. A., Gomes R. N., Bozza M., Weller P. F., Castro-Faria-Neto H. C., Bozza P. T. Lipopolysaccharide-induced leukocyte lipid body formation in vivo: innate immunity elicited intracellular loci involved in eicosanoid metabolism. J. Immunol. 2002;169 6498-6506.

[27]   Moriishi K., Matsuura Y. Exploitation of lipid components by viral and host proteins for hepatitis C virus infection. Front. Microbiol. 2012;3 54.

[28]   Garton N. J., Christensen H., Minnikin D. E., Adegbola R. A., Barer M. R. Intracellular lipophilic inclusions of mycobacteria in vitro and in sputum. Microbiology 2002;148 2951-2958.

[29]   Russell D. G. Who puts the tubercle in tuberculosis? Nat. Rev. Microbiol. 2007;5 39-47.

[30] Kurup G., Mahadevan P. R. Cholesterol metobolism of macrophages in relation to the presence of *Mycobacterium leprae*. J. Biosci. 1982;4 307–316.

[31] Athenstaedt K., Zweytick D., Jandrositz A., Kohlwein S. D., Daum G. Identification and characterization of major lipid particle proteins of the yeast *Saccharomyces cerevisiae*. J. Bacteriol. 1999;181 6441-6448.

[32] Wan H. C., Melo R. C., Jin Z., Dvorak A. M., Weller P. F. Roles and origins of leukocyte lipid bodies: proteomic and ultrastructural studies. Faseb J. 2007;21 167-178.

[33] Beller M., Riedel D., Jänsch L., Dieterich G., Wehland J., Jäckle H., Kühnlein R. P. Characterization of the Drosophila lipid droplet subproteome. Mol. Cell. Proteomics. 2006;5 1082-1094.

[34] D'Avila H., Maya-Monteiro C. M., Bozza P. T. Lipid bodies in innate immune response to bacterial and parasite infections. Int. Immunopharmacol. 2008;8 1308-1315.

[35] Beller M., Thiel K., Thul P. J., Jäckle H. Lipid droplets: a dynamic organelle moves into focus. FEBS Lett. 2010;584 2176-2182.

[36] Murphy D. J. The dynamic roles of intracellular lipid droplets: from archaea to mammals. Protoplasma 2011;15 15.

[37] Tauchi-Sato K., Ozeki S., Houjou T., Taguchi R., Fujimoto T. The surface of lipid droplets is a phospholipid monolayer with a unique fatty acid composition. J. Biol. Chem. 2002;277 44507-44512.

[38] Job C. K. *Mycobacterium leprae* in nerve lesions in lepromatous leprosy. An electron microscopic study. Arch. Pathol. 1970;89 195-207.

[39] Tanigawa K., Suzuki K., Nakamura K., Akama T., Kawashima A., Wu H., Hayashi M., Takahashi S., Ikuyama S., Ito T., Ishii N. Expression of adipose differentiation-related protein (ADRP) and perilipin in macrophages infected with *Mycobacterium leprae*. FEMS Microbiol. Lett. 2008;289 72-79.

[40] Alvarez H. M., Steinbüchel A. Triacylglycerols in prokaryotic microorganisms. Appl. Microbiol. Biotechnol. 2002;60 367-376.

[41] Barksdale L., Kim K. S. *Mycobacterium*. Bacteriol. Rev. 1977;41 217-372.

[42] Christensen H., Garton N. J., Horobin R. W., Minnikin D. E., Barer M. R. Lipid domains of mycobacteria studied with fluorescent molecular probes. Mol. Microbiol. 1999;31 1561-1572.

[43] Wältermann M., Stöveken T., Steinbüchel A. Key enzymes for biosynthesis of neutral lipid storage compounds in prokaryotes: properties, function and occurrence of wax ester synthases/acyl-CoA: diacylglycerol acyltransferases. Biochimie 2007;89 230-242.

[44] Burdon K. L. Fatty material in bacteria and fungi revealed by staining dried, fixed slide preparations. J. Bacteriol. 1946;52 665-678.

[45] Deb C., Lee C. M., Dubey V. S., Daniel J., Abomoelak B., Sirakova T. D., Pawar S., Rogers L., Kolattukudy P. E. A novel *in vitro* multiple-stress dormancy model for *Mycobacterium tuberculosis* generates a lipid-loaded, drug-tolerant, dormant pathogen. PLoS One 2009;4 e6077.

[46] Daniel J., Maamar H., Deb C., Sirakova T. D., Kolattukudy P. E. *Mycobacterium tuberculosis* uses host triacylglycerol to accumulate lipid droplets and acquires a dormancy-like phenotype in lipid-loaded macrophages. PLoS Pathog. 2011;7 e1002093.

[47] Deb C., Daniel J., Sirakova T. D., Abomoelak B., Dubey V. S., Kolattukudy P. E. A novel lipase belonging to the hormone-sensitive lipase family induced under starvation to utilize stored triacylglycerol in *Mycobacterium tuberculosis*. J. Biol. Chem. 2006;281 3866-3875.

[48] Daniel J., Deb C., Dubey V. S., Sirakova T. D., Abomoelak B., Morbidoni H. R., Kolattukudy P. E. Induction of a novel class of diacylglycerol acyltransferases and triacylglycerol accumulation in *Mycobacterium tuberculosis* as it goes into a dormancy-like state in culture. J. Bacteriol. 2004;186 5017-5030.

[49] Low K. L., Rao P. S., Shui G., Bendt A. K., Pethe K., Dick T., Wenk M. R. Triacylglycerol utilization is required for regrowth of *in vitro* hypoxic nonreplicating *Mycobacterium bovis* bacillus Calmette-Guerin. J. Bacteriol. 2009;191 5037-5043.

[50] Rohde K., Yates R. M., Purdy G. E., Russell D. G. *Mycobacterium tuberculosis* and the environment within the phagosome. Immunol. Rev. 2007;219 37-54.

[51] Peters W., Ernst J. D. Mechanisms of cell recruitment in the immune response to *Mycobacterium tuberculosis*. Microbes Infect. 2003;5 151–158.

[52] Flynn J. L., Chan J. Immunology of tuberculosis. Annu. Rev. Immunol. 2001;19 93–129.

[53] Cáceres N., Tapia G., Ojanguren I., Altare F., Gil O., Pinto S., Vilaplana C., Cardona P. J. Evolution of foamy macrophages in the pulmonary granulomas of experimental tuberculosis models. Tuberculosis (Edinb) 2009;89 175-182.

[54] Dubos R. J., Middlebrook G. Media for tubercle bacilli. Am. Rev. Tuberc. 1947;56 334-345.

[55] Neyrolles O., Hernandez-Pando R., Pietri-Rouxel F., Fornes P., Tailleux L., Barrios Payan J. A., Pivert E., Bordat Y., Aguilar D., Prevost M. C., Petit C., Gicquel B. Is adipose tissue a place for *Mycobacterium tuberculosis* persistence? PLoS One 2006;1 e43.

[56] Jain M., Petzold C. J., Schelle M. W., Leavell M. D., Mougous J. D., Bertozzi C. R., Leary J. A., Cox J. S. Lipidomics reveals control of *Mycobacterium tuberculosis* virulence lipids via metabolic coupling. Proc. Natl. Acad. Sci. U S A 2007;104 5133-5138.

[57] Pandey A. K., Sassetti C. M. Mycobacterial persistence requires the utilization of host cholesterol. Proc. Natl. Acad. Sci. U S A 2008;105 4376-4380.

[58] Klepp L. I., Forrellad M. A., Osella A. V., Blanco F. C., Stella E. J., Bianco M. V., Santangelo M. D., Sassetti C., Jackson M., Cataldi A. A., Bigi F., Morbidoni H. R. Impact

of the deletion of the six mce operons in *Mycobacterium smegmatis*. Microbes Infect. 2012;7-8 590-599.

[59] Williams D. L., Torrero M., Wheeler P. R., Truman R. W., Yoder M., Morrison N., Bishai W. R., Gillis T. P. Biological implications of *Mycobacterium leprae* gene expression during infection. J. Mol. Microbiol. Biotechnol. 2004;8 58-72.

[60] Akama T., Tanigawa K., Kawashima A., Wu H., Ishii N., Suzuki K. Analysis of *Mycobacterium leprae* gene expression using DNA microarray. Microb. Pathog. 2010;49 181-185.

[61] Suzuki K., Takeshita F., Nakata N., Ishii N., Makino M. Localization of CORO1A in the macrophages containing *Mycobacterium leprae*. Acta Histochem. Cytochem. 2006;39 107-112.

[62] Gatfield J., Pieters J. Essential role for cholesterol in entry of mycobacteria into macrophages. Science. 2000;288 1647-1650.

[63] Anand P. K., Kaul D. Downregulation of TACO gene transcription restricts mycobacterial entry/survival within human macrophages. FEMS Microbiol. Lett. 2005;250 137-144.

[64] Takayama K., Wang C., Besra G. S. Pathway to synthesis and processing of mycolic acids in *Mycobacterium tuberculosis*. Clin. Microbiol. Rev. 2005;18 81-101.

[65] Glickman M. S. The mmaA2 gene of *Mycobacterium tuberculosis* encodes the distal cyclopropane synthase of the alpha-mycolic acid. J. Biol. Chem. 2003;278 7844-7849..

[66] Glickman M. S., Cox J. S., Jacobs W. R., Jr. A novel mycolic acid cyclopropane synthetase is required for cording, persistence, and virulence of *Mycobacterium tuberculosis*. Mol. Cell. 2000;5 717-727.

[67] Kalscheuer R., Steinbüchel A. A novel bifunctional wax ester synthase/acyl-CoA:diacylglycerol acyltransferase mediates wax ester and triacylglycerol biosynthesis in *Acinetobacter calcoaceticus* ADP1. J. Biol. Chem. 2003;278 8075-8082.

[68] Sirakova T. D., Dubey V. S., Deb C., Daniel J., Korotkova T. A., Abomoelak B., Kolattukudy P. E. Identification of a diacylglycerol acyltransferase gene involved in accumulation of triacylglycerol in *Mycobacterium tuberculosis* under stress. Microbiology 2006;152 2717-2725.

[69] Low K. L., Shui G., Natter K., Yeo W. K., Kohlwein S. D., Dick T., Rao S. P., Wenk M. R. Lipid droplet-associated proteins are involved in the biosynthesis and hydrolysis of triacylglycerol in *Mycobacterium bovis* bacillus Calmette-Guerin. J. Biol. Chem. 2010;285 21662-21670.

[70] Deb C., Daniel J., Sirakova T. D., Abomoelak B., Dubey V. S., Kolattukudy P. E. A novel lipase belonging to the hormone-sensitive lipase family induced under starvation to utilize stored triacylglycerol in *Mycobacterium tuberculosis*. J. Biol. Chem. 2006;281 3866-3875. Epub 2005 Dec 3813.

[71] Elamin A. A., Stehr M., Spallek R., Rohde M., Singh M. The *Mycobacterium tuberculosis* Ag85A is a novel diacylglycerol acyltransferase involved in lipid body formation. Mol. Microbiol. 2011;81 1577-1592.

[72] Canaan S., Maurin D., Chahinian H., Pouilly B., Durousseau C., Frassinetti F., Scappuccini-Calvo L., Cambillau C., Bourne Y. Expression and characterization of the protein Rv1399c from *Mycobacterium tuberculosis*. A novel carboxyl esterase structurally related to the HSL family. Eur. J. Biochem. 2004;271 3953-3961.

[73] Mishra K. C., de Chastellier C., Narayana Y., Bifani P., Brown A. K., Besra G. S., Katoch V. M., Joshi B., Balaji K. N., Kremer L. Functional role of the PE domain and immunogenicity of the *Mycobacterium tuberculosis* triacylglycerol hydrolase LipY. Infect. Immun. 2008;76 127-140.

[74] Singh V. K., Srivastava V., Singh V., Rastogi N., Roy R., Shaw A. K., Dwivedi A. K., Srivastava R., Srivastava B. S. Overexpression of Rv3097c in *Mycobacterium bovis* BCG abolished the efficacy of BCG vaccine to protect against *Mycobacterium tuberculosis* infection in mice Vaccine 2011;29 4754-4760.

[75] Daleke M. H., Cascioferro A., de Punder K., Ummels R., Abdallah A. M., van der Wel N., Peters P. J., Luirink J., Manganelli R., Bitter W. Conserved Pro-Glu (PE) and Pro-Pro-Glu (PPE) protein domains target LipY lipases of pathogenic mycobacteria to the cell surface via the ESX-5 pathway. J. Biol. Chem. 2011;286 19024-19034.

[76] Côtes K., Dhouib R., Douchet I., Chahinian H., de Caro A., Carriere F., Canaan S. Characterization of an exported monoglyceride lipase from *Mycobacterium tuberculosis* possibly involved in the metabolism of host cell membrane lipids. Biochem. J. 2007;408 417-427.

[77] Lun S., Bishai W. R. Characterization of a novel cell wall-anchored protein with carboxylesterase activity required for virulence in *Mycobacterium tuberculosis*. J. Biol. Chem. 2007;282 18348-18356.

[78] Zheng X., Guo J., Xu L., Li H., Zhang D., Zhang K., Sun F., Wen T., Liu S., Pang H. Crystal structure of a novel esterase Rv0045c from *Mycobacterium tuberculosis*. PLoS One 2011;6 e20506.

[79] McKinney J. D., Honer zu Bentrup K., Muñoz-Elías E. J., Miczak A., Chen B., Chan W. T., Swenson D., Sacchettini J. C., Jacobs W. R., Jr., Russell D. G. Persistence of *Mycobacterium tuberculosis* in macrophages and mice requires the glyoxylate shunt enzyme isocitrate lyase. Nature 2000;406 735-738.

[80] Muñoz-Elías E. J., McKinney J. D. *Mycobacterium tuberculosis* isocitrate lyases 1 and 2 are jointly required for in vivo growth and virulence. Nat. Med. 2005;11 638-644.

[81] Ensign S. A. Revisiting the glyoxylate cycle: alternate pathways for microbial acetate assimilation. Mol. Microbiol. 2006;61 274-276.

[82] Williams K. J., Boshoff H. I., Krishnan N., Gonzales J., Schnappinger D., Robertson B. D. The *Mycobacterium tuberculosis* beta-oxidation genes echA5 and fadB3 are dispensable for growth in vitro and in vivo. Tuberculosis (Edinb) 2011;91 549-555.

[83] Kornberg H. Krebs and his trinity of cycles. Nat. Rev. Mol. Cell. Biol. 2000;1 225-228.

[84] Brennan P. J. *Mycobacterium leprae* - The outer lipoidal surface J. Biosci. 1984;6 685–689.

[85] Fisher C. A., Barksdale L. Cytochemical reactions of human leprosy bacilli and mycobacteria: ultrastructural implications. J. Bacteriol. 1973;113 1389-1399.

[86] Sakurai I., Skinsnes O. K. Lipids in leprosy. 2. Histochemistry of lipids in human leprosy. Int Int. J. Lepr. 1970;38 389-403.

[87] Kaplan G., Van Voorhis W. C., Sarno E. N., Nogueira N., Cohn Z. A. The cutaneous infiltrates of leprosy. A transmission electron microscopy study. J. Exp. Med. 1983;158 1145-1159.

[88] Hunter S. W., Brennan P. J. A novel phenolic glycolipid from *Mycobacterium leprae* possibly involved in immunogenicity and pathogenicity. J. Bacteriol. 1981;147 728-735.

[89] Guenin-Mace L., Simeone R., Demangel C. Lipids of pathogenic Mycobacteria: contributions to virulence and host immune suppression. Transbound. Emerg. Dis. 2009;56 255-268.

[90] Ng V., Zanazzi G., Timpl R., Talts J. F., Salzer J. L., Brennan P. J., Rambukkana A. Role of the cell wall phenolic glycolipid-1 in the peripheral nerve predilection of *Mycobacterium leprae*. Cell. 2000;103 511-524.

[91] Puzo G. The carbohydrate- and lipid-containing cell wall of mycobacteria, phenolic glycolipids: structure and immunological properties. Crit. Rev. Microbiol. 1990;17 305-327.

[92] Cruz D., Watson A. D., Miller C. S., Montoya D., Ochoa M. T., Sieling P. A., Gutierrez M. A., Navab M., Reddy S. T., Witztum J. L., Fogelman A. M., Rea T. H., Eisenberg D., Berliner J., Modlin R. L. Host-derived oxidized phospholipids and HDL regulate innate immunity in human leprosy. J. Clin. Invest. 2008;118 2917-2928.

[93] Kumar R., Bhakuni V. *Mycobacterium tuberculosis* isocitrate lyase (MtbIcl): role of divalent cations in modulation of functional and structural properties. Proteins 2008;72 892-900.

[94] Höner Zu Bentrup K., Miczak A., Swenson D. L., Russell D. G. Characterization of activity and expression of isocitrate lyase in *Mycobacterium avium* and *Mycobacterium tuberculosis*. J. Bacteriol. 1999;181 7161-7167.

[95] Sharma V., Sharma S., Hoener zu Bentrup K., McKinney J. D., Russell D. G., Jacobs W. R., Jr., Sacchettini J. C. Structure of isocitrate lyase, a persistence factor of *Mycobacterium tuberculosis*. Nat. Struct. Biol. 2000;7 663-668.

[96]   Yoshimoto R., Fujita Y., Kakino A., Iwamoto S., Takaya T., Sawamura T. The discovery of LOX-1, its ligands and clinical significance. Cardiovasc. Drugs Ther. 2011;25 379-391.

[97]   Collot-Teixeira S., Martin J., McDermott-Roe C., Poston R., McGregor J. L. CD36 and macrophages in atherosclerosis. Cardiovasc. Res. 2007;75 468-477.

[98]   Palanisamy G. S., Kirk N. M., Ackart D. F., Obregon-Henao A., Shanley C. A., Orme I. M., Basaraba R. J. Uptake and accumulation of oxidized low-density lipoprotein during *Mycobacterium tuberculosis* infection in guinea pigs. PLoS One 2012;7 e34148.

[99]   Philips J. A., Rubin E. J., Perrimon N. Drosophila RNAi screen reveals CD36 family member required for mycobacterial infection. Science 2005;309 1251-1253.

[100] Leelahavanichkul A., Bocharov A. V., Kurlander R., Baranova I. N., Vishnyakova T. G., Souza A. C., Hu X., Doi K., Vaisman B., Amar M., Sviridov D., Chen Z., Remaley A. T., Csako G., Patterson A. P., Yuen P. S., Star R. A., Eggerman T. L. Class B scavenger receptor types I and II and CD36 targeting improves sepsis survival and acute outcomes in mice. J. Immunol. 2012;188 2749-2758.

[101] Mattos K. A., Oliveira V. G. C., D'Avila H., Rodrigues L. S., Pinheiro R. O., Sarno E. N., Pessolani M. C. V., Bozza P. T. TLR6-driven lipid droplets in *Mycobacterium leprae*-infected Schwann cells: Immunoinflammatory platforms associated with bacterial persistence. J. Immunol. 2011;187 2548-2558.

[102] Mattos K. A., D'Avila H., Rodrigues L. S., Oliveira V. G., Sarno E. N., Atella G. C., Pereira G. M., Bozza P. T., Pessolani M. C. Lipid droplet formation in leprosy: Toll-like receptor-regulated organelles involved in eicosanoid formation and *Mycobacterium leprae* pathogenesis. J. Leukoc. Biol. 2010;87 371-384.

[103] D'Avila H., Melo R. C., Parreira G. G., Werneck-Barroso E., Castro-Faria-Neto H. C., Bozza P. T. *Mycobacterium bovis* bacillus Calmette-Guerin induces TLR2-mediated formation of lipid bodies: intracellular domains for eicosanoid synthesis in vivo. J. Immunol. 2006;176 3087-3097.

[104] Almeida P. E., Silva A. R., Maya-Monteiro C. M., Töröcsik D., D'Avila H., Dezsö B., Magalhães K. G., Castro-Faria-Neto H. C., Nagy L., Bozza P. T. *Mycobacterium bovis* bacillus Calmette-Guérin infection induces TLR2-dependent peroxisome proliferator-activated receptor gamma expression and activation: functions in inflammation, lipid metabolism, and pathogenesis. J. Immunol. 2009;183 1337-1345.

[105] Underhill D. M. Toll-like receptors: networking for success. Eur. J. Immunol. 003;33 1767-1775.

[106] Korf J., Stoltz A., Verschoor J., De Baetselier P., Grooten J. The *Mycobacterium tuberculosis* cell wall component mycolic acid elicits pathogen-associated host innate immune responses. Eur. J. Immunol. 2005;35 890-900.

[107] Johnson R., Streicher E. M., Louw G. E., Warren R. M., van Helden P. D., Victor T. C. Drug resistance in *Mycobacterium tuberculosis*. Curr. Issues Mol. Biol. 2006;8 97-111.

[108] Belisle J. T., Vissa V. D., Sievert T., Takayama K., Brennan P. J., Besra G. S. Role of the major antigen of *Mycobacterium tuberculosis* in cell wall biogenesis. Science. 1997;276 1420-1422.

[109] Ronning D. R., Vissa V., Besra G. S., Belisle J. T., Sacchettini J. C. *Mycobacterium tuberculosis* antigen 85A and 85C structures confirm binding orientation and conserved substrate specificity. J. Biol. Chem. 2004;279 36771-36777..

[110] Armitige L. Y., Jagannath C., Wanger A. R., Norris S. J. Disruption of the genes encoding antigen 85A and antigen 85B of *Mycobacterium tuberculosis* H37Rv: effect on growth in culture and in macrophages. Infect. Immun. 2000;68 767-778.

[111] Jackson M., Raynaud C., Laneelle M. A., Guilhot C., Laurent-Winter C., Ensergueix D., Gicquel B., Daffe M. Inactivation of the antigen 85C gene profoundly affects the mycolate content and alters the permeability of the *Mycobacterium tuberculosis* cell envelope. Mol. Microbiol. 1999;31 1573-1587.

[112] Sanki A. K., Boucau J., Ronning D. R., Sucheck S. J. Antigen 85C-mediated acyl-transfer between synthetic acyl donors and fragments of the arabinan. Glycoconj. J. 2009;26 589-596..

[113] Mizuguchi Y., Udou T., Yamada T. Mechanism of antibiotic resistance in *Mycobacterium intracellulare*. Microbiol. Immunol. 1983;27 425-431.

[114] Mdluli K., Slayden R. A., Zhu Y., Ramaswamy S., Pan X., Mead D., Crane D. D., Musser J. M., Barry C. E., 3rd Inhibition of a *Mycobacterium tuberculosis* beta-ketoacyl ACP synthase by isoniazid. Science 1998;280 1607-1610.

[115] Kremer L., Dover L. G., Morbidoni H. R., Vilcheze C., Maughan W. N., Baulard A., Tu S. C., Honore N., Deretic V., Sacchettini J. C., Locht C., Jacobs W. R., Jr., Besra G. S. Inhibition of InhA activity, but not KasA activity, induces formation of a KasA-containing complex in mycobacteria. J. Biol. Chem. 2003;278 20547-20554. Epub 22003 Mar 20524.

[116] Takayama K., Schnoes H. K., Armstrong E. L., Boyle R. W. Site of inhibitory action of isoniazid in the synthesis of mycolic acids in *Mycobacterium tuberculosis*. J. Lipid Res. 1975;16 308-317.

[117] Wilming M., Johnsson K. Spontaneous formation of the bioactive form of the tuberculosis drug isoniazid. Angew. Chem. Int. Ed. Engl. 1999;38 2588-2590.

[118] Schroeder E. K., de Souza N., Santos D. S., Blanchard J. S., Basso L. A. Drugs that inhibit mycolic acid biosynthesis in *Mycobacterium tuberculosis*. Curr. Pharm. Biotechnol. 2002;3 197-225.

[119] Johansson P., Wiltschi B., Kumari P., Kessler B., Vonrhein C., Vonck J., Oesterhelt D., Grininger M. Inhibition of the fungal fatty acid synthase type I multienzyme complex. P. Natl. Atl. Acad. Sci. USA 2008;105 12803-12808.

[120] Luckner S. R., Liu N., am Ende C. W., Tonge P. J., Kisker C. A slow, tight binding inhibitor of InhA, the enoyl-acyl carrier protein reductase from *Mycobacterium tuberculosis*. J. Biol. Chem. 2010;285 14330-14337.

[121] Kremer L., Douglas J. D., Baulard A. R., Morehouse C., Guy M. R., Alland D., Dover L. G., Lakey J. H., Jacobs W. R., Jr., Brennan P. J., Minnikin D. E., Besra G. S. Thiolactomycin and related analogues as novel anti-mycobacterial agents targeting KasA and KasB condensing enzymes in *Mycobacterium tuberculosis*. J. Biol. Chem. 2000;275 16857-16864.

[122] Douglas J. D., Senior S. J., Morehouse C., Phetsukiri B., Campbell I. B., Besra G. S., Minnikin D. E. Analogues of thiolactomycin: potential drugs with enhanced anti-mycobacterial activity. Microbiology (Reading, England) 2002;148 3101-3109.

[123] Brown A. K., Taylor R. C., Bhatt A., Futterer K., Besra G. S. Platensimycin activity against mycobacterial beta-ketoacyl-ACP synthases. PLoS One 2009;4 e6306.

[124] Slayden R. A., Lee R. E., Barry C. E., 3rd Isoniazid affects multiple components of the type II fatty acid synthase system of *Mycobacterium tuberculosis*. Mol. Microbiol. 2000;38 514-525.

[125] Kremer L., Dover L. G., Morbidoni H. R., Vilcheze C., Maughan W. N., Baulard A., Tu S. C., Honore N., Deretic V., Sacchettini J. C., Locht C., Jacobs W. R., Jr., Besra G. S. Inhibition of InhA activity, but not KasA activity, induces formation of a KasA-containing complex in mycobacteria. J. Biol. Chem. 278 20547-20554.

[126] McMurry L. M., McDermott P. F., Levy S. B. Genetic evidence that InhA of *Mycobacterium smegmatis* is a target for triclosan. Antimicrob. Agents Ch. 1999;43 711-713.

[127] Sullivan T. J., Truglio J. J., Boyne M. E., Novichenok P., Zhang X., Stratton C. F., Li H. J., Kaur T., Amin A., Johnson F., Slayden R. A., Kisker C., Tonge P. J. High affinity InhA inhibitors with activity against drug-resistant strains of *Mycobacterium tuberculosis*. ACS chemical biology 2006;1 43-53.

[128] Alahari A., Trivelli X., Guerardel Y., Dover L. G., Besra G. S., Sacchettini J. C., Reynolds R. C., Coxon G. D., Kremer L. Thiacetazone, an antitubercular drug that inhibits cyclopropanation of cell wall mycolic acids in mycobacteria. PLoS One 2007;2 e1343.

Chapter 5

Pathophysiology of Tuberculosis

Ruiru Shi and Isamu Sugawara

Additional information is available at the end of the chapter

1. Introduction

1.1. Inflammatory process of tuberculosis

When many infectious units of 1-3 bacilli are inhaled, a phenotypically hardy bacillus is likely to be among them. In addition, the alveolar macrophages apparently vary in their capacity to destroy bacilli [1]. Staining for acid-fast bacilli is very useful for demonstrating *M. tuberculosis* (A). Fig. 1 reveals histologic manifestation of tuberculosis over the time course. Histologically, tuberculosis displays exudative inflammation (B), proliferative inflammation (D) and productive inflammation (C) depending on the time course. Using animal experiments and an inhalation exposure system, the pathologic condition of the infected animals was followed up for one year. Exudative inflammation was observed for the first 10 days. Thereafter, granulomas, which corresponded to foci of proliferative inflammation, were formed. Cavity formation was not recognized in animal tuberculosis, except for rabbits. Using rabbit models, Dr. Arthur Dannenberg described the pathology of tuberculosis in detail [2, 3]. There are five stages: onset, symbiosis, early stages of caseous necrosis, interplay of cell-mediated immunity and tissue damaging delayed-type hypersensitivity, and liquefaction and cavity formation. In stage 1, tubercle bacilli are usually destroyed or inhibited by the mature resident alveolar macrophages that ingest them. If bacilli are not destroyed, they grow and eventually destroy the alveolar macrophages. In stage 2, bacilli grow logarithmically within the immature nonactivated macrophages. These macrophages enter a tubercle from the bloodstream. This stage is termed symbiosis because bacilli multiply locally without apparent damage to the host, and macrophages accumulate and divide. In stage 3, the stage at which caseous necrosis first occurs, the number of viable bacilli becomes stationary because their growth is inhibited by the immune response to tuberculin-like antigens released from bacilli. Stage 4 is the stage that usually determines whether the disease becomes clinically apparent. Cell-mediated immunity plays a major role in this situation. The cytotoxic delayed- type hypersensitivity immune response kills these macrophages, causing enlargement of the caseous center and progression of the disease. If good cell-mediated immunity develops, a mantle of highly activated macrophages surrounds the caseous necrosis. In stage 5, bacilli evade host defenses. When liquefaction of the caseous center occurs, the bacilli multiply extracellularly, frequently attaining very large numbers. The high local concentration of tuberculin-like products derived from these bacilli causes a tissue-damaging delayed-type hypersensitivity response that erodes the bronchial wall, forming a cavity.

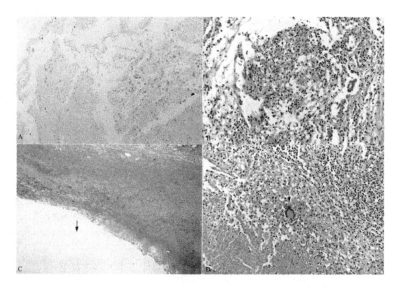

Figure 1. Histologic appearance of tuberculosis A. Staining for acid-fast bacilli, B. exudative stage, C. productive stage with cavity formation (→), D. proliferative stage with a multinucleated giant cell.

2. Clinical manifestations

As the cellular processes occur, tuberculosis may develop differently in each patient, according to the status of the patient's immune system. Stages include latency, primary disease, primary progressive disease, and extrapulmonary disease. Each stage has different clinical manifestations [4]. *M. tb* organisms can be enclosed but are difficult to completely eliminate [5]. Persons with latent tuberculosis have no signs or symptoms of the disease, do not feel sick, and are not infectious [5]. However, viable bacilli can persist in the necrotic material for years or even a lifetime [6], and if the immune system later becomes compromised, as it does in many critically ill patients, the disease can be reactivated. Primary pulmonary tuberculosis is often asymptomatic. Although it essentially exists subclinically, some self-limiting findings might be noticed. Associated paratracheal lymphadenopathy may occur because the bacilli spread from the lungs through the lymphatic system. Active tuberculosis develops in only 5% to 10% of persons exposed to *M. tb*. Fig. 2 shows typical chest X-ray before (A) and after (B) chemotherapy. Fatigue, malaise, weight loss, low-grade fever, night sweats, cough, sputum, are the main symptoms. The sputum may also be streaked with blood. Hemoptysis can be due to destruction of a patent vessel located in the wall of the cavity [7]. Extrapulmonary disease occurs in more than 20% of patients. The most serious location is the central nervous system, where infection may result in meningitis, which could be fatal in most cases. Another fatal form is infection of the blood stream by mycobacteria, this form is called disseminated or military tuberculosis. The most common extrapulmonary tuberculosis is lymphatic tuberculosis. Other possible locations include bones, joints, pleura, and genitourinary system [4].

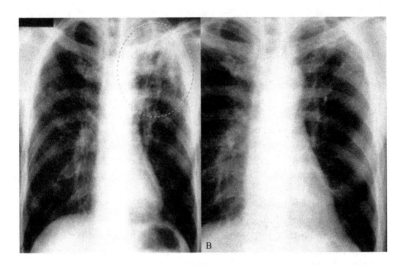

Figure 2. Chest X-ray of pulmonary tuberculosis and cured Tuberculosis A. before chemotherapy with rifampicin, isoniazide, ethambutol and pyrazinamide, B. after chemotherapy. Apical shadow (dotted circle) disappears.

3. T cell activation against *Mycobacterium tuberculosis*

In human, a TB index case may infect a contact person through cough and expectoration, so the lung is the primary route of infection and often the main tissue exhibiting TB. Infectious droplet nuclei are deposited in the alveolar spaces of the contact person where *Mycobacterium tuberculosis (M. tb)* can be phagocytosed by alveolar macrophages, epithelial cells, dendritic cells (DC) and neutrophils [8, 9]. Alveolar macrophages and DC are then believed to transport *M. tb* to local lymph nodes where T cell activation occurs and expand. Activation of the phagocytic host cell is much required to limit growth of *M. tb*; as in the absence of activation, disease outcome is extremely poor. Effective phagocyte activation requires a specific cellular response, as infected hosts lacking specific components of the acquired response have a poor outcome [10]. While acquired cellular protection is expressed rapidly following systemic challenge with *M. tb*, it is less rapid in the lung. Slow expression of protection in the lung allows mycobacteria to grow and modulate the infection site. Until recently it has not been clear whether the slow response to aerosol delivery of bacteria resulted from limited availability of antigen or inhibition of antigen-presentation by *M. tb*. Several studies show that the first T cell activation occurs in the draining lymph node (DLN) of the lung 8–10 days following initial challenge. The activation of T cells correlated temporally with the arrival of bacteria and availability of antigen in the DLN, however conditions for T cell activation were unique to the draining lymph nodes as the presence of antigen-producing bacteria in the lung and spleen did not result in initial activation of T cells [11, 12]. While delivery of lipopolysaccharide (LPS) to the MTB-infected lung failed to accelerate T cell priming [11], increasing the bacterial dose did accelerate the response modestly suggesting that both antigen burden and refractory cells serve to slow the response. So, protective memory cells will not become activated until they see antigen, i.e. more than 8 days post infection. Once T cells become activated they differentiate into effector T cells that migrate to the lung. By day 14 of infection, when activated T cells first arrive in the lung, bacteria are within alveolar macrophages, myeloid DC and neutrophils [11]. T cells can recognize antigen within the mycobacterially-infected lung but the antigen presentation is not optimal. It takes time for the protective T cells to reach sufficient numbers to stop bacterial growth. T cells can be divided into two subsets, Th1 and Th2, on the basis of the cytokines they produce. In tuberculosis, Th1 plays a major role in defense against tuberculosis. Th1 cells suppress Th2 cells. CD4 + T cells have unambiguously been identified as the most important lymphocyte subset for mediating protection.CD4 T lymphocytes differentiate in the peripheral tissues to adopt a variety of fates such as the Th-1 cells, which produce interferon (IFN)-γ to down-regulate Th2 responses and Th-2 cells, which produce interleukin (IL)-4. CD8 T lymphocytes produce predominantly IFN-γ. Though CD4 response is greater than the CD8 response, the latter can provide protection in the absence of CD4 help [13]. During active TB there is a local pulmonary immune response characterized by α/β T cells and strongly enhanced *M. tuberculosis* antigen-specific Th1 responses, with large amounts of locally secreted IFN-γ [14].

4. Animal models of tuberculosis

A wide variety of animal models have been used to test new vaccines and drugs [15]. Mice can harbor high numbers of *M. tb* within lung tissue without showing clinical signs [16]. Mice do not cough nor form cavitary lesions, making them a poor model for transmission studies [17]. Fibrous capsules are not observed histologically, which can affect the validity of antibiotic studies, as *M. tb* would be more easily accessed by drugs in the mouse lung. In addition, because of their short life span, mice are poor models for the study of latent infection. Rat TB also showed similar pathophysiology to murine TB [31]. Guinea pigs develop robust DTH response to mycobacterial antigens and, after infection with *M. tb*, reproduce many of the aspects of human infection, such as caseous and mineralized granulomas, primary and hemato-genous pulmonary lesions, fibrous capsule formation, and dissemination [19], however, pulmonary lesions in guinea pig contain a high proportion of granulocytes, particularly eosmophils, which are not common features of human disease [20]. The rabbit is the only common laboratory animal in which the disease closely resembles the typical chronic cavitary type found in the majority of human beings [21, 22]. Rabbits infected with *M. tb* mount a moderate DTH response and form caseous granulomas and cavitary lesions [23-25]. Rabbits, including currently available inbred strains, are relatively resistant to *M. tb*, however, requiring the inhalation of 500 to 3000 bacilli to form one grossly visible tubercle at 5 weeks postinfection [23]. Most rabbits will also overcome disease completely, with few culturable bacilli [24]. This model is useful in the study of latent or paucibacillary TB states, however, without the use of antibiotics as in the Cornell model. Rabbits do need to be experimentally immunosuppressed as they will not spontaneously reativate disease [26]. There are minimal immune reagents, however, for this model, and the larger size of rabbits makes them more costly to use. There are inbred strains of rabbits, such as the Lurie and Thorbecke rabbits, which are more susceptible to *M. tb* infection. This susceptibility has been linked to suppressed macrophage antimycobacterial activity, decreased MHC Class 2 expression, and impaired development of type 4 hypersensitivity [27]. Other animal models, such as nonhuman primates, which are susceptible to *M. tb* and full spectrum of granuloma types can be observed [28], have not been widely used. Using mycobacterial inoculation into trachea, at necropsy, all unvaccinated monkeys (*Macaca fascicularis* and *Macaca mulatta*) exhibited extensive bilateral lung pathology characterized by the presence of multiple granulomas. These granulomas exhibited conglomeration to larger caseous areas, especially in the hilar region [55].

5. Alveolar macrophages in tuberculosis

When tubercle bacilli reach alveoli, they are phagocytosed by resident alveolar macrophages. Though tubercle bacilli are killed byalveolar macrophages, tubercle bacilli can also kill macrophages through apoptosis. What is the fate of tubercle bacilli once they enter the phagosomes of macrophages? Alveolar macrophages of aerially infected guinea pigs were collected by bronchoalveolar lavage. At 12 days after infection, one out of 10,000 alveolar macrophages of various sizes contained many tubercle bacilli [31]. This indicates that certain alveolar macrophages permit M. tuberculosis to replicate in the phagosomes, although most of tubercle bacilli are killed by activated alveolar macrophages. It will be of great interest to examine the survival mechanism of *M. tuberculosis* at the single-cell level, but we still do not know why macrophages targeted by tubercle bacilli cannot kill the bacilli.

IFN-γ knockout mice were infected with avirulent H37Ra or BCG Pasteur, multinucleated giant cells were recognized in the granulomatous lesions. The lesions also contained tubercle bacilli and consisted of multinucleated cell clusters, being immunopositive with anti-Mac-3 antibody. The alveolar macrophages were transformed into multinucleated ginat cells. We subsequently infected various cytokine-konockout mice with *M. tb*, but no Langerhans' multinucleated giant cells were recognized in the granulomas. Therefore, it seems that formation of multinucleated giant cells requires optimal combinations and concentrations of various cytokines, and the level of IFN-γ, at least, has to be significantly low.

6. Roles of cytokines, neutrophils, NK cells, NKT cells and γδT cells

IFN-γ and TNF have long been implicated as regulators of T cell responses in mycobacterial disease [29]. The technique of gene targeting (knockout) has swept through biomedical research. IFN-γ, TNF-α, IRF-1, NF-IL6, NF-κB p50, STAT 1 and STAT 4 knockout mice succumbed to *M. tuberculosis* infection over time. There appears to be a cytokine and transcription factor hierarchy in experimental tuberculosis. The results indicate that these molecules play major roles in defense against the disease, IFN-γ and TNF-α being the leading players in this respect [30].

The role of neutrophils in the development of tuberculosis remained unknown for a long time. We utilized LPS-induced transient neutrophilia in the lungs [31]. LPS (50μg/ml) was administered intratracheally to male Fischer rats, which were then infected with *M. tuberculosis* via an airborne route. Intratracheal injection of LPS significantly blocked the development of pulmonary granulomas and significantly reduced the number of pulmonary colony-forming units (CFU). Treatment with amphotericin B (an LPS inhibitor) or neutralizing anti-rat neutrophil antibody reversed the development of pulmonary lesions. LPS-induced transient neutrophilia prevented early mycobacterial infection. The timing of LPS administration was important. When given intratracheally at least 10 days after aerial infection, LPS did not prevent the development of tuberculosis. Neutrophils obtained by bronchoalveolar lavage killed M. tuberculosis bacilli. These results indicate clearly that neutrophils participate actively in defense against early-phase tuberculosis.

Natural killer (NK) cells are innate lymphocytes which are a first line of defense against infection. NK cells can kill autologous infected cells without prior sensitization, and are believed to play a pivotal role in innate immunity to microbial pathogens. In mouse model, NK cells are activated and produce IFN-γ during the early response to pulmonary tuberculosis [31] and NK cell-produced IFN-γ regulates the anti-mycobacterial resistance mediated by neutrophils [32]. However animal models do not give a clear answer to whether NK cells is important in *M. tb* infection in vivo. Depletion of NK cells had no effect on bacterial replication in the lung of immunocompetent mice [33], suggesting that NK cells may be redundant in the presence of intact adaptive immunity. Surprisingly, IFN-γ knockout mice, which are impaired in their ability to clear mycobacteria, cleared them as effectively as wild-type mice when NK cells were depleted, suggesting that NK cells can inhibit protective immunity [34].

Human NK cells use the NKp46, the natural cytotoxicity receptors (NCRs) and NKG2D receptors to lyse *M. tuberculosis*-infected monocytes and alveolar macrophages [35], through damage of infected cells and secretion of cytokines, such as IFN-γ [36]. Inhibitory receptors of NK cells include killer immunoglobulin-like receptors (KIRs) and the NKG2A:CD94 dimer and NK cell activation can also be triggered by loss of inhibitory ligands from the cell surface. In addition, NK cells can also be activated by cytokines, including type I interferons, IL-12 and IL-18. NK cells are a potent and early source of cytokines, particularly IFN- γ, but they can also produce Th2-associated cytokines, such as IL-5 and IL-13, and the regulatory cytokine IL-10 [37]. NK cell NKp46 expression and cytotoxicity are reduced in freshly isolated peripheral blood mononuclear cells (PBMCs) from tuberculosis patients, which may be attributable to suppression by monocytes and IL-10. Recent studies have found that NK cells produce IL-22 [38], which was induced by IL-15 and DAP-10, an adaptor protein that is known to be involved in NK cell activation, in response to *M. tuberculosis*. Rohan Dhiman *et al.* also found that IL-22 can restrict growth of *M. tuberculosis* in macrophages by enhancing phagolysosomal fusion [39]. Nonetheless to fully understand the importance of NK cells in *M. tb* infection it may be necessary to differentiate their contributions at different stages of disease.

Certain T subsets, such as NKT cells and $\gamma\delta$ T cells, have features of innate immune cells including a partially activated phenotype, a rapid response following detection of infected cells, and the modulation of other cell types. Together with NK cells, these cell subsets are functionally defined as innate lymphocytes.CD1d-restricted invariant NKT (iNKT) cells are a conserved subset of T cells that express an invariant T cell receptor (TCR) α chain (Vα24-Jα18 in humans, and Vα14-Jα18 in mice) paired with TCR β chains encoded by one or a few Vβ gene segments (Vβ11 in humans, and predominantly Vβ2, 7 and 8 in mice). These cells show different phenotypes and functions [40].Many iNKT cells are CD4+, and they have been mainly associated with the induction of Th2 cytokines such as IL-4, IL-5, IL-13. This subset is believed to play a prominent role in suppression of autoimmune or chronic inflammatory diseases, and in promoting allergic conditions such as asthma. Few iNKT cells are CD8+, and most of those express only the CD8α subunit, which means that they likely express only CD8$\alpha\alpha$ homodimers. An additional fraction of iNKT cells are negative for both CD4 and CD8 (DN T cells). They have been found to produce predominantly IFN-γ and other Th1-associated cytokines. Studies of human iNKT cells have shown that they have the ability to kill *M. tuberculosis* organisms within infected macrophages, possibly through their production of the peptide granulysin [41]. Jin S. Im *et al.* [42] found that the percentages of iNKT cells among total circulating T cells in TB patients were not significantly different compared to those in healthy controls. However, TB patients showed a selective reduction of the proinflammatory CD4–CD8– (DN) iNKT cells with a proportionate increase in the CD4+ iNKT cells. The mouse model of tuberculosis has been used by Sada-Ovalle et al to find that iNKT cells have a direct bactericidal effect on *M. tuberculosis*, and protect mice against aerosol *M.TB* infection [43]. Their activation requires CD1d expression by infected macrophages as well as IL-12 and IL-18. In addition, pharmacological activation of iNKT cells with the synthetic ligand aGalCer often enhances host resistance to infection. iNKT cell use several mechanisms to modify host immunity. These include induction of DC maturation, secondary activation of effector cells (NK cells) or recruitment of inflammatory cells to the site of infection [44, 45]. Thus, by being an early producer of IFN-γ and suppressing intracellular bacterial growth, iNKT cells function as an important part of the early immune response against *M. tb* that affect both the innate and the adaptive arms of the immune response.

Antigen-specific γ/δ T cells represent an early innate defense that may play a role in antimycobacterial immunity. Studies done in humans and animal models have demonstrated complex patterns of γ/δ T cell immune responses during early mycobacterial infections and chronic TB. Like α/β T lymphocytes, γ/δ T cells carry antigen TCR that vary in the physical properties of their ligand-binding sites. γ/δ T cells are frequently activated by a variety of pathogens including *M. tb* [46]. Mice lacking γ/δ T cells succumb more rapidly than control mice following intravenous challenge with virulent *M. tb*; however, such a difference has not been observed following infection by the aerosol route. *γ/δ* T cells constitute a whole system of functionally specialized subsets that have been implicated in the innate responses against tumors and pathogens, the regulation of immune responses, cell recruitment and activation, and tissue repair [47]. Human alveolar macrophages and monocytes can serve as antigen presentation cells (APCs) for *γ/δ* T cells. Furthermore, the predominance of Vγ9Vδ2 T cells in TB disease has been confirmed [48]. When MTB-activated CD4+ and *γ/δ* T cells from healthy tuberculin-positive donors were analyzed for cytokine production in response to MTB-infected monocytes, both groups secreted large amounts of IFN-*γ* [49]. Previous studies have also demonstrated an increased proliferative activity of Vγ9Vδ2 T cells from patients with TB [50], but reduced production of IFN-*γ*, compared with that of healthy tuberculin-positive donors [51]. Additionally, Dieli *et al.* reported that decrease of Vγ9Vδ2 T cell effector functions involves not only IFN-*γ* production but also expression of granulysin [52]. Fig. 3 shows interaction of cells and cytokines involved in tuberculosis.

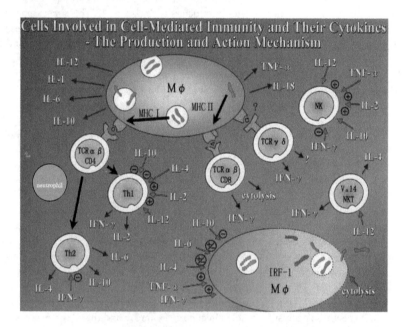

Figure 3. Cytokine and cellular network in tuberculosis +. Production of cytokine, -. No production of cytokine.

7. Conclusion

Tuberculosis is an international public health problem. It is becoming evident that *M. tb* infection is a dynamic state with a wide spectrum of pathology. An improved understanding of the immunopathogenesis of TB can facilitate the design of effective vaccines, new drug candidates and evaluation of their efficacy [53]. Understanding latent tuberculosis can also be the key to improve diagnostic and novel treatment strategies [54].

Author details

Ruiru Shi[1] and Isamu Sugawara[2]

1 Sino-US Tuberculosis Research Center and Clinical Laboratory Department of Henan Provincial Chest Hospital, Zhengzhou, Henan, China

2 Center of Tuberculosis Diagnosis and Treatment, Shanghai Pulmonary Hospital, Tongji University School of Medicine, Shanghai, China

References

[1] Dye, C, & Williams, B. G. The population dynamics and control of tuberculosis. *Science* (2010). , 328, 856-861.

[2] Dannenberg AM JrBurstone M, Walter PC, et al. A histochemical study of phagocytic and enzymatic functions of rabbit mononuclear and polymorphonuclear exudate cells and alveolar macrophages. Survey and quantitation of enzymes, and states of cellular activation. *J Cell Biol* (1963). , 17, 465-486.

[3] Dannenberg AM: Pathogenesis of human pulmonary tuberculosisInsights from the rabbit model. ASM Press, Washington, DC. (2006).

[4] Knechel, N. A. tuberculosis: Pathophysiology, clinical features, and diagnosis. *Crit Care Nurse* (2009). , 2, 34-43.

[5] Goyot-revol, V, Innes, J. A, Hackforth, S, Hinks, T, & Lalvani, A. regulatory T cells are expanded in blood and disease sites in patients with tuberculosis. *Am J Resp Crit Care Med* (2006). , 173, 803-810.

[6] Jensen, P. A, Lambert, L. A, & Iademarco, M. F. Ridzon R; Centers for Disease Control and Prevention. Guidelines for preventing the transmission of *Mycobacterium tuberculosis* in health-care settings. (2005). *MMWR Recomm Rep* 2005;54(RR-17): 1-141

[7] American Thoracic Society and Centers for Disease Control and PreventionDoagnostic standards and classification of tuberculosis in adults and children. *Am J Respir Crit Care Med* (2000). , 161, 1376-1395.

[8]   Tailleux, L, Pham-thi, N, Bergeron-lafaurie, A, et al. DC-SIGN induction in alveolar macrophages defines privileged target host cells for mycobacteria in patients with tuberculosis. *PLoS Med* (2005). e381.

[9]   Kang, P. B, Azad, A. K, Torrelles, J. B, et al. The human macrophage mannose receptor directs Mycobacterium tuberculosis lipoarabinomannan-mediated phagosome biogenesis. J. Exp.Med. (2005). , 202, 987-999.

[10] Cooper, A. Cell mediated immune responses in Tuberculosis. *Ann Rev Immunol* (2009). , 27, 393-422.

[11] Wolf, A, Desvignes, L, Linas, B, Banaiee, N, Tamura, T, Takatsu, K, & Ernst, J. Initiation of the adaptive immune response to *Mycobacterium tuberculosis* depends on antigen production in the local lymph node, not the lungs. *J Exp Med* (2008). , 205, 105-115.

[12] Reiley, W, Calayag, M, Wittmer, S, Huntington, J, Pearl, J, Fountain, J, Martino, C, Roberts, A, Cooper, A, Winslow, G, et al. ESAT-6-specific CD4 T cell responses to aerosol *Mycobacterium tuberculosis* infection are initiated in mediastinal lymph nodes. *Proc Natl Acad Sci USA* (2008). , 105, 10961-10966.

[13] Ngai, P, Mccormick, S, Small, C, Zhang, X, Zganiacz, A, Aoki, N, & Xing, Z. Gamma interferon responses of CD4 and CD8 T-cell subsets are quantitatively different and independent of each other during pulmonary *Mycobacterium bovis* BCG infection. *Infect Immun* (2007). , 75, 2244-2252.

[14] Herrera, M. T, Torres, M, Nevels, D, et al. Compartmentalized bronchoalveolar IFN-gamma and IL-12 response in human pulmonary tuberculosis. *Tuberculosis (Edinb)* (2009). , 89, 38-47.

[15] Ordway, D. J, & Orme, I. M. Animal models of Mycobacteria infection. *Current Protocols in Immunology* (2011). Supple , 94, 1-50.

[16] Mcmurray, D. N. Disease model: pulmonary tuberculosis. *Trends Mol Med* (2001). , 7, 135-137.

[17] Mitchison, D. A. The diagnodis and therapy of tuberculosis during the past 100 years. *Am J Respir Crit Care Med* (2005). , 171, 699-706.

[18] Sugawara, I, Yamada, H, & Mizuno, S. Pathological and immunological profiles of rat tuberculosis. *Int J Exp Pathol* (2004). , 85, 125-134.

[19] Mcmurray, D. N. Guinea Pig Model of Tuberculosis. Washington DC: American Society for Microbiology, (1994).

[20] Ordway, D, Palanisamy, G, Henao-tamayo, M, et al. The cellular immune response to *Mycobacterium tuberculosis* infection in the guinea pig. *J Immunol* (2007). , 179, 2532-2541.

[21] Dannenberg AM JrPathogenesis of tuberculosis : native and acquired resistance in animals and humans. In: Microbiology-(1984). Washington, DC: American Society for Microbiology, 1984; , 344-354.

[22] Dannenberg AM JrCollins FM. Progressive pulmonary tuberculosis is not due to increasing numbers of viable bacilli in rabbits, mice and guinea pigs, but is due to a continuous host response to mycobacterial products. *Tuberculosis* (2001). , 81, 229-242.

[23] Manabe, Y. C, & Dannenberg, A. M. Jr, Tyagi SK, *et al*. Different strains of *Mycobacterium tuberculosis* cause various spectrums of disease in the rabbit model of tuberculosis. *Infect Immun* (2003). , 71, 6004-6011.

[24] Via, L. E, Schimel, D, Weiner, D. M, et al. Infection dynamics and response to chemotherapy in a rabbit model of tuberculosis using F2-Fluoro-Deoxy-d-Glucose positron emission tomography and computed tomography. *Antimicrob Agents Chemother* (2012). , 56, 4391-4397.

[25] Kjellsson, M. C, Via, L. E, Goh, A, et al. Pharmacokinetic evaluation of the penetration of antituberculosis agents in rabbit pulmonary lesions. *Antimicrob Agents Chemother* (2012). , 56, 446-457.

[26] Manabe, Y. C, Kesavan, A. K, Lopez-molina, J, et al. The aerosol rabbit model of TB latency, reactivation and immune reconstitution inflammatory syndrome. *Tuberculosis (Edinb)* (2008). , 88, 187-196.

[27] Mendez, S, Hatem, C. L, Kesavan, A. K, et al. Susceptibility to tuberculosis: composition of tuberculosis granulomas in Thorbecke and outbred New Zealand White rabbits. *Vet Immunol Immunopathol* (2008). , 122, 167-174.

[28] Capuano, S. V, Croix, D. A, Pawar, S, et al. Experimental *Mycobacterium tuberculosis* infection of cynomolgus macaques closely resembles the various manifestations of human *M. tuberculosis* infection. *Infect Immun* (2003). , 71, 5831-5844.

[29] Cooper, A. M, Adams, L. B, Dalton, D. K, Appelberg, R, & Ehlers, S. IFN-γ and NO in mycobacterial disease: new jobs for old hands. *Trends Microbiol* (2002). , 10, 221-226.

[30] Sugawara, I, & Yamada, H. Shi R: Pulmonary tuberculosis in various gene knockout mice with special emphasis on roles of cytokines and transcription factors. *Current Resp Rev* (2005). , 1, 7-13.

[31] Sugawara, I, & Udagawa, T. Yamada H: Rat neutrophils prevent the development of tuberculosis. *Infect Immun* (2004). , 72, 1804-1806.

[32] Feng, C. G, Kaviratne, M, Rothfuchs, A. G, Cheever, A, Hieny, S, Young, H. A, Wynn, T. A, Sher, A, & Cell-derived, N. K. IFN-γ differentially regulates innate resistance and neutrophil response in T cell-deficient hosts infected with *Mycobacterium tuberculosis*. *J Immunol* (2006). , 177, 7086-7093.

[33] Junqueira-kipnis, A. P, Kipnis, A, Jamieson, A, Juarrero, M. G, Diefenbach, A, Raulet, D. H, Turner, J, & Orme, I. M. NK cells respond to pulmonary infection with *Mycobacterium tuberculosis*, but play a minimal role in protection. *J Immunol* (2003). , 171, 6039-6045.

[34] Woolard, M. D, Hudig, D, Tabor, L, Ivey, J. A, & Simecka, J. W. NK Cells in gamma-interferon-deficient mice suppress lung innate immunity against Mycoplasma spp. *Infect Immun* (2005). , 73, 6742-6751.

[35] Doolan, D. L, & Hoffman, S. L. IL-12 and NK cells are required for antigen-specific adaptive immunity against malaria initiated by CD8+ T cells in the *Plasmodium yoelii* model. *J Immunol* (1999). , 163, 884-892.

[36] Vankayalapati, R, Garg, A, Porgador, A, Griffith, D. E, Klucar, P, Safi, H, Girard, W. M, Cosman, D, Spies, T, & Barnes, P. F. Role of NK cell activating receptors and their ligands in the lysis of mononuclear phagocytes infected with an intracellular bacterium. *J Immunol* (2005). , 175, 4611-4617.

[37] Maroof, A, Beattie, L, Zubairi, S, Svensson, M, Stager, S, & Kaye, P. M. Posttranscriptional regulation of IL-10 gene expression allows natural killer cells to express immunoregulatory function. *Immunity* (2008). , 29, 295-305.

[38] Wolk, K, Witte, E, Wallace, E, Docke, W. D, Kunz, S, Asadullah, K, Volk, H. D, Sterry, W, & Sabat, R. IL-22 regulates the expression of genes responsible for antimicrobial defense, cellular differentiation, and mobility in keratinocytes: a potential role in psoriasis. *Eur J Immunol* (2006). , 36, 1309-1323.

[39] Rohan DhimanMohanalaxmi Indramohan, Peter F. Barnes, *et al.* IL-22 Produced by Human NK Cells Inhibits Growth of *Mycobacterium tuberculosis* by Enhancing Phagolysosomal Fusion. *J Immunol* (2009). , 6639-6645.

[40] Swann, J. B, Coquet, J. M, Smyth, M. J, Godfrey, D. I, & Cells, C. D1-r. e. s. t. r. i. c. t. e. d T. and tumor immunity. *Curr Top Microbiol Immunol* (2007). , 314, 293-323.

[41] Gansert, J. L, Kiessler, V, Engele, M, et al. Human NKT cells express granulysin and exhibit antimycobacterial activity. *J Immunol* (2003). , 170, 3154-3161.

[42] Jin, S. Im, Tae-Jin Kang, Seong-Beom Lee, *et al.* Alteration of the relative levels of iNKT cell subsets is associated with chronic mycobacterial infections. *Clin Immunol* (2008). , 127, 214-224.

[43] Sada-ovalle, I, Chiba, A, Gonzales, A, et al. Innate invariant NKT cells recognize *Mycobacterium tuberculosis*-infected macrophages, produce interferon-gamma, and kill intracellular bacteria. *PloS Pathog* (2007). e1000239

[44] Fujii, S, Shimizu, K, Hemmi, H, & Steinman, R. M. Innate Valpha14(+) natural killer T cells mature dendritic cells, leading to strong adaptive immunity.*Immunol Rev* (2007). , 220, 183-198.

[45] Nakamatsu, M, Yamamoto, N, Hatta, M, Nakasone, C, Kinjo, T, et al. Role of interferon-gamma in Valpha14+ natural killer T cell-mediated host defense against Streptococcus pneumoniae infection in murine lungs. *Microbes Infect* (2007). , 9, 364-374.

[46] Behar, S. M, & Boom, W. H. Unconventional T Cells. In: Kaufmann SHE, Britton WJ, eds. Handbook of Tuberculosis. Weinheim: Wiley-VCH. (2008). , 157-183.

[47] Girardi, M. Immunosurveillance and immunoregulation by γδ T cells. *J Invest Dermatol* (2006). , 126(1), 25-31.

[48] De Libero, G, Casorati, G, Giachino, C, et al. Selection by two powerful antigens may account for the presence of the major population of human peripheral γ/δ T cells. *J Exp Med* (1991). , 1311-1322.

[49] Gioia, C, Agrati, C, & Goletti, D. *et al.* Different cytokine production and effector/ memory dynamics of αβ+ or γδ+ T cell subsets in the peripheral blood of patients with active pulmonary tuberculosis. *Int J Immunopathol Pharmacol* (2003). , 247-252.

[50] Dieli, F, Friscia, G, & Di, C. Sano *et al.* Sequestration of T lymphocytes to body fluids in tuberculosis: reversal of anergy following chemotherapy. *J Infect Dis* (1999). , 225-228.

[51] Sanchez, F. O, Rodriguez, J. I, Agudelo, G, & Garcia, L. F. Immune responsiveness and lymphokine production in patients with tuberculosis and healthy controls. *Infect Immun* (1994). , 5673-5678.

[52] Dieli, F, Sireci, G, & Caccamo, N. *et al.* Selective depression of interferon-γ and granulysin production with increase of proliferative response by Vδ2 T cells in children with tuberculosis. *J Infect Dis* (2002). , 9

[53] Russell, D. G, & Barry, C. E. [rd], Flynn JL. Tuberculosis: What we do not know can, and does, hurt us. *Science* (2010). , 328, 852-856.

[54] Esmail, H, & Barry, C. E. [rd], and Wilkinson RJ. Understanding latent tuberculosis: the key to improved diagnosis and novel treatment strategies. *Drug Discovery Today* (2012). , 17, 514-521.

[55] Sugawara, I, Sun, L, Mizuno, S, et al. Protective efficacy of recombinant BCG Tokyo (Ag85A) in rhesus monkeys (*Macaca mulatta*) infected intratracheally with H37Rv Mycobacterium tuberculosis. *Tuberculosis* (2009). , 89, 62-67.

Chapter 6

Tuberculosis Pharmacogenetics: State of The Art

Raquel Lima de Figueiredo Teixeira,
Márcia Quinhones Pires Lopes,
Philip Noel Suffys and Adalberto Rezende Santos

Additional information is available at the end of the chapter

1. Introduction

The interindividual variability in the metabolism of xenobiotics and drug response is extensive and many factors are involved with this variation including genetic composition, gender, age, co-administration of medication, individual physiology, pathophysiology and presence of other environmental factors (alcohol consumption, smoking, eating habits).

To produce their therapeutic effects, the drug must be present in appropriate concentrations at its site of action. Although the therapeutic concentrations are dependent on the given dose, they will also depend on the magnitude and rate of absorption, distribution, biotransformation, and excretion. Pharmacokinetics studies the course and distribution of drug and its metabolites in different tissues, covering the mechanisms of absorption, transport, metabolism and excretion. In addition, pharmacodynamics concentrates on the biochemical and physiological effects of drugs and their mechanism of action. Proteins involved in drug effects are defined as target molecules and include not only (direct) receptors, but also proteins associated with mechanism of action such as e.g. signal transducer proteins [1].

After its administration, a drug is absorbed and then distributed throughout the body, requiring the coordinated functioning of various proteins, including metabolic enzymes, trafficking proteins, receptor proteins, and others. Medication can enter the body as either active drugs or as inactive prodrugs. Most drugs are metabolized in the liver to make them more soluble for subsequent elimination through the kidneys or intestines. Prodrugs require metabolic conversion, also called biotransformation, to liberate the active compound. Complete biotransformation of any one drug typically requires several different enzymes. [2]. Genetic variability has been described to have effect on drug absorption and metabolism and its interactions with the receptors. This forms the basis for slow and rapid drug absorption, poor, efficient or ultrarapid drug metabolism and poor or efficient receptor interactions [3]. The consequences of such variations can lead to adverse drug reaction and/or terapeutic failure.

In this context, pharmacogenetics is the study of genetic variations associated with individual variability in drug response, including differences in efficacy, drug-drug interactions, and the relative risk of an adverse response to drugs. It includes the study of genetic polymorphisms that could affect the expression or activity of drug transporters, drug metabolizing enzymes and drug receptors [2-4].

It's estimated that 99.9% of the human genome sequence between individuals is identical and genetic differences in polulations are called mutations if they are present in less than 1% and polymorphisms when present in at least 1% of a population. A single-nucleotide polymorphism (SNP) involves a replacement of one nucleotide base with any one of the other three and occuring at approximately one out of every 1,000 bases in the human genome [5].

A mutation or polymorphism in genes that encode metabolic enzymes, carriers or receptors can affect the drug pharmacokinetics and pharmacodinamics leading to undesired therapeutic effects. The identification of these genetic markers which predicted if a person responds well or not to a specific drug could help to select the right medication in right dosage, maximizing the eficacy and preventing or reducing the adverse drug reactions.

2. Problem statement

TB is an important global public health problem but has cure in almost 100% of the new cases if correct quimiotherapy is applied. The American Thoracic Society (ATS) treatment guidelines recommend an initial phase for TB treatment which consists of rifampicin 10 mg/kg (maximum 600 mg), isoniazid 5 mg/kg (maximum 300 mg), pyrazinamide 15–30 mg/kg (maximum 2 g), and ethambutol 15–20 mg/kg (maximum 1.6 g) given daily for 8 weeks, followed by a continuous phase of isoniazid 15 mg/kg (maximum 900 mg) and rifampicin 10 mg/kg (maximum 600 mg) administered 2–3 times/week for 18 weeks [6]. The use of fixed-dose combination (FDC) tablets containing anti-TB drugs has been recommended by the World Health Organization (WHO) as an additional measure to improve treatment adherence by reducing the number of tablets to be taken. The principal disadvantages of combining three or more drugs in one tablet include (a) the possibility of overdosage or underdosage resulting from a prescription error, (b) changes in the bioavailability of rifampicin and (c) difficulties in determining which drug is responsible for adverse effects [7].

Isoniazid (INH) is an important drug in the TB treatment and was introduced in chemotherapic scheme since 1952. It is the hidrazine of isonicotinic acid and shows cytotoxic activity for *Mycobacterium tuberculosis* both in rest (during latency) and proliferation phases. This drug enters easily in macrophague cells to kill bacilli in multiplication and is specific for mycobacteria [1].

INH-induced adverse reactions include fever, nausea, vomiting, hepatotoxicity, skin reactions, gastrointestinal and neurological disorders. Only in the early 1970s, the occurrence of severe liver injury as a side effect of this drug was recognized, resulting in the death of some patients [8]. Among the first-line anti-TB drugs, INH is the main associated with drug-induced hepatotocixity with a frequency ranging from 1 to 30% in different populations [9]. Other drugs causing liver injury are mainly reported in combination with INH [10, 11]. Drug-induced hepatotoxicity is defined as a serum alanine aminotransferase (ALT) level three times greater than the upper limit of normal (ULN) with clinical symptoms or five times the ULN without symptoms. In both cases treatment should be interrupted and, generally, a modified or alternative regimen is introduced [9]. Because these adverse reactions do not only affect morbidity and mortality rate but also lead to treatment interruptions, failure and relapse, adverse reactions contribute to the spread of the disease and the emergence of multidrug resistence (MDR).

Adverse Drug Reactions (ADRs) are common causes of hospitalization and lead to large costs to society. There are two main financial burdens due to illnesses caused by ADRs: that of treating and that of avoiding them [12]. The occurrence of serious and fatal ADRs has been extensively studied in hospitalized patients and a meta-analysis of prospective studies in approximately forty hospitals in the United States of America (USA) suggests that 6-7% of hospitalized patients suffer from serious ADRs and 0.32% of patients develop fatal ADRs [13]. This results in approximately 100,000 deaths annually in the U.S. and an annual cost of over a hundred billion dollars to the society due to prolonged hospitalization and reduced productivity [3, 13]. Furthermore, it has been estimated that ADRs are responsible for up to 7% of all admissions in hospitals in the United Kindown (UK) and 13% in medical clinics in Sweden [3], which shows the magnitude of this problem in the context of chemotherapy and drug development. Additionally, in France, a 10-year study in the Liver Unit of Hôpital Beaujon in Paris showed that among all patients hospitalized with acute hepatitis, 10% were due to adverse reaction to drugs and the prevalence of drug hepatotoxicity in patients older than fifty years exceeded 40%. In Japan and other Eastern countries, drugs are responsible for about 10-20% of cases of fulminant hepatitis [14].

Liver injury is the most common ADR and the main complication during chemotherapy since liver is the central organ for the biotransformation and excretion of most drugs and xenobiotics [14-17]. There are basically six mechanisms involving primarily the hepatocyte injury. The reactions of mono-oxygenase cytochrome P450 (CYP450) with certain drugs generate toxic metabolites that bind to intracellular proteins, leading to calcium homeostasis pump dysfunction with consequent disruption of actin fibers and cell lysis. Some drugs affect transport proteins in the cell membrane interrupting the flow of bile and then causing cholestasis. Several reactions involving CYP P450 can promote binding of the drug to the enzyme, with consequent exposure of this complex on the cell surface for recognition by T cells and antibody production as part of the autoimmune response. Finally, certain drugs may promote hepatic injury mediated by programmed cell death (apoptosis) or being capable of inhibiting respiration and/ or mitochondrial beta-oxidation [17].

Xenobiotics are usually lipophilic and this facilitates their transport in association with lipoproteins in the blood stream and their penetration of lipid membranes and entrance into organs. However, physicochemical properties of drug molecules difficult their removal from the organism by biliary or renal excretion and therefore, these substances require enzymatic conversion to water soluble compounds [1]. The xenobiotics metabolization, often through multiple pathways, can generate metabolites that are more toxic than the substrate and through their interaction with target macromolecules such as DNA, RNA, proteins and receptors, generate the toxic effects. The organ affected is generally that reponsible for drug metabolization or excretion of metabolites [1].

The enzyme systems responsible for the biotransformation of many drugs are located in the endoplasmic reticulum of the liver (microsomal fraction). Such enzymes are also present in the kidneys, lungs and gastrointestinal epithelium, although at a lower concentration [1]. The metabolic modification in biotransformation usually takes place in two consecutive steps and results in the loss of biological activity. Phase I reactions convert the xenobiotic into a metabolite with higher polarity by oxidation, reduction or hydrolysis and generates a pharmacologically inactive or less active, or in the case of a pro-drug, more active molecule. This metabolite is than either eliminated or go through Phase II reactions (so-called synthesis or conjugation reactions), involving binding to a primary metabolite or endogenous substrate such as glucuronate, sulfate, acetate, amino acids or glutathione (tripeptide). Such enzymatic reactions include glucuronidation, methylation, sulfation, acetylation, conjugation with glutathione and conjugation with glycine [1].

The risk for developing hepatotoxicity is associated both with genetic and acquired factors. The acquired factors include: age, gender, nutritional habits, drug abuse, pregnancy and extrahepatic disease. Genetic variations in isoenzymes involved in drug biotransformation can result in abnormal reactions leading to toxic effects [14,17]. In the case of INH in particular, advanced age is a risk factor for hepatotoxicity whereas deficiency in the ability of N-acetylation represent a genetic risk factor for liver injury.

INH is administered orally and rapidly absorbed through the gastrointestinal tract passing through the liver by the portal venous system before reaching the general circulation where is metabolized by a process known as the first pass effect with reduction of its biodiponibility. About 75% to 95% of the INH is excreted by the kidneys during the first 24 hours, mainly as the metabolic forms acetyl-isoniazid and isonicotinic acid [1].

In the liver, INH is metabolized to acetylisoniazid by N-acetyltransferase 2 (NAT2), followed by hydrolysis to acetylhydrazine and then oxidized by cytochrome P4502E1 (CYP2E1) to hepatotoxic intermediates [18, 19]. These metabolites can destroy hepatocytes either by interfering with cell homeostasis or by triggering immunologic reactions in which reactive metabolites that are bound to hepatocyte plasma proteins may act as haptens [17]. The other metabolic pathway to generate toxic metabolites is direct hydrolysis of INH to hydrazine, a potent hepatotoxin. NAT2 is also responsible for converting acetylhydrazine to diacetylhydrazine, a nontoxic component [18, 20, 21] (Figure 1). Glutathione S-transferase (GST), an important phase II detoxification enzyme, is thought to play a protective role as an intracellular free radical scavenger, which conjugates glutathione with toxic metabolites that are generated from CYP2E1 [22]. Sulphydryl conjugation facilitates the elimination of metabolites from the body and reduces the toxic effect [23] (Figure 1).

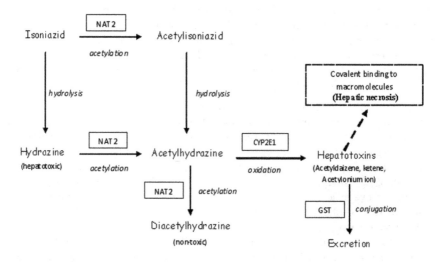

Figure 1. Schematic representation of the INH metabolism. The major enzymes involved in this pathway are indicated in boxes [20, 24].

In the last few years, an increasing number of studies have suggested that genetic polymorphisms in *NAT2*, *CYP2E1* and *GST* genes would be associated with susceptibility to drug-induced hepatotoxicity during TB treatment. The present work focused in an overview of the role of such polymorphisms in occurence of liver injury induced by anti-TB drugs, and by INH in particular.

3. State of the art

3.1. N-acetyltransferase 2

NAT2, the main enzyme responsible for the metabolism and inactivation of INH in humans, is a Phase II enzyme that catalyzes the transfer of the acetyl group from the cofactor acetyl coenzyme A (acetyl-CoA) to the nitrogen terminal of the drug. Variations in activity of NAT2 were discovered over 50 years ago when observing interindividual differences in the metabolism of INH and the level of drug-induced toxicity in TB patients. NAT2 is encoded by the *NAT2* gene and according family genetic studies, variability of NAT2 was directly related to the emergence of different phenotypes of acetylation [25].

The molecular study of human N-acetyltransferases revealed the presence of three genetic loci, two very homologous encoding the enzymes NAT1 and NAT2, and a third including the pseudogene *pNAT* (Figure 2). These loci are located on chromosome 8 between 170-360Kb at 8p22 [26]. The *pNAT* is a pseudogene containing a premature stop codon, and is not transcribed. *NAT1* and *NAT2* genes consist of 873 bp, are intronless, and encode proteins of 34 kDa. Protein sequence homology between both enzymes is 81% while that between their respective genes is 87%. Both enzymes have N-acetylation, O-acetylation and NO-transfer in different xenobiotics and carcinogens but differ considerably in their tissue distribution and expression levels during embryonic development [26-28].

Both *NAT1* and *NAT2* are polymorphic genes and SNPs in their coding region can alter the enzymatic activity [29, 30] and are the basis of the three major genetically determined phenotypes, being rapid, intermediate and slow acetylators, which are inherited as a codominant trait [31, 32]. The reference *NAT2*4* allele (without mutations / wild-type) and 66 variants were identified and classified in human populations depending on the combination of up to four SNPs present throughout the *NAT2* coding region [33]. So far, over 30 SNPs have been identified in this region, including several rare mutations described in different populations [34]. Among these, the seven most frequent are the 191 G>A (R64Q), 282 C>T (silent), 341 T>C (I114T), 481 C>T (silent), 590 G>A (R197Q), 803 A>G (K268R) and 857 G>A (G286T) SNPs identified in different human populations [35]. *NAT2* alleles containing the 191G>A, 341T>C, 590G>A or 857G>A SNPs are associated with slow acetylator *NAT2* alleles [33].

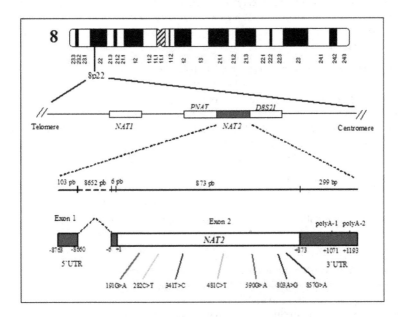

Figure 2. Schematic representation of *NAT* genes on human chromosome 8p22. Distribution of the seven most common SNPs in *NAT2*. D8S21 represents a polymorphic marker situated in the *NAT2* locus [26, 36].

Presence of different SNPs in *NAT2* can be easily determined by genotyping procedures such as PCR-RFLP [37], allele specific PCR [38] or direct sequencing [39]. To achieve the *NAT2* genotype of each individual and predict the phenotype, the haplotype of both chromosomes is usually reconstructed using the statistic software (PHASEv2.1.1[40, 41]). Using haplotype data, many studies have reported the frequencies of the different acetylation profiles among ethnically different populations showing the high diversity around the world. In Asians and Ameridians, the fast acetylator phenotype is more frequent [42-44] whereas in Euro-descend-ants slow acetylators account for 50% of the study population [37,45]. The molecular basis for such discrepancy is that the most common *NAT2* allele in Euro-descendants is very rare in Asians and may represent a different selective advantage within the gene pools of these separate populations. Description of new alleles of *NAT2* is still ocurring in recent studies [34].

In an attempt to establish an association between acetylation profiles and development of disease, cohort or case-control studies have been performed using of genotyping and pheno-typing tools. Evidence was found for an association between the slow acetylator predicted phenotype and developing urinary bladder cancer, while rapid acetylators seem more susceptible to development of colon cancer. For a review, see [27, 46].

For many years, INH has been considered the main cause of hepatotoxicity during TB treatment and association studies between the acetylation phenotypes and susceptibility to liver-related ADRs have been performed. Two early studies conducted in oriental populations investigated the association of the acetylator phenotype with INH induced hepatotoxicity and observed an increased risk of developing hepatotoxicity by INH among the slow acetilators [47, 48]. This observation was confirmed in several other studies performed in different populations [49-52].

Several studies reported the absence of a relationship between acetylation status and hepato-toxicity during TB treatment [53-55] but some, suggested the rapid acetylators as more susceptible to side effects [55, 56]. Reasons for these different findings range from genotyping methods to ethnicity. In some studies, NAT2 acetylation phenotypes were determined by an enzymatic method leading to possible misclassification of the acetylation status [53, 56, 57]. Indeed, it is difficult to compare the accuracy of different NAT phenotyping methods or different cut-off points using the same phenotyping method. In addition, for genotyping, investigators sometimes select a small number of SNPs to define the acetylation status [54, 55]. Since the frequencies of *NAT2* alleles are different among worldwide populations and new alleles are been identified in some countries, investigators need to characterize such alleles in their own study population in order to choose appropriate SNPs for genotyping and classify the acetylation status of individuals, otherwise overestimation of slow acetylators may be obtained, contributing to a spurious results in the association study.

Recently, a study with an admixed population showed that *NAT2* is a genetic factor for predisposition to anti-TB drug-induced hepatitis. In this case, *NAT2* genes were well charac-terized by direct sequencing and their genotypes achieved by haplotype reconstruction using the PHASE software. In addition, functional unknown genotypes were disconsidered and others confounding variables for hepatotocixity were taken into account. The incidence of elevated levels of serum transaminases was significantly higher in slow acetylators than those of the rapid/intermediate type. These results corroborate with the current hypothesis that the acetylator status may be a risk factor for the hepatic side effects of isoniazid [58].

Finally, a meta-analysis was conducted to solve the problem of inadequate statistical power and controversial results based on accumulated data with small sample size [59]. Data from 14 studies performed between 2000 and 2011 were pooled and showed that TB patients with a slow acetylator genotype had a higher risk of anti-tuberculosis drug induced hepatotocixity than patients with rapid or intermediate acetylation ($p < 0.001$). Moreover, subgroup analyses indicate that both Asians and non-Asians slow acetylators develop anti-tuberculosis drug induced hepatotocixity more frequently. Additionally, there were statistically significant associations between NAT2*5/*7, NAT2*6/*6, NAT2*6/*7 and NAT2*7/*7 and the risk of anti-TB drug induced hepatotocixity [59].

As a final consideration, NAT acetylates more slowly not only isoniazid but also acetylhydrazine, the immediate precursor of toxic intermediates, to the harmless diacetylhydrazine [60, 61]. This protective acetylation is further suppressed by INH competition. Therefore, slow acetylators may be prone to higher accumulation rates of INH toxic metabolites. Another important route to generate toxic intermediates is the direct hydrolysis of unacetylated INH [62], producing hydrazine that also induces hepatic injury [62, 63]. Pharmacokinetic studies showed that the serum concentration of hydrazine was significantly higher in slow acetylators than in rapid acetylators, probably due to the high INH concentration. The high amount of INH disposed of through this pathway is likely to lead to enhanced hydrolysis to hydrazine, since the rate of metabolic conversion of INH to acetylisoniazid is lower in slow than in rapid acetylators [64, 65]. All of these drug-disposal processes may support the finding that slow acetylators are prone to INH-induced hepatitis. We therefore conclude that screening of patients for the *NAT2* genetic polymorphisms can prove clinically useful for the prediction and prevention of anti-tuberculosis drug induced hepatotoxicity.

3.2. CYP450

Cytochromes P450 (CYP450) are hemoproteins and form the most important enzymatic group for Phase I biotransformation. The main activity of isozymes of CYP450 system is oxidation and they are located in the smooth endoplasmic reticulum, mainly in liver cells. However, these mono-oxygenases are also localized in the intestine, pancreas, brain, lung, kidney, bone marrow, skin, ovary and testicles [66]. The CYP450 proteins are clustered into families and subfamilies according to the similarity between the amino acid sequences: where family members have $\geq 40\%$ identity in amino acid sequence, members of the same subfamily share $\geq 55\%$ identity [67].

The CYP450s are responsible for the metabolization of several endogenous substrates and the synthesis of hydrophobic lipids such as cholesterol, steroid hormones, bile acids and fatty acids. Moreover, some enzymes of P450 complex metabolize exogenous substances including drugs, environmental chemicals and pollutants as well as products derived from plants. The metabolism of exogenous substances by CYP450 usually results in detoxification of the xenobiotic; however, the reactions triggered by such enzymes can lead to generation of toxic metabolites that contribute to the increased risk of developing cancers and other toxic effects [68].

The complete sequencing of the human genome revealed the presence of about 115 genes of CYP450, including 57 active genes and 58 pseudogenes [67]. They belong to families 1-3 and are responsible for 70-80% of Phase I-dependent metabolism of clinically used drugs. Other families of CYPs are involved in metabolism of endogenous components [66]. The CYP2 constitutes the largest family of isoenzymes and comprises one third of all human CYPs. Genes encoding these enzymes are polymorphic and the frequency distribution of allelic variants in different ethnic groups differs. Overall, four phenotypes based on genotypes can be identified: (i) poor metabolizers who present low enzymatic activity, (ii) intermediate metabolizers, usually heterozygous for a defective allele, (iii) rapid metabolizers, who have two normal alleles and (iv) ultrarapid metabolizers, who have several gene copies [69].

The enzyme CYP2E1 is expressed mainly in the liver but can be found in other organs such as kidney, gastrointestinal tract and brain and involved in oxidation of substrates such as ethanol and the metabolism of many drugs and pre-carcinogens. Besides ethanol, CYP2E1 can be induced by various drugs such as INH but also by hydrocarbons, benzene, chloroform and various organic solvents [70].

The activity of CYP2E1 is also modulated by polymorphisms in several locations of its gene and more activity of this enzyme may increase the synthesis of hepatotoxins. Two polymorphisms upstream of the CYP2E1 transcriptional start site are characterized by Pst I and Rsa I digestion and appear to be in complete linkage disequilibrium (Figure 3). These two polymorphisms are located in a putative HNF-q binding site and thus may play a role in the regulation of CYP2E1 transcription and subsequent protein expression [71]. Genotypes of CYP2E1 are classified as being *1A/*1A, *1A/*5 or *5/*5 by Rsa I based restriction analysis. The polymorphism detectable by Dra I (7632 T>A) is located in intron 6 and characterizes the allelic variant CYP2E1*6. The other polymorphism is an insertion/deletion of 96 bp (CYP2E1*1D and *1C alleles) that regulates the expression of the gene [72]. Some studies have shown that allelic variants CYP2E1 *5, *6 and *1D would increase enzyme activity [71, 73]. However, other authors did not confirm any relationship with these polymorphisms with CYP2E1 activity [74].

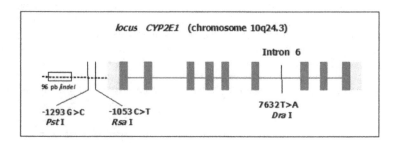

Figure 3. Polymorphic and corresponding restriction enzyme cutting sites at CYP2E1 [24].

Several studies have described the involvement of polymorphisms in CYP2E1 in cancer development but results are controversial. The studies showed that the frequency of SNP -1053 C>T in the promoter region varies significantly in different ethnic groups. The mutant allele is present with a frequency of 2-8% in Euro-descendants but varies in Asia from 25 to 36% [75].

In 2003, Huang and coworkers showed an association of the wild-type genotype *1A/*1A with risk of developing liver damage induced by isoniazid in adult TB patients, regardless of their profile of acetylation (OR 2.52; 95% CI 1.26 to 5.05) [76]. Later, Vuilleumier and colleagues showed association between this CYP and isoniazid-induced hepatotoxicity, without hepatitis, during chemoprophylaxis for TB (OR 3.4; 95% CI 1.1 to 12; p = 0.02). The risk of having high levels of liver enzymes was 3.4-fold higher when compared with all other CYP2E1 genotypes [55]. Another study on Indian children with TB showed association between risk of hepatotoxicity and polymorphisms in CYP2E1, despite of low sample size [77]. However, a study with on a Korean population found no relationship between hepatic adverse effects with genotype *1A/*1A of CYP2E1 during anti-TB treatment [51]. Lack of association between this CYP and antituberculosis drug-induced liver injury was also observed in Brazil [58]. The discrepancy of these results may be due to differences in the frequencies of CYP2E1*1A and CYP2E1*5 alleles among the populations and the different criteria to define hepatotoxicity used.

Finally, CYP2E1 converts acetyl hydrazine into hepatotoxins like acetyldiazene, ketene and acetylonium ion. The reaction of acetyl hydrazine (at high levels) with CYP2E1 leads to covalent binding of these secondary metabolites with intracellular proteins (Figure 1). As a consequence, intracellular changes occur resulting in loss of ionic gradients and decrease of ATP levels and consequent disruption of actin followed by cell lysis. Further studies in different populations and with a larger sample size are needed to determine the true influence of CYP2E1 gene polymorphisms on the occurrence of liver injury during treatment for TB.

3.3. Glutathione S-transferases

Glutathione S-transferases constitute a superfamily of multifunctional ubiquitous enzymes that play an important role in cellular detoxification by protecting macromolecules against reactive electrophilic attack. The GSTs are Phase II enzymes that catalyze the nucleophilic attack of glutathione (GSH) into components that contain an electrophilic carbon, nitrogen or sulfur atom. The combination of the GSH with these compounds often leads to formation of less reactive and more water soluble products, more easily excreted by the body [23, 78].

Glutathione transferases are of great interest to pharmacologists and toxicologists, since they are drug targets for the treatment of asthma and cancer, in addition to metabolize drugs, insecticides, herbicides, carcinogens and products of oxidative stress. Polymorphisms in GST genes are often correlated with susceptibility to various cancers, as well as alcoholic liver disease [23, 78-81].

In humans, eight gene families of soluble (or cytosolic) GSTs have been described: alpha (α) located on chromosome 6, mu (μ) on chromosome 1, theta (θ) on chromosome 22, pi (π) on chromosome 11; zeta (ζ) on chromosome 14, sigma (σ) on chromosome 4; kappa (κ) (chromosomal location not given) and omega (Ω) on chromosome 10 [80]. This classification is based on amino acid sequences, substrate specificity, chemical affinity, protein structure and enzyme kinetics. These enzymes are highly expressed in the liver and constitute up to 4% of total soluble proteins but can be seen in several other tissues [82]. GSTs have an overlap of specific substrates and the deficiency in one isoform can be compensated by other isoforms. Glutathione S-transferase mu (GSTM), glutathione S-transferase theta (GSTT) and glutathione S-transferase Pi (GSTP) have been the most studied isoform [83-88].

The subfamily GST mu is encoded by five genes arranged in tandem (5_-GSTM4-GSTM2-GSTM1-GSTM5-GSTM3-_3), forming a 100 kb gene cluster on chromosome 1p13.3 (Figure 4). Polymorphisms have been identified and clinical consequences of genotypes resulting from combinations of alleles GSTM1*0, GSTM1*A, and GSTM1*B have been widely investigated [78, 81, 89, 90]. Individuals who possess the homozygous null for GSTM1 (GSTM1*0/GSTM1*0) do not express this protein. Thus, the absence of this gene can cause an increased accumulation of reactive metabolites in the body, increasing the interaction with cellular macromolecules and tumor initiation process. GSTM1*A and GSTM1*B differ in only one base in exon 7 and encode monomers that form active dimers. The catalytic activity of these enzymes are very similar [91].

The GSTM1 gene is flanked by two almost identical 4.2-kb regions. GSTM1*0 originates from homologous recombination between the two repeat regions which results in a 16 Kb deletion containing the entire gene GSTM1 (Figure 4). GSTM1 is precisely excised leaving the adjacent GSTM2 and GSTM5 genes intact [78]. In a study of liver specimens of 168 autopsied Japanese subjects, observed was that the GSTM1*0 null allele was more frequent in livers with hepatitis and hepatocellular carcinoma compared to control livers [92].

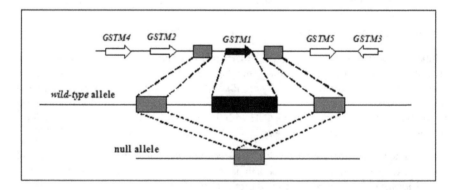

Figure 4. Structural localization of 100 kb gene cluster encoding the GST mu subfamily (chromosome 1p13.3). The figure indicates the homologous recombination event that can happen causing the null allele (GSTM1*0 - no GSTM1). Figure adapted from [78].

The subfamily GST theta consists of two genes, GSTT1 and GSTT2, located on chromosome 22q11.2 and separated by approximately 50 Kb (Figure 5). Analysis of the 119 Kb portion containing these genes revealed two regions flanking *GSTT1*, HA3 and HA5, with more than 90% homology. HA3 and HA5 contain two identical 403-bp repeats and the occurence of *GSTT1*0* allele is probably caused by homologous recombination between the two regions [78]. In humans, *GSTT1* is also expressed in erythrocytes and probably plays a global role in early detoxification of xenobiotics and carcinogens.

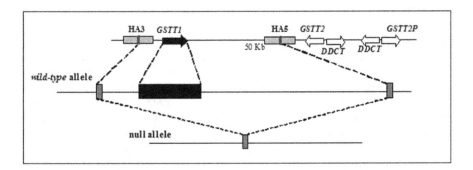

Figure 5. Structural localization of gene cluster encoding the GST subfamily theta (chromosome 22q11.2). The *GSTT1* null allele (*GSTT1*0*) arises by homologous recombination of the left and right 403-bp repeats, which results in a 54-kb deletion containing the entire *GSTT1* gene. Figure adapted from [78].

Deficiencies in the GST activity due to the null genotypes of *GSTM1* and *GSTT1* may modulate susceptibility to the development of hepatotoxicity induced by drugs and xenobiotics. Furthermore, it was observed that the frequencies of *GSTT1*0* and *GSTM1*0* alleles vary within different ethnic groups [78, 82]. Liver injury induced by INH has been associated with the depletion of glutathione content and reduction of GST activity in an animal model for hepatotoxicity by anti-TB drugs [22].

In 2001, Roy and colleagues demonstrated that individuals, homozygous for the null *GSTM1*, had a relative risk of 2.12 for developing hepatotoxicity induced by anti-TB drugs. However, these authors found no association of the *GSTT1* null genotype with this side effects [54]. Similarly, another study in the Thai population found that only the *GSTM1* null genotype increases the risk of liver injury (OR 2.23, 95% CI 1.07 to 4.67) [93]. The opposite was observed by Leiro and colleagues: individuals with the *GSTT1* null genotype had an increased risk of developing hepatotoxicity induced by anti-TB drugs and no significant association was observed between GSTM1*0/*0 genotype and liver injury [94]. These studies suggest a protective effect of glutathione S-transferases to the hepatotoxic effects of isoniazid.

On the other hand, recent studies in different population showed no relationship between GSTM1*0/*0 or GSTT1*0/*0 genotypes and liver injury during anti-TB treatment [58, 95, 96]. In a population-based prospective antituberculosis treatment coort in China, a more robust case-control study was conducted and there was no statistically significant association between null genotypes and hepatotoxicity induced by anti-TB drugs [97].

These controversal results may be due to the small sample size in many studies and the different frequencies of the null genotypes. New populations should be evaluated with large sample size to see which of these polymorphisms can be used as genetic markers for the risk of side effects during anti-TB treatment.

4. Conclusion

The concept of personalized medicine is not really new, but it has been receiving increasing attention in recent years for improval of drug regulation and medical guidelines. There is considerable interindividual variability in metabolism, partly due to human differences on a genetic level. Genetic polymorphisms in drug-metabolizing enzymes can affect enzyme activity and may cause differences in treatment response or drug toxicity, for example, due to an increased formation of reactive metabolites. Such polymorphisms may explain differences in incidence of anti-TB drugs induced hepatotoxicity between different populations.

Genotyping cannot completely predict the phenotype on an individual level because of to the additional contribution of epigenetic, endogenous and environmental factors. However, pharmacogenetics is able to add important information in many cases where therapeutic drug scheme is inappropriate or not sufficient. Nowadays, we can cite three examples of personalized medicine application in clinical practice, (i) AIDS treatment (abavir / skin hypersensitivity / HLA-B*5701), (ii) anticoagulation (warfarin / bleeding / CYP2C9) and (iii) treatment of acute lymphoblastic leukemia (azathioprine / treatment resistence / TPMT) [98].

Although limited information exists regarding isoniazid concentrations that cause toxic reactions, it has been proposed to adjust isoniazid dosage depending on individuals acetylator status: a lower dosage for slow acetylators to reduce the risk of liver injury and a higher isoniazid dosage for fast acetylators to increase the early bactericidal activity and thereby lower the probability of treatment failure [50]. However, more robust clinical prospective studies are needed to evaluate the real contribution of these different polyporphirms in the occurence of liver side effects during anti-TB treatment. Future studies should include larger sample size, different ethnic population, simultaneous analysis of different genetic markers, different degrees of liver injury and consideration of possible confounding factors.

Author details

Raquel Lima de Figueiredo Teixeira*, Márcia Quinhones Pires Lopes, Philip Noel Suffys and Adalberto Rezende Santos

*Address all correspondence to: raquelft@ioc.fiocruz.br

Laboratory of Molecular Biology Applied to Mycobacteria – Oswaldo Cruz Institute – Fiocruz, Rio de Janeiro, Brazil

References

[1] Hardman, JG., Limbird LE, Molinoff PB, Ruddon RW, Goodman AG. Goodman and Gilman's The Pharmacological Basis of Therapeutics. 9th ed. New York, NY: McGraw-Hill, 1996.

[2] Prows CA, Prows DR. Medication Selection by genotype: How genetics is changing drug prescribing and efficacy. American Journal of Nursing 2004; 104 60-70.

[3] Ingelman-Sundberg M. Pharmacogenetics: an opportunity for a safer and more efficient pharmacotherapy. Journal of Internal Medicine 2001; 250 186-200.

[4] Roses AD. Pharmacogenetics place in modern medical science and practice. Life Sciences 2002; 70 1471-1480.

[5] Sachidanandam R, Weissman D, Schmidt SC, Kakol JM, Stein LD, Marth G, Sherry S, Mullikin JC, Mortimore BJ, Willey DL, Hunt SE, Cole CG, Coggill PC, Rice CM, Ning Z, Rogers J, Bentley DR, Kwok PY, Mardis ER, Yeh RT, Schultz B, Cook L, Davenport R, Dante M, Fulton L, Hillier L, Waterston RH, McPherson JD, Gilman B, Schaffner S, Van Etten WJ, Reich D, Higgins J, Daly MJ, Blumenstiel B, Baldwin J, Stange-Thomann N, Zody MC, Linton L, Lander ES, Altshuler D. International SNP Map Working Group. A map of human genome sequence variation containing 1.42 million single nucleotide polymorphisms. Nature 2001; 409(6822) 928-33.

[6] Hall II RG, Leff RD, Gumbo T. Treatment of Active Pulmonary Tuberculosis in Adults: Current Standards and Recent Advances: Insights from the Society of Infectious Diseases Pharmacists. Pharmacotherapy 2009; 29(12) 1468–1481.

[7] Blomberg B, Fourie B. Fixed-dose combination drugs for tuberculosis: application in standardised treatment regimens. Drugs 2003;63(6) 535-53.

[8] Garibaldi RA, Drusin RE, Ferebee SH, Gregg MB. Isoniazid-associated hepatitis. Report of an outbreak. American Review of Respiratory Disease. 1972; 106 357-365.

[9] Saukkonen JJ, Cohn DL, Jasmer RM, Schenker S, Jereb JA, Nolan CM, Peloquin CA, Gordin FM, Nunes D, Strader DB, Bernardo J, Venkataramanan R, Sterling TR. An Official ATS Statement: Hepatotoxicity of Antituberculosis Therapy. American Journal of Respiratory and Critical Care Medicine 2006; 174 935–952.

[10] Xue HY, Hou YN, Liu HC. The general investigation of the increased hepatotoxicity caused by isoniazid in combination with rifampin. Chinese Journal Modern Applied Pharmacy 2002; 19 463–465.

[11] Tostmann A, Boeree MJ, Aarnoutse RE, Lange WC, van der Ven AJ, Dekhuijzen R. Antituberculosis drug-induced hepatotoxicity: concise up-to-date review. Journal of Gastroenterology and Hepatology 2007; 6 1440–1446.

[12] Lundkvist J, Jonsson B. Pharmacoeconomics of adverse drug reactions. Fundamental and Clinical Pharmacology 2004; 18 275-280.

[13] Hug H, Bagatto D, Dannecker R, Schindler R, Horlancher O, Gut J. ADRIS – The adverse drug reactions information scheme. Pharmacogenetics. 2003; 13:767-772.

[14] Larrey D. Epidemiology and individual susceptibility to adverse drug reactions affecting the liver. Seminars in Liver Disease 2002; 22 145155.

[15] Bagheri H, Michel F, Lapeyre-Mestre M, Lagier E, Cambus JP, Valdiguié P, Montastruc JL. Detection and incidence of drug-induced injuries in hospital: a prospective analysis from laboratory signal. British Journal of Clinical Pharmacology 2000; 50 479-484.

[16] Bissell DM, Gores GJ, Laskin DL, Hoofnagle JH. Drug-induced liver injury: mechanisms and test systems. Hepatology 2001; 33 1009-1013.

[17] Lee WM. Drug-induced hepatotoxicity. New England Journal of Medicine 2003; 349 474-485.

[18] Nelson SD, Mitchell JR, Timbrell JA, Snodgrass WR, Corcoran GB. Isoniazid and iproniazid: activation of metabolites to toxic intermediates in man and rat. Science 1976; 193(4256) 901-903.

[19] Timbrell JA, Mitchell JR, Snodgrass WR, Nelson SD. Isoniazid hepatotoxicity: the relationship between covalent binding and metabolism in vivo. Journal of Pharmacology and Experimental Therapeutics 1980; 213 364-369.

[20] Mitchell JR, Snodgrass WR, Gillette JR. The Role of Biotransformation in Chemical-Induced Liver Injury. Environmental Health Perspectives 1976; 15 27-38.

[21] Woodward KN, Timbrell JA. Acetylhidrazine hepatotoxicity: the role of covalent binding. Toxicology 1984; 30 65-74.

[22] Sodhi CP, Rana SV, Mehta SK, Vaiphei K, Attri S, Thakur S, Mehta S. Study of oxidative stress in isoniazid-induced hepatic injury in young rats with and without protein-energy malnutrition. Journal of Biochemical and Molecular Toxicology 1996; 11 139-146.

[23] Hayes JD, Flanagan JU, Jowsey IR. Glutathione transferases. Annual Review of Pharmacology and Toxicology 2005; 45 51-88.

[24] Roy PD, Majumder M, Roy B. Pharmacogenomics of anti-TB drugs-related hepatotoxicity. Pharmacogenomics 2008; 9 311-321.

[25] Evans DAP. N-acetyltransferase. Pharmacology & Therapeutics 1989; 42:157-234

[26] Sim E, Payton M, Noble M, Minchin R. An update on genetic, structural and functional studies of arylamine N-acetyltransferases in eucaryotes and procaryotes. Human Molecular Genetics 2000; 9 2435-41.

[27] Hein DW, Doll MA, Fletland AJ, Leff MA, Webb SJ, Xiao GH, Devanaboyina US, Nangju NA, Feng Y. Molecular genetics and epidemiology of the NAT1 and NAT2 acetylation polymorphisms. Cancer Epidemiology, Biomarkers and Prevention 2000; 9 29-42.

[28] Hein DW. Molecular genetics and function of NAT1 and NAT2: role in aromatic amine metabolism and carcinogenesis. Mutation Research 2002; 506-507 65-77.

[29] Fretland AJ, Leff MA, Doll MA, Hein DW. Functional characterization of human N-acetyltransferase 2 (NAT2) single nucleotide polymorphisms. Phamacogenetics 2001; 11 207-215.

[30] Zang Y, Doll MA, Zhao S, States JC, Hein DW. Functional characterization of single-nucleotide polymorphisms and haplotypes of human N-acetyltransferase 2. Carcinogenesis 2007; 28 1665-1671.

[31] Parkin DP, Vandenplas S, Botha FJ, Vandenplas ML, Seifart HI, van Helden PD, van der Walt BJ, Donald PR, van Jaarsveld PP. Trimodality of isoniazid elimination: phenotype and genotype in patients with tuberculosis. American Journal of Respiratory and Critical Care Medicine 1997; 155 1717-1722.

[32] Chen B, Zhang WX, Cai WM. The influence of various genotypes on the metabolic activity of NAT2 in Chinese population. European Journal of Clinical Pharmacology 2006; 62 355-359.

[33] Consensus Human Arylamine N-Acetyltransferase Gene Nomenclature www.louisville.edu/medschool/pharmacology/NAT.html (accessed 15 August 2012).

[34] Teixeira RL, Silva Jr FP, Silveira AR, Cabello PH, Mendonça-Lima L, Rabahi MF, Kritski AL, Mello FC, Suffys PN, de Miranda AB, Santos AR. Sequence analysis of NAT2 gene in Brazilians: identification of undescribed single nucleotide polymorphisms and molecular modeling of the N-acetyltransferase 2 protein structure. Mutation Research 2010; 683 43-49.

[35] García-Martín E. Interethnic and intraethnic variability of NAT2 single nucleotide polymorphisms. Current Drug Metabolism 2008; 9 (6) 487-497.

[36] Boukouvala S, Sim E. Structural Analysis of the Genes for Human Arylamine N-Acetyltransferases and Characterisation of Alternative Transcripts. Basic & Clinical Pharmacology & Toxicology 2005; 96 343–351.

[37] Cascorbi I, Drakoulis N, Brockmoller J, Maurer A, Sperling K, Roots I. Arylamine N-acetyltransferase (NAT2) mutations and their allelic linkage in unrelated Caucasian individuals: Correlation with phenotypic activity. American Journal of Human Genetics 1995; 57 581-592.

[38] Lin HJ, Han CY, Lin BK, Hardy S. Slow acetylator mutations in the human polymorphic N-acetyltransferase gene in 786 Asians, blacks, Hispanics, and whites: applica-

tion to metabolic epidemiology. American Journal of Human Genetics 1993; 52(4) 827-34.

[39] Teixeira RL, Miranda AB., Pacheco AG, Lopes MQ, Fonseca-Costa J, Rabahi MF, Melo HM, Kritski AL, Mello FC, Suffys PN, Santos AR. Genetic profile of the arylamine N-Acetyltransferase 2 coding gene among individuals from two different regions of Brazil. Mutatation Ressearch 2007; 624 31-40.

[40] Stephens M, Smith NJ, Donnelly P. A new statistical method for haplotype reconstruction from population data. American Journal of Human Genetics 2001; 68 978-989.

[41] Stephens M, Donnelly P. A comparison of Bayesian methods for haplotype reconstruction. American Journal of Human Genetics 2003; 73 1162-1169.

[42] Xie HG, Xu ZH, Ou-Yang DS, Shu Y, Yang DL, Wang JS, Yan XD, Huang SL, Wang W, Zhou HH. Meta-analysis of phenotype and genotype of NAT2 deficiency in Chinese populations. Pharmacogenetics 1997; 7(6) 503-14.

[43] Sekine A, Saito S, Iida A, Mitsunobu Y, Higuchi S, Harigae S, Nakamura Y. Identification of single-nucleotide polymorphisms (SNPs) of human N-acetyltransferase genes NAT1, NAT2, AANAT, ARD1 and L1CAM in the Japanese population. Journal of Human Genetics 2001; 46 314-319.

[44] Jorge-Nebert LF, Eichelbaum M, Griese EU, Inaba T, Arias TD. Analysis of six SNPs of NAT2 in Ngawbe and Embera Amerindians of Panama and determination of the Embera acetylation phenotype using caffeine. Pharmacogenetics 2002; 12 39–48.

[45] Cascorbi I, Brockmoller J, Mrozikiewicz PM, Muller A, Roots I. Arylamine N-acetyltransferase activity in man. Drug Metab Rev 1999; 31 489–502.

[46] Hein, D. N-acetyltransferase 2 genetic polymorphism: Effects of carcinogen and haplotype on urinary bladder cancer risk. Oncogene 2006; 25(11) 1649–1658.

[47] Ohno M, Yamaguchi I, Yamamoto I, Fukuda T, Yolota S, Maekura R, Ito M, Yamamoto Y, Ogura T, Maeda K., Komuta K, Igarashi T, Azuma J. Slow N-acetyltransferase 2 genotype affects the incidence of isoniazid and rifampicin-induced hepatotoxicity. International Journal of Tuberculosis Lung Disease. 2000; 4 256-261.

[48] Huang YS, Chern HD, Su WJ, Wu JC, Lai SL, Yang SY, Chang FY, Lee SD. Polymorphism of the N-acetyltransferase 2 gene as a susceptibility risk factor for antituberculosis drug-induced hepatitis. Hepatology 2002; 35 883-889.

[49] Kinzig-Schippers M, Tomalik-Scharte D, Jetter A, Scheidel B, Jakob V, Rodamer M, Cascorbi I, Doroshyenko O, Sörgel F, Fuhr U. Should we use N-acetyltransferase type 2 genotyping to personalize isoniazid doses? Antimicrobial Agents and Chemotherapy 2005; 49 1733–1738.

[50] Shimizu Y, Dobashi K, Mita Y, Endou K, Moriya S, Osano K, Koike Y, Higuchi S, Yabe S, Utsugi M, Ishizuka T, Hisada T, Nakazawa T, Mori M. DNA microarray gen-

otyping of N-acetyltransferase 2 polymorphism using carbodiimide as the linker for assessment of isoniazid hepatotoxicity. Tuberculosis 2006; 86(5) 374-81.

[51] Cho HJ, Koh WJ, Ryu YJ, Ki CS, Nam MH, Kim JW, Lee SY. Genetic polymorphisms of NAT2 and CYP2E1 associated with antituberculosis drug-induced hepatotoxicity in Korean patients with pulmonary tuberculosis. Tuberculosis 2007; 87:551-556.

[52] Higuchi N, Tahara N, Yanagihara K, Fukushima H, Suyama N, Inoue Y, Miyazaki Y, Kobayashi T, Yoshiura K, Niikawa N, Wen CY, Isomoto H, Shikuwa S, Omagari K, Mizuta Y, Kohno S, Tsukamoto K. NAT2*6A, a haplotype of the N-acetyltransferase 2 gene, is an important biomarker for risk of anti-tuberculosis drug-induced hepatotoxicity in Japanese patients with tuberculosis. World J Gastroenterology 2007; 13 6003-6008.

[53] Singh J, Arora A, Garg PK, Thakur VS, Pande JN, Tandon RK. Antituberculosis treatment-induced hepatotoxicity: role of predictive factors. Postgraduate Medical Journal 1995; 71 359-362.

[54] Roy B, Chowdhury A, Kundu S, Santra A, Dey B, Chakraborty M, Majumder PP. Increased risk of antituberculosis drug-induced hepatotoxicity in individuals with gluthatione S-transferase M1 "null" mutation. Journal of Gastroenterology and Hepatology 2001; 16 1033-1037.

[55] Vuilleumier N, Rossier MF, Chiappe A, Degoumois F, Dayer P, Mermillod B, Nicod L, Desmeules J, Hochstrasser D. CYP2E1 genotype and isoniazid-induced hepatotoxicity in patients treated for latent tuberculosis. European Journal of Clinical Pharmacology 2006; 62 423-429.

[56] Mitchell JR, Thorgeisson UP, Black M Timbrell JA, Snodgrass WR, Potter WZ, Jollow HR, Keiser HR. Increased incidence of isoniazid hepatitis in rapid acetylators: possible relation to hydralazine metabolites. Clinical Pharmacology & Therapeutics 1975; 18 70–79.

[57] Yamamoto T, Suou T, Hirayama C. Elevated serum aminotransferase induced by isoniazid in relation to isoniazid acetylator phenotype. Hepatology 1986; 6 295–298.

[58] Teixeira RL, Morato RG, Cabello PH, Muniz LM, Moreira Ada S, Kritski AL, Mello FC, Suffys PN, Miranda AB, Santos AR. Genetic polymorphisms of NAT2, CYP2E1, GST enzymes and the occurrence of antituberculosis drug-induced hepatitis in Brazilian TB patients. Memórias do Instituto Oswaldo Cruz 2011; 106(6) 716-24.

[59] Wang PY, Xie SY, Hao Q, Zhang C, Jiang BF. NAT2 polymorphisms and susceptibility to anti-tuberculosis drug-induced liver injury: a meta-analysis. The International Journal of Tuberculosis and Lung Disease 2012; 16(5) 589-95.

[60] Ellard GA, Gammon PT. Pharmacokinetics of isoniazid metabolism in man. Journal of Pharmacokinetics and Biopharmaceutics 1976; 4 83-113.

[61] Lauterburg BH, Smith CV, Todd EL, Mitchell JR. Pharmacokinetics of the toxic hydrazine metabolites formed from isoniazid in humans. J Pharmacol Exp Ther 1985; 235 566-570.

[62] Timbrell JA, Wright JM, Baillie TA. Monoacetylhydrazine as a metabolite of isoniazid in man. Clinical Pharmacology & Therapeutics 1977; 22 602-608.

[63] Timbrell JA, Mitchell JR, Snodgrass WR, Nelson SD. Isoniazid hepatotoxicity: the relationship between covalent binding and metabolism in vivo. Journal of Pharmacology and Experimental Therapeutics 1980; 213 364-369.

[64] Sarma GR, Immanuel C, Kailasam S, Narayana ASL, Venkatesan P. Rifampin-induced realese of hydrazine from isoniazid: a possible cause of hepatitis during treatment of tuberculosis with regimens containing isoniazid and rifampin. American Review of Respiratory Disease 1986; 133 1072-1075.

[65] Fukino K, Sasaki Y, Hirai S, Nakamura T, Hashimoto M, Yamagishi F, Ueno K. Effects of NAT2, CYP2E1 and GST genotypes on the serum concentrations of isoniazid and metabolites in tuberculosis patients. The Journal of Toxicological Sciences 2008; 33 187-95.

[66] Wijnen PAHM, Op Den Buijsch RAM, Drent M, Kuipers PMJC, Neef C, Bast A, Bekers O, Koek GH. Review article: the prevalence and clinical relevance of cytochrome P450 polymorphisms. Alimentary Pharmacology & Therapeutics 2007; 26 Supl: 211-219.

[67] The CYP 450 nomenclature. http://drnelson.uthsc.edu/CytochromeP450.html (accessed 15 August 2012).

[68] Nebert DW, Russell DW. Clinical importance of the cytovhromes P450. Lancet 2002; 360 1155-1162.

[69] Ingelman-Sundberg M. Pharmacogenetics of cytochrome P450 and its applications in drug therapy: the past, present and future. Trends in Pharmacological Sciences 2004; 25 193-200.

[70] Caro AA, Cederbaum AI. Oxidative stress, toxicology, and pharmacology of CYP2E1. Annual Review of Pharmacology and Toxicology 2004; 44 27-42.

[71] Watanabe J, Hayashi S, Kawajiri K. Different regulations and expression of the human CYP2E1 gene due to the Rsa I polymorphism in the 5`flanking region. The Journal of Biochemistry 1994; 116 321-326.

[72] CYP2E1 allele nomenclature. www.cypalleles.ki.se/cyp2e1.htm (accessed 15 August 2012).

[73] Carriere V, Berthou F, Baird S, Belloc C, Beaune P, Waziers ID. Human cytochrome P4502E1 (CYP2E1): from genotype to phenotype. Pharmacogenetics 1996; 6 203-211.

[74] Powell H, Kitteringham NR, Pirmohamed M, Smith DA, Perk BK. Expression of cytochorme P-4502E1 in human liver: assessment by mRNA, genotype and phenotype. Pharmacogenetics 1998; 8 411-421.

[75] Neuhaus T, Ko YD, Lorenzen K, Fronhoffs S, Harth V, Bröde P, Vetter H, Bolt HM, Pesch B, Brüning T. Association of cytocrome P450 2E1 polymorphisms and head and neck squamous cell cancer. Toxicology 2004; 151 273-282.

[76] Huang YS, Chern HD, Su WJ, Wu JC, Chang SC, Chiang CH, Chang FY, Lee SD. Cytochome P450 2E1 genotype and the susceptibility to antituberculosis drug-induced hepatitis. Hepatology 2003; 37 924-930.

[77] Roy B, Ghosh SK, Sutraghar D, Sikdar N, Mazumder S, Barman S. Predisposition of antituberculosis drug induced hepatotoxicity by cytochrome P450 2E1 genotype and haplotype in pediatric patients. Journal of Gastroenterology and Hepatology 2006; 21 781-786.

[78] Parl FF. Glutathione S-transferase genotypes and cancer risk. Cancer Letters 2005; 221 123-129.

[79] Strange RC, Jones PW, Fryer AA. Glutathione S-transferase: genetics and role in toxicology. Toxicology Letters 2000; 112-113 357–363.

[80] Strange RC, Spiteri MA, Ramachandran S, Fryer AA. Glutathione-S-transferase family of enzymes. Mutation Research 2001; 482 21–26.

[81] Coughlin SS, Hall IJ. Glutathione S-transferase polymorphisms and risk of ovarian cancer: A HuGE review. Genetics Medicine 2002; 4 250–257.

[82] Landi S. Mammalian class theta GST and differential susceptibility to carcinogens: a review. Mutation Research 2000; 463 247–283.

[83] Pemble S, Schroeder KR, Spencer SR, Meyer DJ, Hallier E, Bolt HM, Brian Ketterer, Taylor JB. Human glutathione S-transferase Theta (GSTT1): cDNA cloning and the characterization of a genetic polymorphism. Biochemical Journal 1994; 300 271-276.

[84] Geisler SA, Olshan AF. GSTM1, GSTT1, and the Risk of Squamous Cell Carcinoma of the Head and Neck: A Mini-HuGE Review. American Journal of Epidemiology 2001; 154 95–105.

[85] Henrion-Caude A, Roussey C, Housset M, Flahault C, Fryer A, Chadelat AA, Strange RC, Clement A. Liver disease in pediatric patients with cystic fibrosis is associated with glutathione S-transferase P1 polymorphism. Hepatology 2002; 36 913-917.

[86] Vineis P, Veglia F, Anttila S, Benhamou S, Clapper ML, Dolzan V, Ryberg D, Hirvonen A, Kremers P, Le Marchand L, Pastorelli R, Rannug A, Romkes M, Schoket B, Strange RC, Garte S, Taioli E. CYP1A1, GSTM1 and GSTT1 polymorphisms and lung cancer: a pooled analysis of gene-gene interactions. Biomarkers 2004; 9 298-305.

[87] Raimondi S, Paracchini V, Autrup H, Barros-Dios JM, Benhamou S, Boffetta P, Cote ML, Dialyna IA, Dolzan V, Filiberti R, Garte S, Hirvonen A, Husgafvel-Pursiainen K,

Imyanitov EN, Kalina I, Kang D, Kiyohara C, Kohno T, Kremers P, Lan Q, London S, Povey AC, Rannug A, Reszka E, Risch A, Romkes M, Schneider J, Seow A, Shields PG, Sobti RC, Sørensen M, Spinola M, Spitz MR, Strange RC, Stücker I, Sugimura H, To-Figueras J, Tokudome S, Yang P, Yuan JM, Warholm M, Taioli E. Meta- and Pooled Analysis of GSTT1 and Lung Cancer: A HuGE-GSEC Review. American Journal of Eepidemiology 2006; 164 1027–1042

[88] Holley SL, Fryer AA, Haycock JW, Grubb SEW, Strange RC, Hoban PR. Differential effects of glutathione S-transferase pi (GSTP1) haplotypes on cell proliferation and apoptosis. Carcinogenesis 2007; 28 2268-2273.

[89] Brockmöller J, Kerb R, Drakoulis N, Staffeldt B, Roots I. Glutathione S-transferase M1 and its variants A and B as host factors of bladder cancer susceptibility: a case-control study. Cancer Research 1994; 54 4103-4111.

[90] Cotton SC, Sharp L, Little J, Brockton N. Glutathione S-transferase polymorphisms and colorectal cancer: a HuGE review. American Journal of Epidemiology 2000; 151 7-32.

[91] Widersten M, Pearson WR, Engström A, Mannervik B. Heterologous expression of the allelic variant mu-class glutathione transferases mu and psi. Biochemical Journal 1991; 276 519-524.

[92] Harada S, Abei M, Tanaka N, Agarwal DP, Goedde HW. Liver glutathione S-transferase polymorphism in Japanese and its pharmacogenetic importance. Human Genetics 1987; 75 322-325.

[93] Huang YS. Genetic polymorphisms of drug-metabolizing enzymes and the susceptibility to antituberculosis drug-induced liver injury. Expert Opinion on Drug Metabolism & Toxicology 2007; 3 1-8.

[94] Leiro V, Fernandez-Villar A, Valverde D, Constenla L, Vazquez R, Pineiro L, González-Quintela A. Influence of glutathione S-transferase M1 and T1 homozygous null mutations on the risk of antituberculosis drug-induced hepatotoxicity in Caucasian population. Liver International 2008; 28 835-839.

[95] Chatterjee S, Lyle N, Mandal A, Kundu S. GSTT1 and GSTM1 gene deletions are not associated with hepatotoxicity caused by antitubercular drugs. Journal of Clinical Pharmacy and Therapeutics 2010; 35(4) 465-70.

[96] Sotsuka T, Sasaki Y, Hirai S, Yamagishi F, Ueno K. Association of isoniazid-metabolizing enzyme genotypes and isoniazid-induced hepatotoxicity in tuberculosis patients. In Vivo 2011; 25(5) 803-12.

[97] Tang SW, Lv XZ, Zhang Y, Wu SS, Yang ZR, Xia YY, Tu DH, Deng PY, Ma Y, Chen DF, Zhan SY. CYP2E1, GSTM1 and GSTT1 genetic polymorphisms and susceptibility to antituberculosis drug-induced hepatotoxicity: a nested case-control study. Journal of Clinical Pharmacy and Therapeutics 2012 doi: 10.1111/j.1365-2710.2012.01334.x.

[98] Cascorbi I. The promises of personalized medicine. European Journal of Clinical Pharmacology 2010; 66 749–754.

Chapter 7

Influence of the Interferon–Gamma (IFN–γ) and Tumor Necrosis Factor Alpha (TNF–α) Gene Polymorphisms in TB Occurrence and Clinical Spectrum

Márcia Quinhones Pires Lopes,
Raquel Lima de Figueiredo Teixeira,
Antonio Basilio de Miranda, Rafael Santos Pinto,
Lizânia Borges Spinassé,
Fernanda Carvalho Queiroz Mello,
José Roberto Lapa e Silva, Philip Noel Suffys and
Adalberto Rezende Santos

Additional information is available at the end of the chapter

1. Introduction

Tuberculosis (TB) is a major public concern and is the most important single infectious cause of mortality and morbidity worldwide. According the World Health Organization (WHO) records, in 2009, there were an estimated 9.4 million new cases, 14 million prevalent cases, and approximately 1.7 million deaths by TB [1]. Additionally, approximately one third of the world's population is infected with the causative bacterium, *Mycobacterium tuberculosis* (*Mtb*), and is at risk for developing active tuberculosis. Interestingly, while approximately 9 million people develop active TB each year, the majority remain asymptomatically (latently) infected with the pathogen presumably due to a protective immune response. Without intervention, approximately five to ten percent of those latently infected will develop overt disease and the potential to transmit *Mtb* to others [2].

Familial clustering data, twin studies and complex segregation analysis have all suggested a strong genetic component in the human susceptibility to the chronic mycobacterial diseases [3-7] but also a complex picture of geographic heterogeneity in genetic effects on the different mycobacterial infections is involved [8, 9]. Several non-HLA genes have been implicated in TB susceptibility. However, the discrepant data reported may be attributed to a number of different factors, such as the types of studies, ethnicity, genetic background, and clinical status of patients with tuberculosis that may be associated with a particular genetic profile. The interaction among lung cells with pro and anti-inflammatory mediators during the infection with *Mtb* have been deeply investigated [10]. Among involved cytokines, the key role of interferon-gamma (IFN-γ) and tumor necrosis factor (TNF-α) in eliciting an inflammatory response against *Mtb* have been emphasized [11-13].

In human studies, the crucial role of TNF-α in protective host immunity against reactivation of latent TB was highlighted by the observation that the relapse and severe course of TB is over-represented in rheumatoid arthritis patients following the use of anti-TNF-α antibodies [14]. Concerning the IFN-γ, it is well established that deficiency in IFN-γ gene expression is associated with severe impairment of resistance to infections, in particular those that are normally killed by activated macrophages [15, 16]. Low synthesis of this cytokine has been associated with active tuberculosis [17]. However, on the contrary of TNF-α, the Interferon gamma conding gene (*IFNG*) is highly conserved and few single nucleotide polymorphisms (SNPs) are found in the intragenic region. Several case-control studies to evaluate association of SNPs in these genes with TB have produced mixed results, with little consensus in most cases on whether any TNF polymorphisms are actually associated with active TB disease [18, 19].

In the present study we aimed to analyse the existing promoter variability of the *IFNG* and *TNF-α* genes by partial mapping of this region in samples from Brazilians, followed by an association study of the identified SNPs and TB outcome after infection with *Mtb*.

2. Method used

2.1. Study population

In a case-control design, five hundred consanguineously unrelated individuals admitted at the University Hospital Complex: Thoracic Institute/ClementinoFraga University Hospital from Federal University of Rio de Janeiro-UFRJ were enrolled in this study after signing informed consent approved by the local Ethics Committee of HUCFF-UFRJ.

Demographic, clinical, and microbiological data as well as the HIV status of the subjects (age > 18 years old) were collected. Active TB cases (n=265) were defined as those after a positive culture confirmation in clinical specimen or with clinical, radiographic and laboratory improvement according to the American Thoracic Statements.They comprised 265 TB patients to be used for the descriptive genetic analysis. For the association study, TB-HIV comorbity was considered as an exclusion criteria and sample size was reduced as follow: 140 TB patients, being 121 with pulmonary TB (PTB) and 19 extrapulmonary forms of TB (TBE). The mean age of TB patients was ± 51 years (range 18-84 years) including 73 males and 67 females.

For the control group, a complete questionnaire to document TB risk factors since baseline testing was used. Individuals were eligible as controls if they had no previous TB history, consanguinity and negative HIV status. In formations concerning Tuberculin Skin Test (TST) response were available for all controls. They comprised 235 individuals, to be used for descriptive genetic analysis. For the association study, after application of the exclusion criteria, 154 individuals were included in this group, of which, 96 were TST positive (TST+) and 58 TST negative (TST-). The mean age in this group was ± 50 (range 18 - 82 years) and included 55 males and 99 females.

Sample Collection and handling

A volume of 3 mL of venous blood was collected from each volunteer and stored at -20°C. Genomic DNA was isolated from 100 µL of frozen whole blood using the FlexiGene DNA Kit (Qiagen Inc., USA), according to the manufacturer's specifications. After extraction, DNA samples were stored at -20°C.

2.2. *IFNG* and *TNF–α* genotyping

Genotyping of the proximal portion of the promoter region in *TNF-α* and *IFNG* genes was achieved by direct sequencing of PCR products. Two sets of primers for PCR amplification and sequencing of *IFNG*, DNA fragment of 863bp, (IFN-EF: 5' GGAACTCCCCCTGG-GAATATTCT 3`, IFNER: 5'AGCTGATCAGGTCCAAAGGA3', IFNIF: 5 'CGAAGTGGGGAGGT ACAAAA 3' and IFNIR: 5' CCCAGGAAACTGCTACTCTG 3'), and *TNF-α*, DNA fragment of 855bp (TNFEF: 5'CAGGACCTCCAGGTATGGAA3', TNFER: 5' TAGCTGGTCCTCTGCTGTCC3', TNFIF: 5'CCTGCATCCTGTCTGGAAGT 3' and TNF-IR: 5'TTTCAACCCCTGTGTGTTCG 3') were designed by using the Primer3 software [20].

For PCR-mediated DNA amplification of *IFNG*, 100 ng of genomic DNA were added to a 50µL reaction mixture containing 200ng of each primer (IFN-EF and IFN-ER), 0.2mM of each dNTPs, 2.0mM $MgCl_2$ and 1U *Taq* DNA polymerase (Invitrogen by Life Technologies, USA) and submitted to an initial denaturation at 94°C for 5 min., followed by 35 cycles of 1 min. at 94°C, 1 min. at 65.3°C and 1 min at 72°C. Final extension was performed for 5 min. at 72°C. Likewise, for amplification of the 855pb *TNF-α* fragment, 100ng of genomic DNA were added to a 25µL reaction mixture containing 200ng of each primer (TNF-EF and TNF-ER), 2mM $MgCl_2$, 0.2mM of each dNTPs and 0.5U of *Taq* gold DNA polymerase (PE Applied BioSystems) and submitted to initial denaturation at 94°C for 15 min, followed by 35 cycles of 1 min. at 94°C, 1 min. at 65.9°C and 1 min at 72°C with a final extension at 72°C for 5 min. Evaluation of PCR products was done by electrophoresis on 1.2% agarose gel followed by ethidium bromide staining.

For sequencing, PCR products were purified with ChargeSwitch Kit (Invitrogen Life Technologies), according to the manufacturer's recommendations. Sequencing of the amplified fragments was performed in both DNA strands using a combination of the internal and external primers using ABI PRISM Big Dye Terminator v. 3.1 Kit (PE Applied BioSystems), according to the manufacturer's recommendations, on an ABI PRISM 3730 DNA Analyser (PE

Applied BioSystems). All singletons and even new/rare mutation identified were confirmed by re-amplification and re-sequencing.

2.3. Computational analysis

The SNPs identification in each individual sample was achieved after alignment of the generated sequences with the GenBank reference sequences AF3757790 and AB088112 for *IFNG* and *TNF-α* respectively. Transcription starting site sequence definition adopted for both genes considered as starting point, the first nucleotide immediately preceding position (-1) out of mRNA. Sequence analysis was carried out through SeqScapev. 2.6 software (Applied Biosystem). Haplotype reconstruction was achieved through the use of PHASE Vs. 2.1.1 software [21, 22].

2.4. Statistical analysis

Pair-wise linkage disequilibrium was tested for the loci studies. The Hardy-Weinberg equilibrium using χ^2 test. Statistics were performed in XLSTAT 2008.7 (Addinsoft Software Inc - New York USA). The magnitude of the associations was estimated by odds ratio values and the coefficient of associations. All tests were performed at the 0.05 level of significance by Epi Info version 3.5.1 2008 (Centers for Disease Control and Prevention, USA).

3. Results

In this work, a partial mapping of the promoter regions of *IFNG* and *TNF-α* genes was performed by direct PCR sequencing approach in 265 TB patients and 235 healthy controls residents in Rio de Janeiro, Brazil. Sequencing approach allowed the identification of new SNPs and consequently new haplotypes for both genes. Expected genotype frequencies were calculated from respective single allele frequencies and were consistent with Hard Weinberg Equilibrium using χ^2test.

3.1. Partial mapping of the *IFNG* promoter region in samples from Brazilians residents in Rio de Janeiro

Sequence analysis of the proximal portion of *IFNG* promoter region (863 bp upstream of the transcription starting site) revealed the presence of seven SNPs, of which, four were new, and located at positions (-787C>T, -599C>G, -517C>T, and -255A>G). The three remaining SNPs, already deposited in GenBank-Entrez SNP database, were located at positions (-785C>T, -200G>T, reported as (-183 and -179) and -172A>G (reported as -155). Table 1 show the allele and genotype frequencies of the identified SNPs in the whole studied population (500 samples). All SNPs were found in a very low frequency, sometimes as a singleton (-255A>G). In this case, the SNP was confirmed by new PCR amplification and re-sequencing. The two more frequent SNPs were the ones located at positions -599C>G and -200G>T, both with 1.4%. No homozygosity was identified in these positions.

Diagnosis and Management of Tuberculosis

Locus *IFNG*	Genotype	Subjects (n = 500)	Absolute Frequency	Allele frequency
	CC	495	0.99	
-787*	TC	5	.001	0.05
	(f) T	5	–	
	CC	495	0.99	
-785	CT	5	0.01	0.05
	(f) T	5	–	
	CC	487	0.974	
-599*	CG	12	0.024	
	GG	1	0.002	0.014
	(f) G	2	-	
	CC	497	0.994	
-517*	CT	3	0.06	0.003
	(f)T	3	-	
	AA	499	0.998	
-255*	AG	1	0.002	0.001
		1	-	
	(f) G			
	GG	486	0.972	
-200	GT	14	0.028	0.014
	(f) T	14	-	
	AA	498	0.996	
-172	AG	2	0.004	0.002
	(f) G	2		

Table 1. Genotype and allele frequencies of SNPs within *IFNG* promoter in Brazilians from Rio de Janeiro.

3.2. *IFNG* haplotypes characterization

Haplotype reconstruction was achieved from genotyping data by using Phase Vs. 2.1.1 software. A total of eight different haplotypes were characterized with basis on the combination of the seven SNPs identified within the *IFNG* promoter. Table 2 shows the frequencies of the identified haplotypes in the total population. The haplotype 4 was the, more frequent among the whole samples analyzed.

Haplotypes	-787	-785	-599	-517	-255	-200	-172	Frequency
1	C	C	C	C	A	G	A	0.916
2	C	T	C	C	A	G	A	0.010
3	C	C	G	C	A	G	A	0.024
4	C	C	C	C	A	T	A	0.028
5	T	C	C	C	A	G	A	0.010
6	C	C	C	C	G	G	A	0.002
7	C	C	C	C	A	G	G	0.004
8	C	C	C	T	A	G	A	0.006

Table 2. Characterization of the identified haplotypes within *IFNG* proximal promoter region in Brazilians from Rio de Janeiro (n=500).

3.3. Partial mapping of the *TNF–α* promoter region in samples from Brazilians residents in Rio de Janeiro

The partial mapping of the proximal portion (855 bp upstream of the transcription starting site) of *TNF-α* promoter was also performed by direct sequencing of PCR products. Upon analysis of the generated sequences seven SNPs, all described in the literature, and were identified in a total of 500 samples. Table 3 shows the allele and genotype frequencies. With the exception of the most studied SNPs (-238 -308, and -376) presenting frequencies higher than 3%, all others were present in less than one percent.

3.4. *TNF–α*haplotypes characterization

A total of fourteen different haplotypes were characterized. Except for the wild-type, haplotype 1, the higher frequent was the haplotype 3, presenting a mutant variation only at -308 position. As expected, the rare combination presenting polymorphisms only at positions -238 and -308 was present in the sample studied although in a low frequency (Table 4).

Locus	Genotype	Subjects (n=500)	Absolute Frequency	Allele Frequency
	GG	495	0.990	-
-646	GA	5	0.010	-
	A	5	–	0.005
	AA	495	0.990	-
-572	AC	5	0.010	-
	C	5	–	0.005
	CC	499	0.998	–
-422	CT	1	0.002	–
	T	1	–	0.001
	GG	471	0.942	–
-376	GA	28	0.056	–
	AA	1	0.002	–
	A	30	–	0.030
	GG	418	0.836	–
-308	GA	77	0.154	–
	AA	5	0.010	–
	A	87	–	0.087
	GG	489	0.978	–
-244	GA	11	0.022	–
	A	11	–	0.011
	GG	453	0.906	–
-238	GA	44	0.088	–
	AA	3	0.006	–
	A	50	–	0.050

Table 3. Genotype and allele frequencies of SNPs within *TNF-α* promoter in Brazilians from Rio de Janeiro.

Haplotype	-646	-572	-422	-376	-308	-238	-244	Frequency
1	G	A	C	G	G	G	G	0.710
2	G	A	C	**A**	G	G	G	0.006
3	G	A	C	G	**A**	G	G	0.146
4	G	**C**	C	G	G	G	G	0.006
5	G	A	C	G	G	G	**A**	0.020
6	G	A	C	G	G	**A**	G	0.040
7	**A**	A	C	G	G	G	G	0.008
8	G	A	**T**	G	G	G	G	0.002
9	G	A	C	**A**	G	**A**	G	0.044
10	G	A	C	**A**	**A**	**A**	G	0.060
11	G	A	C	**A**	**A**	G	G	0.002
12	G	A	C	G	**A**	G	**A**	0.002
13	G	A	C	G	**A**	**A**	G	0.004
14	G	**C**	C	G	**A**	G	G	0.004

Table 4. Haplotypes description and frequencies within *TNF-α* promoter in Brazilians from Rio de Janeiro.

3.5. Association of the *IFNG* SNPs and TB outcomes

Association of the identified SNPs variations within the analyzed region of *IFNG* with different TB outcomes (susceptibility *per se*, protection, severity and susceptibility to latent *M. tuberculosis* infection) was assessed based in the comparison of allele, genotype and haplotype frequencies between the stratified groups. The groups used for each evaluation were as follow: a) susceptibility *per se* to TB (TB patients versus TST+ controls), b) disease severity (PTB versus TBE) and c) susceptibility to the latent infection (healthy controls TST+ versus TST-).

As previously stated, for this analysis, the sample size was reduced in groups, (patients and controls) because of the exclusion criteria of TB-HIV co-infection and consanguinity. After exclusions, because of the very low frequency of the -255 A>G and -172 A>G these SNPs were also excluded.

Results of the association study upon comparison of genotype frequencies of the five remaining SNPs between TB patients (TBP/EPTB) versus TST+ controls are shown in Table 5. Only the SNP -200G>T presented a significantly higher frequency of the GT genotype in the control group indicating an association of this genotype with protection to the occurrence of active TB ($\chi^2 = 3.86$, $p = 0.033$, OR = 0.18 CI = 0.03 -1.00). Evaluation of the identified SNPs with the other outcomes did not show any association (data not shown).

Loci	Genotype	Patientes (N=140)	Controls TST+* (N= 96)	χ^2	p-value	OR	IC
-787	CC	138	96	1.383	0.515	#	#
	CT	2	0				
-785	CC	140	94	2.942	0.16	#	0.00<2.79
	CT	0	2				
-599	CC	135	93	0.035	NS	1.15	0.23<6.23
	CG	5	3				
-517	CC	140	93	2.29	0.066	#	0.00<1.52
	CG	0	3				
-200	GG	138	89	3.86	0.033	0.18	0.03<1.00
	GT	2	7				

Table 5. Genotype distribution of the *IFNG* SNPs among TB patients and healthy controls (TST+).

Given that the SNP -200 *IFNG* was the only one that was associated with any of the studied outcomes at genotype level, allele frequency was also tested for the same outcomes. Table 6 shows the comparison of the -200T variant between the stratified groups. The results confirm the association with protection to the occurrence of active TB and, additionally to TBP. Association of the -200T variant was also seen to occurrence of latent infection (p=0.035).

Different outcomes	Groups		SNP IFNG -200		
			P-valor*	OR	IC
Occurrence of TBactive	Pacientes 0.0071	TST+ 0.036	0033	0.19	0.03<1.01
Occurrence pulmonary TB	TBP 0.0082	TST+ 0.036	0.043	0.22	0.033<1.17
disease severity	TBP 0.0082	TBE 0.00	1.00	#	#
latent infection	TST+ 0.036	TST- 0.000	0.035	#	#

Table 6. Distribution of allele frequencies of -200T variant mutant groups according to the different outcomes.

Finally, the more prevalent *IFNG* polymorphisms (-599C>G and -200G>T) were tested against demographic variables, such as, gender and age. No significant association was found after stratified analysis at allele, genotype or haplotype levels (data not shown).

3.6. Association of the *TNF–α* SNPs and TB outcomes

Table 7 summarizes the distribution and comparison of genotype frequencies of each individual SNP among TB patients and TST+ controls. No significant difference was observed. The
evaluation of the possible association of different genotypes of *TNF-α* gene with susceptibility
to the occurrence of TBP or TBE was also carried out separately, however, no association was
found (data not shown).

Locus	Genotype	Patients (N=140)	Controls TST+ (N= 96)	*p-valor*	OR	IC
-646	GG	139	95			
	GA	1	1	1.00	0.68	0.02<25.33
-572	AA	138	95			
	CA	2	1	1.00	1.38	0.10<38.92
-422	CC	140	96			
	CT	0	0	-	-	-
-376	GG	127	93			
	GA	11	3	0.11	3.17	0.81<14.46
	AA	2	0			
-308	GG	118	83			
	GA	19	11	0.78	1.19	0.54<2.67
	AA	3	2			
-244	GG	136	92			
	GA	4	4	0.71	0.68	0.14<3.31
-238	GG	123	88			
	GA	15	8	0.47	1.50	0.58<3.97
	AA	2	0			

Table 7. Genotype distribution of the *TNF*-α SNPs among PTB patients and healthy controls (TST+).

Comparison of the *TNF-α* SNPs frequencies between TBP and TBEis shown in (Table 8). Only
the -572A>C (CA genotype) presented a significant difference between these groups, being
absent among the 121 TBP subjects, (RR = 8.12, CI = 5.20 <12.67 and *p*-value = 0.0175). The results
indicate a risk for disease severity. This association was confirmed upon allele frequency
evaluation (RR = 7.72, CI = 5.69 <10.47 and *p* = 0.0179) data not shown.

Locus	Genotype	PTB N=121	TBE N=19	p-value	RR	IC
-646	GG	120	19	1.00	0.00	0,00<115.2
	GA	1	0			
-572	AA	121	17	0.0175	8.12	5.20<12.67
	AC	0	2			
-422	CC	121	19	-	-	-
	CT	0	0			
-376	GG	111	17			
	GA	10	1	0.506	1.25	0.33<4.79
	AA	0	1			
-308	GG	101	17			
	GA	18	1	0.392	0.63	0.16<2.54
	AA	2	1			
-244	GG	117	19	0.554	#	#
	GA	4	0			
-238	GG	106	17			
	GA	14	1	0.585	0.85	0.22<3.37
	AA	1	1			

Table 8. Genotypes distribution of the *TNF-α* SNPs among TBP and TBE.

The association between the *TNF-α* genotypes with latent infection was also evaluated. No significant difference was found (data not shown).

The final evaluation of independent SNPs with the different TB outcomes was performed based in the allele frequencies comparison for the most common *TNF-α* SNPs (-376G>A, -308G>A, -244G>A and -238G>A). The SNP -376G>A, allele variant -376A, showed a significant association with susceptibility to the occurrence of active TB ($p = 0.035$, OR = 3.57, CI = 0.95 < 15.72) and severity ($p = 0.038$ and RR = 2.68) (Table 9). All other outcomes showed no significant association with any of the variants tested, (data not shown).

Different outcomes	Study Group		SNP TNF-α -376A		
			p-valor	OR	IC
Occurrence of activeTB	Patients (fa) 0.054	TST+ 0.016	0.035	3.57	0.95<15.72
Occurrence of PTB	PTB (fa) 0.041	TST+ 0.016	0.201	2.72	0,68<12.62
Severity of disease	PTB (fa) 0.041	TBE 0.052	0.038	2.68*	1.22<5.86
Latent infection	TST+ (fa) 0.016	TST- 0.017	0.90	0.623	0.12<7.86

Table 9. Distribution of allele frequency of the *TNF-α* -376A variant and association analysis with different outcomes studied.

Table 10 shows the distribution of the 14 identified haplotypes in the different groups used for the association study. No significant difference was observed in the haplotypes frequencies between groups (data not shown) and their distribution was quite homogeneous.

Haplotype	General TB n= 140	PTB n=121	EPTB n=19	Controls PPD+ n=96	Controls PPD- n=58
1	95[67.9%]	82[67.8%]	0	70[72.9%]	40[69%]
2	2[1.4%]	1[0.8%]	0	0	0
3	19[13.6%]	17[14.1%]	2[10.5%]	11[11.5%]	7[12.1%]
4	1[0.7%]	0	1[5.26%]	0	1[1.72%]
5	3[2.1%]	3[2.5%]	0	4[4.2%]	2[3.4%]
6	7[5 %]	6[5%]	1[5.3%]	5[5.2%]	5[8.6%]
7	1[0.7%]	1[0.8%]	0	1[1.1%]	1[1.7%]
9	9[6%]	8[6.6%]	1[5.3%]	3[3.1%]	2[3.4%]
11	1[0.7%]	1[0.8%]	0	1[1.1%]	0
12	1[0.7%]	1[0.8%]	0	0	0
13	1[0.7%]	1[0.8%]	0	0	0
14	1[0.71%]	0	1[5.26%]	1[1.04%]	0

Table 10. Frequency of *TNF-α* haplotypes in the different groups studied

After the genotyping of all samples and evaluation of the possible association with the different TB outcomes, the most frequent polymorphisms (-376G>A; -308G>A; -244G>A and -238G>A) were tested in a stratified analysis against the demographic variables gender and age. No significant differences were found for gender or age (data not shown).

4. Discussion

It is well known that to *M. tuberculosis*, ethiologic agent of human TB can cause a broad spectrum of effects ranging from no infection to different clinical disease phenotypes [2, 16, 23-25]. However, the reasons for individual or ethnic differences in acquiring infection, active disease, disease severity, and different clinical outcomes have not been completely clarified. It has long been realized that many human diseases arise from the complex interplay between environmental exposures and host genetics susceptibilities [26]. In addition, several genetic factors have also been associated with different outcomes: host susceptibility *per se* the occurrence of active TB, disease severity and / or protection for the occurrence of active disease [27-33].

The establishment of an efficient immune response involves many different molecules, among which, cytokines and their receptors play an extremely important role. Thus, any genetic alteration leading to changes in the regulation of gene expression may reflect this response. It is known that the interindividual variation in the production of these molecules is directly related to the genetic "background". Literature data have clearly demonstrated that genetic variability of the genes encoding these molecules can affect the regulation of gene expression positively or negatively influencing the final yield of the molecule in question. In the last decade, several single nucleotide polymorphisms (SNPs) in the regulatory region of different cytokine genes have been described and associated with susceptibility, severity or protection for a growing number of diseases of different etiologies including tuberculosis [7, 34-35].

Among the possible genetic variations associated with an increased risk of developing TB, there are several polymorphisms, mainly SNPs, in genes coding for cytokines, cytokine receptors and several other molecules such as vitamin D receptor, NRAMP1 (SLC11A1), HLA genes, etc.

The immune defense against *M. tuberculosis* is complex and involves the interaction between T CD4+, T CD8+ lymphocytes, macrophages, and monocytes along with the production of cytokines, such as interferon-γ (IFN-γ) and tumor necrosis factor-α (TNF-α) [36].

Convincing evidence indicating the importance of IFN-γ in particular, in the control of mycobacterial infections has been found in both experimental and clinical studies [37-38].

Among the mainly important cytokines involved in TB progress after infection with *M. tuberculosis*, TNF-α plays a key role. It is also a potent proinflammatory cytokine acting in protection against intracellular pathogens [39-40].

The genetic variability of *TNF-α* and *IFNG* has been described in the last decade [41-46] including association studies with tuberculosis. However, the frequencies of the polymorphisms already described varies according to the ethnicity of the population studied, hampering the better interpretation of the value of association studies. Unfortunately, most of these are performed in ethnically homogeneous populations, and therefore, many of the associations described for a particular allelic variant in a certain gene may not represent genetic risk factor in other populations. In Brazil, a country characterized by ethnically mixed population, there are few data regarding the frequency of single nucleotide polymorphisms in these genes (*IFNG,TNF-α*) and the few existing studies refers to one or two SNPs only. In view of the importance of the promoter region with respect to regulation of gene expression, the major goal of this work was to proceed a partial mapping of the promoter region of IFNG and *TNF-α* genes (approximately, 800bp upstream of the transcription starting site) through PCR-sequencing approach in samples from TB patients and healthy controls from Rio de Janeiro, Brazil. Subsequently, based on frequencies of the different SNPs found individually for each gene, we performed an association study with different TB outcomes.

4.1. Polymorphisms in the promoter region of IFNG and its association with TB

Characterization of the important portion within the *IFNG*was firstly identified two decades ago bydeletion analysisstudies [47-48]. According to authors, it comprises a highly conserved region from positions -117 to -47 and contains two sub regions that can be complexes with proteins. The sub-proximal region (-90 to -65) shows strong homology to the IL-2 promoter [49]. Several transcription factors activate transcription of IFNG by binding to this region. Conversely, several others inhibit factors binds in other regions affecting transcription. Hence, the interest in investigating the polymorphic sites within IFNG gene promoter, particularly considering the importance of this cytokine in eliciting the immune response.

Here, analysis of the generated sequences identified seven polymorphic sites, four of which were new. The transition C →T, was identified at position-787 from the transcription starting site in five subjects, all heterozygous. The second C → T transition, previously described in the data base of SNPs at position-785 was also found in five individuals, all heterozygous, however, no reference to this SNP was found in the literature. The other three SNPs not yet described, were C to G transition at position -599; C to T at position -517 and A to G at position -255. Finally, two additional SNPs, transition from G to T at position -200 and A to G at position -172, already described and well characterized [45] were found in our population.

One of the main problem found during this mapping was the confirmation of the identified SNPs based on literature data and from different SNPs data bases available online because of the lack of standardization regarding to the reference nucleotide to define the promoter region (transcription starting site nt +1). Many authors describe the SNPs identified in relation to the site of translation or use reference sequences containing sequencing errors leading to misclassification of SNPs (eg SNP-200G>T, originally described as -183 [45], later called as -179 [50] and finally, confirmed in this study as -200). The current name, confirmed in this study is based on the correction of the reference sequence used in previous studies and now available online. These types of errors greatly hampered the beginning of the sequence analysis regarding the identification of novel SNPs.

The frequency of each polymorphism was determined in the study population. As noted in Table 1, the allele frequencies for all the identified SNPs were less than one percent, except for the variants -599G and -200T, both in a frequency of 1.4%.

Functionally, it is known that polymorphisms (-200 and -172) can affect transcription of the IFNG. The region from -213 to -200 induces transcription factor through (AP-1) [51]. A polymorphism at this site (position -200, for example) must change the connection of AP-1 and the promoter activity in T cells. The polymorphism -172 is near to the nuclear factors-activated T-cells site (NFAT site) (-186TAAAGGAAA-178) and should affect the stability of this region [50].

The variant IFNG -200T is highly inducible by TNF-α and binds constitutively to nuclear extracts obtained from T cells, whereas the allele -200G does not respond to TNF-α [50; 52]. The induction of transcriptional activity, when the T allele is present, increases protection against tuberculosis. Our results corroborate these data, since the IFNG -200T variant showed to be associated with protection the occurrence of active TB in our study group (P = 0.033, OR= 0.18, CI= 0.03 to 1.00).

According Bream,JH et al., 2002 [50], the promoter region of IFNG is highly conserved, suggesting that these cytokine production variations are probably due to difference in binding to regulatory factors instead of polymorphisms in the gene, which is consistent with our results. Only seven SNPs were found in our population, five of which were at a low frequency. The polymorphisms found with a higher frequency were the -200G>T and -599C>G, the latter being located between two putative binding sites of transcription factors. As this is not yet a SNP described in the literature, functional studies are needed to better understand their functional role. The SNP -200 is of great interest for association studies. However, this polymorphism was not found in Caucasians or Indian populations, suggesting that different selective forces may be operating in different ethnic or racial groups. These data corroborate the evidence that IFN-γ is very important in the immune response and that mutations that interfere with their production may influence the outcome of active tuberculosis as shown by authors [28,31,53-54], and therefore, a selective force lead the gene to be so conserved.

4.2. Polymorphisms within the promoter region of *TNF–α* and their association with TB

TNF-α is a proinflammatory and immunoregulaty cytokine which plays a key role in the initiation, regulation and perpetuation of host defense against infections, but is fatal in excess. As this molecule plays an important role against a variety of pathogens involving different patterns of risks and benefits, it is expected that several genetic elements are involved in its control and production.

The levels of circulating TNF-α are regulated at transcriptional and post-transcriptional levels and several polymorphisms within the promoter region of TNF-α have been associated with altered circulating levels of this cytokine.

In humans, the *TNF-α* gene is located within the complex involving the human leukocyte antigens (HLA), a highly polymorphic region on chromosome 6p21.3 and hence, many of *TNF-α* polymorphisms are in linkage disequilibrium with the HLA genes. Because of differences in the distribution of HLA alleles we might expect variations in associations between polymorphisms of *TNF-α* and various conditions in different geographical areas.

The human genome analysis showed that the level of variations in the genome is approximately one SNP/1.71Kb [55]. However, the *TNF-α* promoter has higher density of SNPs. Despite this level of variation, the regions involved in gene regulation are highly conserved in humans [56-58].

In our work, we perform the mapping of the first 800pb promoter region, through direct sequencing of the amplified PCR product in 500 DNA samples from individuals living in the metropolitan area of Rio de Janeiro, Brazil and found seven polymorphisms previously described in the literature, most of which well characterized. However, according allele frequencies, only the variants -376A, -308A, -238A and -244A were present in more than one percent (0.030, 0.087, 0.011 and 0.050) respectively. The influence of these SNPs in binding of transcription factors have not been fully explored, most of the studies are focused on the association of one or two SNPs with different diseases. The SNPs -376, -308 and -238 have been the most studied but, the results of functional studies performed so far for SNPs -308 and -238 are controversial. It is believed that the variant -308A is associated with an increased transcription rate, leading to an increased production of TNF-α [59] and the variant-238A with a decreased rate of transcription. Regarding the SNP-376G>A different studies show that this polymorphism is located in a region of multiple interactions between proteins and DNA, and that the minor allele acts in the recruitment of proteins OCT1 for this region. According Knight et al (1999) [60] there is a significant interaction between variant -376A and the OCT-1 protein, this variant binds the proteins while the variant -376G does not. The authors report also by tests with the reporter gene system, that this mutant variant moderately increases the basal levels of TNF-α and associate the same with a relative risk of 4 to cerebral malaria. The problem is that the linkage disequilibrium is strong in this area and it is difficult to study the function of an isolated SNP. In some Caucasian populations -376A allele variant is liked to -308G and -238A [60-61], what is not observed in the African Gambia. Thus, association between the linked allelic variants on TNF-α production and diseases has been studied. According, Hajeer& Hutchinson (2001), the combined allele variants -238G, -308A and -376G are associated with high TNF-α levels [62].

A large number of studies have investigated the association between polymorphisms in the promoter region of the gene for TNF-α and tuberculosis. Results vary according to the different populations studied, finding no association [63-72] or a positive association [26, 29, 73-75]. In our analysis of the single SNP association, TB was associated with the -376G>A. In this case, we observed an association of the minor allele -376A with the outcome of susceptibility *per se* the occurrence of active TB (p= 0.035, OR 3.57, IC 0.95 <15.72) and an increased relative risk for the occurrence of extrapulmonary TB (p= 0.038, OR 2.68, IC 1.22 < 5.86). The association of this allele variant with the occurrence of TB and an increased relative risk for the development of extrapulmonary TB is intriguing. Given the influence of this allele with increased expression of TNF-α, one would expect an association with the protection. One possible explanation for this observation may be the small sample size in the stratified groups. The large confidence intervals (CI) for both outcomes could be a reflection of the small sample size.

The PCR-sequencing approach (gold standard) used for the mapping these genes practically discard the possibility of genotyping errors and all mutants found for all SNPs evaluated were confirmed twice by new PCR and resequencing. Another possibility would be due to the strong linkage disequilibrium observed in this region of the gene promoter of TNF-α. It is possible that other allelic variant (eg, 238A), as opposed to the functional role of variant -376A is canceling the same level of control of gene expression.

An important aspect of this study relates to the ethnic characteristics of the studied population. Brazilian population is characterized by mixture of ethnicities and the results obtained here contribute for a global understanding of the influence of genetic factors in TB outcomes. Usually, most of the studies on this field are made with ethnically homogeneous populations. A study conducted by Baena et al., 2002 [76] clearly shows the importance of ethnic difference in the association study of SNPs in *TNF-α* promoter with disease. According authors, the -857 SNP is a marker for Amerindians. In that study, SNPs in *TNF-α* promoter were also used to identify markers of ancestry, understanding that this region was well characterized previously with primates and humans. Several studies [77-81] have shown that some polymorphisms as -238; - 244 and -308 are in association with the HLA genes and in addition, the SNPs -308 [77]; -863 and -857 [81], are markers of Caucasians. The -238 SNP was found in three populations studied, although it has also been found in Caucasians [78] and Asian [80]. Instead, the -376 SNP was not detected in any of the non-African analyzed and were found with the -238.

These data demonstrate the importance of taking into account the "background" of the frequencies of SNPs of TNF-α in studies of gene-disease association.

Association studies of genetic factors with infectious diseases are difficult to conduct because of the multi factorial nature of these diseases that includes host, pathogen and environmental variables in different proportions for each disease. This multi factorial nature of TB stresses the importance to look for haplotypes in the association studies. The fact that our population is so mixed allowed us to find mutations that do not exist in other populations, such as the -308, for example, which is relatively rare in Asians and American Indians. Data from the genotyping of a large number of SNPs for different samples revealed that the human genome has a block structure haplotype [82-83] and configuration of a haplotype sometimes is more important than a single SNP genotype to determine phenotype [84]. Moreover, the construction of a haplotype block is useful for identifying SNPs that isolates would not influence the phenotype [85].

5. Conclusions

In conclusion, this study showed that the proximal part of the promoter region of *IFNG* is highly conserved, as seen in previous publications and the identified SNPs were in very low frequency. The -200T allele variant was associated with protection occurring active TB, and pulmonary TB. In addition, this variant was also associated with latent infection. Concerning *TNF-α*, the high genetic variability was confirmed, but only the -376G>A SNP showed an association with susceptibility *per se* to TB occurrence and increased risk for the occurrence of extrapulmonary TB.

The data presented here shows the reality of a population with characteristics of high ethnic miscegenation, provides the different SNPs identified enabling the realization of real sample calculation for any association studies that may be idealized with these targets and other conditions for this population and finally, provides haplotype that can be used in other studies of association with other diseases.

Acknowledgements

We thank all subjects involved in the study and the Platform-genome DNA sequencing RPT01A PDTIS/FIOCRUZ.

This work was supported by FAPERJ/Pronex:Proc: E-26/170.0003/2008 and FAPERJ Pensa Rio: E-26/110.288/2007.

Author details

Márcia Quinhones Pires Lopes[1*], Raquel Lima de Figueiredo Teixeira[1],
Antonio Basilio de Miranda[2], Rafael Santos Pinto[1], Lizânia Borges Spinassé[1],
Fernanda Carvalho Queiroz Mello[3], José Roberto Lapa e Silva[3], Philip Noel Suffys[1] and
Adalberto Rezende Santos[1]

*Address all correspondence to: mqlopes@yahoo.com.br

1 Laboratory of Molecular Biology Applied to Mycobacteria – Oswaldo Cruz Institute –
Fiocruz, Av. Brasil, Rio de Janeiro, RJ, Brazil

2 Laboratory of Computational and Systems Biology – Oswaldo Cruz Institute – Fiocruz,
Rio de Janeiro, Brazil

3 Medical School - Hospital Complex HUCFF-IDT - Federal University of Rio de Janeiro
(UFRJ), Rio de Janeiro, Brazil

References

[1] World Health Organization ((2010). Global tuberculosis control 2010Switzerland:
WHO Press.

[2] Horsburgh CR JrPriorities for the treatment of latent tuberculosis infection in the
United States. N. Engl. J. Med. (2004). , 350(20), 2060-7.

[3] Bellamy, R, Beyers, N, Mcadam, K. P, Ruwende, C, Gie, R, Samaai, P, et al. Genetic
susceptibility to tuberculosis in Africans: a genome-wide scan. Proc. Natl. Acad. Sci.
U.S.A. (2000). , 97(14), 8005-9.

[4] Frodsham, A. J. Hill AVS. Genetics of infectious diseases. Hum. Mol. Genet. (2004).
Spec R(2), 187-194.

[5] Ottenhoff THMVerreck FAW, Hoeve MA, van de Vosse E. Control of human host
immunity to mycobacteria. Tuberculosis (Edinb). (2005).

[6] Möller, M, De Wit, E, & Hoal, E. G. Past, present and future directions in human genetic susceptibility to tuberculosis. FEMS Immunol. Med. Microbiol. (2010). , 58(1),
3-26.

[7] Ottenhoff THMNew pathways of protective and pathological host defense to mycobacteria. Trends in microbiology [Internet]. (2012). jul 9 [2012 ago 30]; Available de:
http://www.ncbi.nlm.nih.gov/pubmed/22784857

[8]   Miller, E. N, Jamieson, S. E, Joberty, C, Fakiola, M, Hudson, D, Peacock, C. S, et al. Genome-wide scans for leprosy and tuberculosis susceptibility genes in Brazilians. Genes Immun. (2004)., 5(1), 63-7.

[9]   Malik, S, & Schurr, E. Genetic susceptibility to tuberculosis. Clin. Chem. Lab. Med. (2002)., 40(9), 863-8.

[10] Kaplan, G, Post, F. A, Moreira, A. L, Wainwright, H, Kreiswirth, B. N, Tanverdi, M, et al. Mycobacterium tuberculosis growth at the cavity surface: a microenvironment with failed immunity. Infect. Immun. (2003)., 71(12), 7099-108.

[11] Ottenhoff THMVerreck FAW, Lichtenauer-Kaligis EGR, Hoeve MA, Sanal O, van Dissel JT. Genetics, cytokines and human infectious disease: lessons from weakly pathogenic mycobacteria and salmonellae. Nat. Genet. (2002)., 32(1), 97-105.

[12] van de Vosse EHoeve MA, Ottenhoff THM. Human genetics of intracellular infectious diseases: molecular and cellular immunity against mycobacteria and salmonellae. Lancet Infect Dis. (2004)., 4(12), 739-49.

[13] Zganiacz, A, Santosuosso, M, Wang, J, Yang, T, Chen, L, Anzulovic, M, et al. TNF-alpha is a critical negative regulator of type 1 immune activation during intracellular bacterial infection. J. Clin. Invest. (2004)., 113(3), 401-13.

[14] Keane, J, Gershon, S, Wise, R. P, Mirabile-levens, E, Kasznica, J, Schwieterman, W. D, et al. Tuberculosis associated with infliximab, a tumor necrosis factor alpha-neutralizing agent. N. Engl. J. Med. (2001)., 345(15), 1098-104.

[15] Oppenheim, J. J. Cytokines: past, present, and future. Int. J. Hematol. (2001)., 74(1), 3-8.

[16] Jurado, J. O, Pasquinelli, V, Alvarez, I. B, Peña, D, Rovetta, A. I, Tateosian, N. L, et al. IL-17 and IFN-γ expression in lymphocytes from patients with active tuberculosis correlates with the severity of the disease. J. Leukoc. Biol. (2012)., 91(6), 991-1002.

[17] Zhang, M, Lin, Y, Iyer, D. V, Gong, J, & Abrams, J. S. Barnes PF. T-cell cytokine responses in human infection with Mycobacterium tuberculosis. Infect. Immun. (1995)., 63(8), 3231-4.

[18] Selvaraj, P, & Sriram, U. MathanKurian S, Reetha AM, Narayanan PR. Tumour necrosis factor alpha (-238 and-308) and beta gene polymorphisms in pulmonary tuberculosis: haplotype analysis with HLA-A, B and DR genes. Tuberculosis (Edinb) (2001).

[19] Möller, M, & Hoal, E. G. Current findings, challenges and novel approaches in human genetic susceptibility to tuberculosis. Tuberculosis (Edinb). (2010)., 90(2), 71-83.

[20] Primer 3 software http://frodowi.mit.edu/ (accessed 30 August (2012).

[21] Stephens, M, Smith, N. J, & Donnelly, P. A new statistical method for haplotype re-
      construction from population data. American Journal of Human Genetics (2001). ,
      68-978.

[22] Stephens, M, & Donnelly, P. A comparison of Bayesian methods for haplotype recon-
      struction. American Journal of Human Genetics (2003). , 73-1162.

[23] Stead, W. W. Variation in vulnerability to tuberculosis in America today: random, or
      legacies of different ancestral epidemics? Int. J. Tuberc. Lung Dis. (2001). set;, 5(9),
      807-14.

[24] Hoal, E. G. Human genetic susceptibility to tuberculosis and other mycobacterial dis-
      eases. IUBMB Life. (2002). maio;53(4-5):225-9.

[25] [25]Lillebaek, T, Dirksen, A, Baess, I, Strunge, B, Thomsen, V. Ø, & Andersen, A. B.
      Molecular evidence of endogenous reactivation of Mycobacterium tuberculosis after
      33 years of latent infection. J. Infect. Dis. (2002). fev 1;, 185(3), 401-4.

[26] [26]Mcguire, W, Knight, J. C, Hill, A. V, Allsopp, C. E, Greenwood, B. M, & Kwiat-
      kowski, D. Severe malarial anemia and cerebral malaria are associated with different
      tumor necrosis factor promoter alleles. J. Infect. Dis. (1999). jan;, 179(1), 287-90.

[27] [27]Awomoyi, A. A, & Marchant, A. Howson JMM, McAdam KPWJ, Blackwell JM,
      Newport MJ. Interleukin-10, polymorphism in SLC11A1 (formerly NRAMP1), and
      susceptibility to tuberculosis. J. Infect. Dis. (2002). dez 15;, 186(12), 1808-14.

[28] [28]Tso, H. W, Ip, W. K, Chong, W. P, & Tam, C. M. Chiang AKS, Lau YL. Associa-
      tion of interferon gamma and interleukin 10 genes with tuberculosis in Hong Kong
      Chinese. Genes Immun. (2005). jun;, 6(4), 358-63.

[29] [29]Correa, P. A, Gomez, L. M, Cadena, J, & Anaya, J-M. Autoimmunity and tubercu-
      losis. Opposite association with TNF polymorphism. J. Rheumatol. (2005). fev;, 32(2),
      219-24.

[30] [30]Henao, M. I, Montes, C, París, S. C, & García, L. F. Cytokine gene polymorphisms
      in Colombian patients with different clinical presentations of tuberculosis. Tubercu-
      losis (Edinb). (2006). jan;, 86(1), 11-9.

[31] [31]Amim LHLVPacheco AG, Fonseca-Costa J, Loredo CS, Rabahi MF, Melo MH, et
      al. Role of IFN-gamma +874 T/A single nucleotide polymorphism in the tuberculosis
      outcome among Brazilians subjects. Mol. Biol. Rep. (2008). dez;, 35(4), 563-6.

[32] Fan, H-M, Wang, Z, Feng, F-M, Zhang, K-L, Yuan, J-X, Sui, H, et al. Association of
      TNF-alpha-238G/A and 308 G/A gene polymorphisms with pulmonary tuberculosis
      among patients with coal worker's pneumoconiosis. Biomed. Environ. Sci. (2010).
      abr;, 23(2), 137-45.

[33] Anoosheh, S, Farnia, P, & Kargar, M. Association between TNF-Alpha (-857) Gene Polymorphism and Susceptibility to Tuberculosis. Iran Red Crescent Med J. (2011). abr;, 13(4), 243-8.

[34] Casanova, J-L, & Abel, L. Genetic dissection of immunity to mycobacteria: the human model. Annu. Rev. Immunol. (2002). , 20, 581-620.

[35] Möller, M, Flachsbart, F, Till, A, Thye, T, Horstmann, R. D, Meyer, C. G, et al. A functional haplotype in the 3'untranslated region of TNFRSF1B is associated with tuberculosis in two African populations. Am. J. Respir. Crit. Care Med. (2010). fev 15;, 181(4), 388-93.

[36] [36]Barreiro, L. B, & Quintana-murci, L. From evolutionary genetics to human immunology: how selection shapes host defence genes. Nat. Rev. Genet. (2010). jan;, 11(1), 17-30.

[37] [37]Doherty, T. M, Demissie, A, Olobo, J, Wolday, D, Britton, S, Eguale, T, et al. Immune responses to the Mycobacterium tuberculosis-specific antigen ESAT-6 signal subclinical infection among contacts of tuberculosis patients. J. Clin. Microbiol. (2002). fev;, 40(2), 704-6.

[38] [38]Winek, J, Rowinska-zakrzewska, E, Demkow, U, Szopinski, J, Szolkowska, M, Filewska, M, et al. Interferon gamma production in the course of Mycobacterium tuberculosis infection. J. Physiol. Pharmacol. (2008). dez;59Suppl , 6, 751-9.

[39] [39]Knight, J. Polymorphisms in Tumor Necrosis Factor and Other Cytokines As Risks for Infectious Diseases and the Septic Syndrome. Curr Infect Dis Rep. (2001). out;, 3(5), 427-39.

[40] [40]Mohan, V. P, Scanga, C. A, Yu, K, Scott, H. M, Tanaka, K. E, Tsang, E, et al. Effects of tumor necrosis factor alpha on host immune response in chronic persistent tuberculosis: possible role for limiting pathology. Infect. Immun. (2001). mar;, 69(3), 1847-55.

[41] [41]Alfonso, D, & Richiardi, S. PM. An intragenic polymorphism in the human tumor necrosis factor alpha (TNFA) chain-encoding gene. Immunogenetics. (1996). , 44(4), 321-2.

[42] [42]Mira, J. P, Cariou, A, Grall, F, Delclaux, C, Losser, M. R, Heshmati, F, et al. Association of TNF2, a TNF-alpha promoter polymorphism, with septic shock susceptibility and mortality: a multicenter study. JAMA. (1999). ago 11;, 282(6), 561-8.

[43] Giedraitis, V, He, B, & Hillert, J. Mutation screening of the interferon-gamma gene as a candidate gene for multiple sclerosis. Eur. J. Immunogenet. (1999). ago;, 26(4), 257-9.

[44] [44]Bream, J. H, Carrington, M, Toole, O, Dean, S, Gerrard, M, & Shin, B. HD, et al. Polymorphisms of the human IFNG gene noncoding regions. Immunogenetics. (2000). jan;, 51(1), 50-8.

[45] [45]Chevillard, C, Henri, S, Stefani, F, Parzy, D, & Dessein, A. Two new polymorphisms in the human interferon gamma (IFN-gamma) promoter. Eur. J. Immunogenet. (2002). fev;, 29(1), 53-6.

[46] [46]Arora, R, Saha, A, Malhotra, D, Rath, P, Kar, P, & Bamezai, R. Promoter and in-
tron-1 region polymorphisms in the IFNG gene in patients with hepatitis E. Int. J. Immunogenet. (2005). jun;, 32(3), 207-12.

[47] [47]Chrivia, J. C, Wedrychowicz, T, Young, H. A, & Hardy, K. J. A model of human
cytokine regulation based on transfection of gamma interferon gene fragments directly into isolated peripheral blood T lymphocytes. J. Exp. Med. (1990). ago 1;,
172(2), 661-4.

[48] Penix, L, Weaver, W. M, Pang, Y, Young, H. A, & Wilson, C. B. Two essential regulatory elements in the human interferon gamma promoter confer activation specific expression in T cells. J. Exp. Med. (1993). nov 1;, 178(5), 1483-96.

[49] Penix, L. A, Sweetser, M. T, Weaver, W. M, Hoeffler, J. P, Kerppola, T. K, & Wilson,
C. B. The proximal regulatory element of the interferon-gamma promoter mediates
selective expression in T cells. J. Biol. Chem. (1996). dez 13;, 271(50), 31964-72.

[50] [50]Bream, J. H, Carrington, M, Toole, O, Dean, S, Gerrard, M, & Shin, B. HD, et al.
Polymorphisms of the human IFNG gene noncoding regions. Immunogenetics.
(2000). jan;, 51(1), 50-8.

[51] Barbulescu, K. Meyer zumBüschenfelde KH, Neurath MF. Constitutive and inducible
protein/DNA interactions of the interferon-gamma promoter in vivo in [corrected]
CD45RA and CD45R0 T helper subsets. Eur. J. Immunol. (1997). maio;, 27(5),
1098-107.

[52] [52]An, P, Vlahov, D, Margolick, J. B, Phair, J, Brien, O, & Lautenberger, T. R. J, et al.
A tumor necrosis factor-alpha-inducible promoter variant of interferon-gamma accelerates CD4+ T cell depletion in human immunodeficiency virus-1-infected individuals. J. Infect. Dis. (2003). jul 15;, 188(2), 228-31.

[53] Vallinoto ACRGraça ES, Araújo MS, Azevedo VN, Cayres-Vallinoto I, Machado LFA,
et al. IFNG +874T/A polymorphism and cytokine plasma levels are associated with
susceptibility to Mycobacterium tuberculosis infection and clinical manifestation of
tuberculosis. Hum. Immunol. (2010). jul;, 71(7), 692-6.

[54] [54]Rossouw, M, Nel, H. J, Cooke, G. S, Van Helden, P. D, & Hoal, E. G. Association
between tuberculosis and a polymorphic NFkappaB binding site in the interferon
gamma gene. Lancet. (2003). maio 31;, 361(9372), 1871-2.

[55] [55]Cargill, M, Altshuler, D, Ireland, J, Sklar, P, Ardlie, K, Patil, N, et al. Characterization of single-nucleotide polymorphisms in coding regions of human genes. Nat.
Genet. (1999). jul;, 22(3), 231-8.

[56] Falvo, J. V, Uglialoro, A. M, Brinkman, B. M, Merika, M, Parekh, B. S, Tsai, E. Y, et al. Stimulus-specific assembly of enhancer complexes on the tumor necrosis factor alpha gene promoter. Mol. Cell. Biol. (2000). mar;, 20(6), 2239-47.

[57] Tsai, E. Y, Falvo, J. V, Tsytsykova, A. V, Barczak, A. K, Reimold, A. M, Glimcher, L. H, et al. A lipopolysaccharide-specific enhancer complex involving Ets, Elk-1, Sp1, and CREB binding protein and is recruited to the tumor necrosis factor alpha promoter in vivo. Mol. Cell. Biol. (2000). ago;20(16):6084-94., 300.

[58] Tsytsykova, A. V, & Goldfeld, A. E. Inducer-specific enhanceosome formation controls tumor necrosis factor alpha gene expression in T lymphocytes. Mol. Cell. Biol. (2002). abr;, 22(8), 2620-31.

[59] [59]Wilson, A. G, Symons, J. A, Mcdowell, T. L, Mcdevitt, H. O, & Duff, G. W. Effects of a polymorphism in the human tumor necrosis factor alpha promoter on transcriptional activation. Proc. Natl. Acad. Sci. U.S.A. (1997). abr 1;, 94(7), 3195-9.

[60] Knight, J. C, Udalova, I, Hill, A. V, Greenwood, B. M, Peshu, N, Marsh, K, et al. A polymorphism that affects OCT-1 binding to the TNF promoter region is associated with severe malaria. Nat. Genet. (1999). jun;, 22(2), 145-50.

[61] [61]Bayley, J-P. Ottenhoff THM, Verweij CL. Is there a future for TNF promoter polymorphisms? Genes Immun. (2004). ago;, 5(5), 315-29.

[62] Hajeer, A. H, & Hutchinson, I. V. Influence of TNFalpha gene polymorphisms on TNFalpha production and disease. Hum. Immunol. (2001). nov;, 62(11), 1191-9.

[63] [63]Delgado, J. C, Baena, A, Thim, S, & Goldfeld, A. E. Ethnic-specific genetic associations with pulmonary tuberculosis. J. Infect. Dis. (2002). nov 15;, 186(10), 1463-8.

[64] [64]Henao, M. I, Montes, C, París, S. C, & García, L. F. Cytokine gene polymorphisms in Colombian patients with different clinical presentations of tuberculosis. Tuberculosis (Edinb). (2006). jan;, 86(1), 11-9.

[65] [65]Vejbaesya, S, Chierakul, N, Luangtrakool, P, & Sermduangprateep, C. NRAMP1 and TNF-alpha polymorphisms and susceptibility to tuberculosis in Thais. Respirology. (2007). mar;, 12(2), 202-6.

[66] Oh, J-H, Yang, C-S, Noh, Y-K, Kweon, Y-M, Jung, S-S, Son, J. W, et al. Polymorphisms of interleukin-10 and tumour necrosis factor-alpha genes are associated with newly diagnosed and recurrent pulmonary tuberculosis. Respirology. (2007). jul;, 12(4), 594-8.

[67] Kumar, V, Khosla, R, Gupta, V, Sarin, B. C, & Sehajpal, P. K. Differential association of tumour necrosis factor-alpha single nucleotide polymorphism (-308) with tuberculosis and bronchial asthma. Natl Med J India. (2008). jun;, 21(3), 120-2.

[68] Larcombe, L. A, Orr, P. H, Lodge, A. M, Brown, J. S, Dembinski, I. J, Milligan, L. C, et al. Functional gene polymorphisms in canadian aboriginal populations with high rates of tuberculosis. J. Infect. Dis. (2008). out 15;Wu et al., 2008, 198(8), 1175-9.

[69] Wu, F, Qu, Y, Tang, Y, Cao, D, Sun, P, & Xia, Z. Lack of association between cytokine gene polymorphisms and silicosis and pulmonary tuberculosis in Chinese iron miners. J Occup Health. (2008). , 50(6), 445-54.

[70] Ates, O, Musellim, B, Ongen, G, & Topal-sarikaya, A. Interleukin-10 and tumor necrosis factor-alpha gene polymorphisms in tuberculosis. J. Clin. Immunol. (2008). maio;, 28(3), 232-6.

[71] Sharma, S, Rathored, J, Ghosh, B, & Sharma, S. K. Genetic polymorphisms in TNF genes and tuberculosis in North Indians. BMC Infect. Dis. (2010).

[72] Ben-selma, W, Harizi, H, & Boukadida, J. Association of TNF-α and IL-10 polymorphisms with tuberculosis in Tunisian populations. Microbes Infect. (2011). set;Oliveira MM, Silva JCS, Costa JF, Amim LHet al. Single Nucleotide polymorphisms (SNPs) of the TNF-a (-238/-308) gene among TB occurrence. Journal Brasileiro de Pneumologia 2004; 30:461-67., 13(10), 837-43.

[73] Correa, P. A, Gomez, L. M, Cadena, J, & Anaya, J-M. Autoimmunity and tuberculosis. Opposite association with TNF polymorphism. J. Rheumatol. (2005). fev;, 32(2), 219-24.

[74] Correa, P. A, Gómez, L. M, & Anaya, J. M. Polymorphism of TNF-alpha in autoimmunity and tuberculosis]. Biomedica. (2004). jun;24Supp , 1, 43-51.

[75] Amirzargar, A. A, Rezaei, N, Jabbari, H, Danesh, A-A, Khosravi, F, Hajabdolbaghi, M, et al. Cytokine single nucleotide polymorphisms in Iranian patients with pulmonary tuberculosis. Eur. Cytokine Netw. (2006). jun;Baena et al., 2002, 17(2), 84-9.

[76] Baena, A, Leung, J. Y, Sullivan, A. D, Landires, I, Vasquez-luna, N, Quiñones-berrocal, J, et al. TNF-alpha promoter single nucleotide polymorphisms are markers of human ancestry. Genes Immun. (2002). dez;, 3(8), 482-7.

[77] Wilson, A. G, De Vries, N, & Pociot, F. di Giovine FS, van der Putte LB, Duff GW. An allelic polymorphism within the human tumor necrosis factor alpha promoter region is strongly associated with HLA A1, B8, and DR3 alleles. J. Exp. Med. (1993). fev 1;, 177(2), 557-60.

[78] [78]Alfonso, D, & Richiardi, S. PM. A polymorphic variation in a putative regulation box of the TNFA promoter region. Immunogenetics. (1994). , 39(2), 150-4.

[79] [79]Zimmerman, M. R. Pulmonary and osseous tuberculosis in an Egyptian mummy. Bull N Y Acad Med. (1979). jun;, 55(6), 604-8.

[80] [80]Higuchi, T, Seki, N, Kamizono, S, Yamada, A, Kimura, A, Kato, H, et al. Polymorphism of the 5'-flanking region of the human tumor necrosis factor (TNF)-alpha gene in Japanese. Tissue Antigens. (1998). jun;Ugliaro et al., 1998, 51(6), 605-12.

[81] Uglialoro, A. M, Turbay, D, Pesavento, P. A, Delgado, J. C, Mckenzie, F. E, Gribben, J. G, et al. Identification of three new single nucleotide polymorphisms in the human tumor necrosis factor-alpha gene promoter. Tissue Antigens. (1998). out;, 52(4), 359-67.

[82] [82]Collins, A, Lonjou, C, & Morton, N. E. Genetic epidemiology of single-nucleotide polymorphisms. Proc. Natl. Acad. Sci. U.S.A. (1999). dez 21;, 96(26), 15173-7.

[83] [83]Kruglyak, L. Prospects for whole-genome linkage disequilibrium mapping of common disease genes. Nat. Genet. (1999). jun;, 22(2), 139-44.

[84]] Hugot, J. P, Chamaillard, M, Zouali, H, Lesage, S, Cézard, J. P, Belaiche, J, et al. Association of NOD2 leucine-rich repeat variants with susceptibility to Crohn's disease. Nature. (2001). maio 31;, 411(6837), 599-603.

[85] Kamatani, N, Sekine, A, Kitamoto, T, Iida, A, Saito, S, Kogame, A, et al. Large-scale single-nucleotide polymorphism (SNP) and haplotype analyses, using dense SNP Maps, of 199 drug-related genes in 752 subjects: the analysis of the association between uncommon SNPs within haplotype blocks and the haplotypes constructed with haplotype-tagging SNPs. Am. J. Hum. Genet. (2004). ago;, 75(2), 190-203.

Diagnosis and Management of Tuberculosis

Chapter 8

First– and Second–Line Drugs and Drug Resistance

Hum Nath Jnawali and Sungweon Ryoo

Additional information is available at the end of the chapter

1. Introduction

Tuberculosis (TB) is caused by infection with *Mycobacterium tuberculosis*, which is transmitted through inhalation of aerosolized droplets. TB mainly attacks the lungs, but can also affect other parts of the body. TB is highly contagious during the active stage of the disease and can infect an individual through inhalation of as few as 10 *Mycobacterium tuberculosis* (MTB) bacteria. After inhalation, these bacteria are mainly captured by the alveolar macrophages, but they can evade the host immune system and remain in the dormant stage for a long period of time, at which point they can reactivate to a virulent form under immune-compromised conditions of the host. This is possible because *M. tuberculosis* can persist in slow growing as well as in fast growing stages which makes treatment challenging. Almost all of the antibiotics that can be used to treat TB work when the bacteria are actively dividing. In the intensive phase of TB treatment, the antibiotics mainly kill rapidly growing bacteria, which causes rapid sputum conversion, and the eradication of clinical symptoms. However, in order to kill the persistent or slow growing strains of MTB, the continuation phase of the treatment is essential. TB can be treated effectively by using first line drugs (FLD) isoniazid (INH), rifampin (RIF), pyrazinamide (PZA), ethambutol (EMB) and streptomycin (SM). However, this first line therapy often fails to cure TB for several reasons. Relapse and the spread of the disease contribute to the emergence of drug resistant bacteria. The emergence of multidrug resistant TB (MDR-TB), i.e. which is resistant to at least isoniazid (INH) and rifampicin (RIF), is of great concern, because it requires the use of second-line drugs that are difficult to procure and are much more toxic and expensive than FLDs [1]. Therefore, the detection and treatment of drug susceptible or single drug resistant TB is an important strategy for preventing the emergence of MDR-TB [2]. *M. tuberculosis* strains with extensively drug resistant-TB (XDR-TB), that is resistant to either isoniazid or rifampicin (like MDR tuberculosis), any fluoroquinolone, and at least one of three second-line antituberculosis injectable drugs—*i.e.*, capreomycin, kanamycin, and amikacin have also been reported [3].

First- and second-line drugs, minimum inhibitory concentrations (MICs) and mechanisms of drug resistance are presented in Table 1 [4]. Antituberculosis drugs are mainly divided into two parts.

1. First-line antituberculosis drugs- Isoniazid (INH), rifampicin (RIF), ethambutol (EMB), pyrazinamide (PZA) and streptomycin (SM).

2. Second-line antituberculosis drugs- Sub divided into two

    i.   Fluoroquinolones- Ofloxacin (OFX), levofloxacin (LEV), moxifloxacin (MOX) and ciprofloxacin (CIP).

    ii. Injectable antituberculosis drugs- Kanamycin (KAN), amikacin (AMK) and capreomycin (CAP).

    iii. Less-effective second-line antituberculosis drugs- Ethionamide (ETH)/Prothionamide (PTH), Cycloserine (CS)/Terizidone, P-aminosalicylic acid (PAS).

Drug	MIC (mg/L)	Gene	Role of gene product
Isoniazid	0.02–0.2 (7H9/7H10)	katG	catalase/peroxidase
		inhA	enoyl reductase
		ahpC	alkyl hydroperoxide reductase
Rifampicin	0.05–0.1 (7H9/7H10)	rpoB	β-subunit of RNA polymerase
Pyrazinimide	16–50 (LJ)	pncA	PZase
Streptomycin	2–8 (7H9/7H10)	rpsL	S12 ribosomal protein
		rrs	16S rRNA
		gidB	7-methylguanosine methyltransferase
Ethambutol	1–5 (7H9/7H10)	embB	arabinosyl transferase
Fluoroquinolones	0.5–2.0 (7H9/7H10)	gyrA/gyrB	DNA gyrase
Kanamycin	2–4 (7H9/7H10)	rrs	16S rRNA
		eis	aminoglycoside acetyltransferase
Amikacin	2–4 (7H9/7H10)	rrs	16S rRNA
Capreomycin	2-4 (7H9/7H10)	rrs	16S rRNA
		tylA	rRNA methyltransferase
Ethionamide	2.5–10 (7H11)	inhA	enoyl reductase
p-aminosalicylic acid	0.5 (LJ)	thyA	thymidylate synthase A

Table 1. First- and second-line drugs, MICs and mechanisms of drug resistance

2. First-line antituberculosis drugs

2.1. Isoniazid

Isoniazid (INH) is one of the most effective and specific antituberculosis drugs, which has been a key to treatment since its introduction in 1952 [5]. *M. tuberculosis* is highly susceptible to INH (MIC 0.02–0.2 μg/ml). INH is only active against growing tubercle bacilli, and is not active against non-replicating bacilli or under anaerobic conditions. INH enters the mycobacterial cell by passive diffusion [6]. The most significant adverse reactions associated with isoniazid administration are hepatotoxicity and neurotoxicity.

Resistance to isoniazid is a complex process. Mutations in several genes, including *katG*, *ahpC*, and *inhA*, have all been associated with isoniazid resistance. INH is a prodrug that is activated by the mycobacterial enzyme KatG [7]. INH-resistant clinical isolates of *M. tuberculosis* often lose catalase and peroxidase enzyme encoded by *katG* [8], especially in high-level resistant strains (MIC > 5 μg/ml) [9]. Low-level resistant strains (MIC < 1 μg/ml) often still possess catalase activity [9]. Although mutations in *katG* have been shown to be responsible for INH resistance [10], it is not clear whether the regulation of *katG* expression plays a role in INH resistance. The *katG* gene encodes a bifunctional catalase-peroxidase that converts INH to its active form [7]. Activated INH inhibits the synthesis of essential mycolic acids by inactivating the NADH-dependent enoyl-acyl carrier protein reductase encoded by *inhA* [11].

A study by Hazbo´n et al. [12] analysed 240 alleles and found that mutations in *katG*, *inhA* and *ahpC* were most strongly associated with isoniazid resistance. A decrease in or total loss of catalase/peroxidase activity as a result of *katG* mutations are the most common genetic alterations associated with isoniazid resistance [7]. Ser315Thr is the most widespread *katG* mutation in clinical isolates, but there are many mutations that result in inactivation of catalase-peroxidase, with MICs ranging from 0.2 to 256 mg/L.

Mutations in *inhA* or its promoter region are usually associated with low-level resistance (MICs = 0.2 −1 μg/ml) and are less frequent than *katG* mutations [10, 12]. INH-resistant *M. tuberculosis* harboring *inhA* mutations could have additional mutations in *katG*, conferring higher levels of INH resistance [13]. The most common *inhA* mutation occurs in its promoter region (-15C → T) and it has been found more frequently associated with mono-resistant strains [14].

In *M. tuberculosis*, *ahpC* codes for an alkyl hydroperoxidase reductase that is implicated in resistance to reactive oxygen and reactive nitrogen intermediates. It was initially proposed that mutations in the promoter of *ahpC* could be used as surrogate markers for the detection of isoniazid resistance [15]. However, several other studies have found that an increase in the expression of *ahpC* seems to be more a compensatory mutation for the loss of catalase/peroxidase activity rather than the basis for isoniazid resistance [4, 16].

2.2. Rifampicin

Rifampicin (RIF) was introduced in 1972 as an antituberculosis drug and has excellent sterilizing activity. Rifampicin acts by binding to the β-subunit of RNA polymerase (*rpoB*) [17], the enzyme responsible for transcription and expression of mycobacterial genes, resulting in inhibition of the bacterial transcription activity and thereby killing the organism. An important characteristic of rifampicin is that it is active against actively growing and slowly metabolizing (non-growing) bacilli [18]. RIF produces relatively few adverse reactions. It may cause gastro-intestinal upset. Hepatotoxicity occurs less frequently than with isoniazid administration.

Rifampicin MICs ranging from 0.05 to 1 μg/ml on solid or liquid media, but the MIC is higher in egg media (MIC = 2.5–10 μg/ml). Strains with MICs < 1 μg/ml in liquid or agar medium or MICs < 40 μg/ml in Lowenstein-Jensen (LJ) medium are considered RIF-susceptible. The great majority of *M. tuberculosis* clinical isolates resistant to rifampicin show mutations in the gene *rpoB* that encodes the β-subunit of RNA polymerase. This results in conformational changes that determine a low affinity for the drug and consequently the development of resistance [19]. Mutations in a 'hot-spot' region of 81 bp of *rpoB* have been found in about 96% of rifampicin-resistant *M. tuberculosis* isolates. This region, spanning codons 507–533 (numbering according to the *Escherichia coli rpoB* sequence), is also known as the rifampicin resistance-determining region (RRDR) [17]. Mutations in codons 531, 526 and 516 (Ser531Leu, His526Tyr, and Asp516Val) are the most frequently reported mutations in most of the studies [20, 21]. Some studies have also reported mutations outside of the hot-spot region of *rpoB* in rifampicin-resistant *M. tuberculosis* isolates [22].

2.3. Pyrazinamide

Pyrazinamide (PZA) is an important first-line antituberculosis (anti-TB) drug that is used in short-course chemotherapy and is one of the cornerstone drugs in the treatment of MDR-TB [23]. One key characteristic of pyrazinamide is its ability to inhibit semidormant bacilli residing in acidic environments [23]. Pyrazinamide is a structural analogue of nicotinamide and is a pro-drug that needs to be converted into its active form, pyrazinoic acid, by the enzyme pyrazinamidase/nicotinamidase (PZase) [24]. PZA is only active against *M. tuberculosis* at acid pH (e.g., 5.5) [25]. Even at acid pH (5.5), PZA activity is quite poor, with MICs in the range of 6.25–50 μg/ml [26]. Hypersensitivity reactions and gastrointestinal upset may occur with PZA administration.

PZase is encoded in *M. tuberculosis* by the gene *pncA* [27]. Mutations in the *pncA* gene may cause a reduction in PZase activity which may be the major mechanism of PZA resistance in MTB [28, 29]. The mutations of the *pncA* gene in PZA-resistant MTB isolates has been well characterized, however the correlation varies between different geographical areas including missense mutations, one or more base insertions or deletions, and complete deletion [28-32]. Despite the highly diverse and scattered distribution of *pncA* mutations, there is some degree of clustering of mutations within different regions of the *pncA* gene such as at amino acid residues 3–17, 61–85 and 132–142 has been reported [33, 34]. The highly diverse mutation profile in the *pncA* gene observed in PZA-resistant strains is unique among drug-resistance genes in *M. tuberculosis* [28]. While the reason behind this diversity is still unclear, it is thought that this could be due to adaptive mutagenesis or due to deficiency in DNA mismatch repair mechanisms [23]. Most PZA-resistant *M. tuberculosis* strains (72–97%) have mutations in *pncA*; [28, 29, 34, 35] however; some resistant strains do not have *pncA* mutations.

2.4. Ethambutol

Ethambutol (EMB) [dextro-2,2'-(ethylenediimino)di-1-butanol], which is an essential first-line drug in tuberculosis treatment, plays an important role in the chemotherapy of drug-resistant TB [36]. EMB is also an important antimycobacterial drug as it enhances the effect of other companion drugs including aminoglycosides, rifamycins and quinolones. The most common side effects observed with ethambutol are dizziness, blurred vision, color blindness, nausea, vomiting, stomach pain, loss of appetite, headache, rash, itching, breathlessness, swelling of the face, lips or eyes, numbness or tingling in the fingers or toes. Patients taking ethambutol should have their visual acuity and color vision checked at least monthly.

The MICs of EMB for *M. tuberculosis* are in the range of 0.5–2 µg/ml. EMB is a bacteriostatic agent that is active for growing bacilli and has no effect on non-replicating bacilli. EMB interferes with the biosynthesis of cell wall arabinogalactan [37]. It inhibits the polymerization of cell-wall arabinan of arabinogalactan and of lipoarabinomannan, and induces the accumulation of D-arabinofuranosyl-P-decaprenol, an intermediate in arabinan biosynthesis [38, 39].

Arabinosyl transferase, encoded *by embB*, an enzyme involved in the synthesis of arabinogalactan, has been proposed as the target of EMB in *M. tuberculosis* [40] and *M. avium* [41]. In *M. tuberculosis*, *embB* is organized into an operon with *embC* and *embA* in the order *embCAB. embC*, *embB* and *embA* share over 65% amino acid identity with each other and are predicted to encode transmembrane proteins [40]. Mutations in the *embCAB* operon, in particular *embB*, and occasionally *embC*, are responsible for resistance to EMB [40]. Point mutations of the *embABC* gene commonly occurred in *embB* codon 306 [40, 42, 43], and mutations in the *embB306* codon have been proposed as a marker for EMB resistance in diagnostic tests [44]. However, point mutations in the *embB306* locus occur in only 50 to 60% of all EMB-resistant clinical isolates [42, 45-47], and *embB306* mutations can also occur in EMB-susceptible clinical isolates [46, 47]. Five different mutations were uncovered in this codon (ATG→ GTG/CTG/ATA, ATC and ATT), resulting in three different amino acid shifts (Met→ Val, Leu, or Ile) [43]. Although the association between *embB306* mutation and ethambutol resistance or broad drug resistance has been observed in several groups' studies with either clinical or laboratorial isolates [48, 49], the exact role of *embB306* mutations play in the development of ethambutol resistance and multidrug resistance in *M. tuberculosis* is not fully understood. About 35% of EMB-resistant strains (MIC <10 µg/ml) do not have *embB* mutations [39, 45], suggesting that there may be other mechanisms of EMB resistance. Further studies are necessary to identify the potential new mechanisms of EMB resistance.

2.5. Streptomycin

Streptomycin (SM), an aminocyclitol glycoside antibiotic, was the first drug to be used in the treatment of TB, in 1948 [50]. SM kills actively growing tubercle bacilli with MICs of 2–4 µg/ml, but it is inactive against non-growing or intracellular bacilli [23]. The drug binds to the 16S rRNA, interferes with translation proofreading, and thereby inhibits protein synthesis [51, 52]. Ototoxicity and nephotoxicity are associated with SM administration. Vestibular dysfunction is more common than auditory damage. Renal toxicity occurs less frequently than with kanamycin or capreomycin. Hearing and renal function should be monitored in patients getting SM.

Mutations associated with streptomycin resistance have been identified in the genes encoding 16S rRNA (*rrs*) [53] and ribosomal protein S12 (*rpsL*) [54-57]. Ribosomal protein S12 stabilizes the highly conserved pseudoknot structure formed by 16S rRNA [58]. Amino acid substitutions in RpsL affect the higher-order structure of 16S rRNA [51] and confer streptomycin resistance. Alterations in the 16S rRNA structure disrupt interactions between 16S rRNA and streptomycin, a process that results in resistance [59]. Mutations in *rpsL* and *rrs* are the major mechanism of SM resistance [54, 56, 57], accounting for respectively about 50% and 20% of SM-resistant strains [54, 56, 57]. The most common mutation in *rpsL* is a substitution in codon 43 from lysine to arginine [54, 56, 57], causing high-level resistance to SM. Mutation in codon 88 is also common [54, 56, 57]. Mutations of the *rrs* gene occur in the loops of the 16S rRNA and are clustered in two regions around nucleotides 530 and 915 [39, 54, 56, 57]. However, about 20–30% of SM-resistant strains with a low level of resistance (MIC < 32 μg/ml) do not have mutations in *rpsL* or *rrs* [60], which indicates other mechanism(s) of resistance. A mutation in *gidB*, encoding a conserved 7-methylguanosine (m(7)G) methyltransferase specific for 16S rRNA, has been found to cause low-level SM resistance in 33% of resistant *M. tuberculosis* isolates [61]. A subsequent study showed that while Leu16Arg change is a polymorphism not involved in SM resistance, other mutations in *gidB* appear to be involved in low-level SM resistance [62]. In addition, some low-level SM resistance seems to be caused by increased efflux as efflux pump inhibitors caused increased sensitivity to SM, although the exact mechanism remains to be identified [62].

3. Second-line antituberculosis drugs

3.1. Fluoroquinolones

The fluoroquinolones (FQs) have broad-spectrum antimicrobial activity and so are widely used for the treatment of bacterial infections of the respiratory, gastrointestinal and urinary tracts, as well as sexually transmitted diseases and chronic osteomyelitis [63]. In contrast to many other antibiotics used to treat bacterial infections, the FQs have excellent in vitro and in vivo activity against *M. tuberculosis* [64, 65]. FQs include ciprofloxacin, ofloxacin, levofloxacin, and moxifloxacin. So, FQs are currently in use as second-line drugs in the treatment of TB. Adverse effects are relatively infrequent (0.5–10% of patients) and include gastrointestinal intolerance, rashes, dizziness, and headache. Most studies of fluoroquinolone side effects have been based on relatively short-term administration for bacterial infections, but trials have now shown the relative safety and tolerability of fluoroquinolones administered for months during TB treatment in adults.

The cellular target of FQs in *M. tuberculosis* is DNA gyrase, a type II topoisomerase consisting of two A and two B subunits encoded by *gyrA* and *gyrB* genes, respectively [66]. Mutations in a small region of *gyrA*, called quinolone resistance-determining region (QRDR) and, less frequently, in *gyrB* are the primary mechanism of FQ resistance in *M. tuberculosis* [66, 67]. Analysis of QRDR alone by genotypic tests has been suggested as sufficient for rapid identification of vast majority of FQ-resistant *M. tuberculosis* strains as additional targeting of *gyrB* did not enhance the sensitivity significantly [67, 68].

Mutations within the QRDR of *gyrA* have been identified in clinical and laboratory-selected isolates of *M. tuberculosis*, largely clustered at codons 90, 91 and 94 [69-73], with Asp94 being relatively frequent [71, 74]. Codon 95 (Ser95Thr) contains a naturally occurring polymorphism that is not related to fluoroquinolone resistance, as it occurs in both fluoroquinolone-susceptible and fluoroquinolone-resistant strains [75]. A less common involvement is codon 88 [76]. For clinical isolates, *gyrB* mutations appear to be of much rarer occurrence [72, 73]. Generally, two mutations in *gyrA* or concomitant mutations in *gyrA* plus *gyrB* are required for the development of higher levels of resistance [69, 77].

3.2. Aminoglycosides (kanamycin, amikacin and capreomycin)

The aminoglycosides amikacin (AMK)/kanamycin (KAN) and the cyclic polypeptide capreomycin (CAP) are important injectable drugs in the treatment of multidrug-resistant tuberculosis. Although belonging to two different antibiotic families, all exert their activity at the level of protein translation. Renal toxicity occurs from these drugs. Regular monitoring of hearing and renal function is recommended.

AMK and KAN are aminoglycosides that have a high level of cross-resistance between them [78-80]. The cyclic polypeptide CAP is structurally unrelated to the aminoglycosides and thus is a potential candidate to replace AMK or KAN if resistance to either of them is suspected [81, 82]. It has been demonstrated that the risk of treatment failure and mortality increase when CAP resistance emerges among MDR-TB cases [83]. However, cross-resistance in *M. tuberculosis* between AMK/KAN and CAP has been observed in both clinical isolates and laboratory-generated mutants [79, 80, 84, 85].

AMK/KAN and CAP primarily affect protein synthesis in *M. tuberculosis* and resistance to these drugs is associated with changes in the 16S rRNA (*rrs*) [78, 80, 81, 85, 86]. The *rrs* mutation A1401G causes high-level AMK/KAN and low-level CAP resistance. C1402T is associated with CAP resistance and low-level KAN resistance. G1484T is linked to high-level AMK/KAN and CAP resistance [79, 80, 84, 86]. Low-level resistance to kanamycin has been correlated to mutations in the promoter region of the *eis* gene encoding aminoglycoside acetyltransferase, the enhanced intracellular survival protein, Eis [87].

Resistance to the cyclic peptide capreomycin has also been associated with mutations in *tlyA* [86]. The gene *tlyA* encodes a putative 2′-O-methyltransferase (TlyA) that has been suggested to methylate nucleotide C1402 in helix 44 of 16S rRNA and nucleotide C2158 in helix 69 of 23S rRNA in *M. tuberculosis* [81, 88]. Capreomycin binds to the 70S ribosome and inhibits mRNA–tRNA translocation [89]. It is believed that TlyA methylation enhances the antimicrobial activity of capreomycin [81] and that disruption of *tlyA* leads to capreomycin resistance because the unmethylated ribosome is insensitive to the drug [81, 86, 88]. The identified mechanism of capreomycin resistance on the basis of in vitro selected mutants has found that *tlyA* mutations were common [80, 86] whereas infrequent in clinical isolates of *M. tuberculosis* [79, 80].

3.3. Ethionamide/prothionamide

Ethionamide (ETH, 2-ethylisonicotinamide) is a derivative of isonicotinic acid and has been used as an antituberculosis agent since 1956. The MICs of ETH for *M. tuberculosis* are 0.5–2 μg/ml in liquid medium, 2.5–10 μg/ml in 7H11 agar, and 5–20 μg/ml in LJ medium. Ethionamide and the similar drug prothionamide (PTH, 2-ethyl-4-pyridinecarbothioamide) act as pro-drugs, like isoniazid. Which is activated by EtaA/EthA (a mono-oxygenase) [90, 91] and inhibits the same target as INH, the InhA of the mycolic acid synthesis pathway [92]. Once delivered into the bacterial cell, ethionamide undergoes several changes. Its sulfo group is oxidized by flavin monooxygenase, and the drug is then converted to 2-ethyl-4-aminopyridine. The intermediate products formed before 2-ethyl-4-aminopyridine seem to be toxic to mycobacteria, but their structures are unknown (may be highly unstable compounds). Mutants resistant to ethionamide are cross-resistant to prothionamide. ETH frequently causes gastrointestinal side effects, such as abdominal pain, nausea, vomiting and anorexia. It can cause hypothyroidism, particularly if it is used with *para*-aminosalicylic acid.

3.4. *p*-Amino salicylic acid

p-Amino salicylic acid (PAS) was one of the first antibiotics to show anti-TB activity and was used to treat TB in combination with isoniazid and streptomycin [93]. Later, with the discovery of other more potent drugs including rifampicin, its use in first line regimens was discontinued. PAS is still useful as part of a treatment regimen for XDR TB although its benefit is limited and it is extremely toxic. Thymidylate synthase A, encoded by *thyA*, an enzyme involved in the biosynthesis of thymine, has been proposed recently as the target of PAS in *M. bovis* BCG [94]. Most common mutation in *thyA* was Thr202Ala, though few susceptible isolates also showed the same mutation [95]. However, its mechanism of action was never clearly elucidated. The most common adverse reactions associated with PAS are gastrointestinal disturbances.

3.5. Cycloserine

Cycloserine (CS) is an antibiotic that is used to treat TB. The exact mechanism of action of cycloserine is unknown, but it is thought to prevent the tuberculosis bacteria from making substances called peptidoglycans, which are needed to form the bacterial cell wall. This results in the weakening of bacteria's cell wall, which then kills the bacteria. Cycloserine possesses high gastric tolerance (compared with the other drugs) and lacks cross-resistance to other compounds. But it causes adverse psychiatric effects; [96, 97] which is its main drawback. So, psychiatric interrogation is necessary before prescribing cycloserine drug. Cycloserine is one of the cornerstones of treatment for MDR and XDR tuberculosis [96, 97, 98]. Terizidone (a combination of two molecules of cycloserine) might be less toxic [96, 97], although studies of this drug are scarce.

4. Conclusions

Despite all the advances made in the treatment and management, TB still remains as one of the main public health problems that have plagued mankind for millennia. The challenges posed by *M. tuberculosis* infection, through its interaction with the immune system and its mechanisms for evasion, require many more breakthroughs to make a significant impact on the worldwide tuberculosis problem. The introduction of MDR and XDR strains of *M. tuberculosis* poses several problems in mycobacterial genetics and phthisiotherapy. Among the response priorities, rapid detection of anti-tuberculosis drug resistance, use of appropriate regimens for treatment, and new drug development are of paramount importance. However, regarding the dynamics of TB transmission, and also in view of rational development of new anti-TB drugs, it is extremely important to extend our knowledge on the molecular basis of drug resistance and all its complexity. It is necessary to clarify the association between specific mutations and the development of MDR-TB or the association between drug resistance and fitness. This would allow better evaluation of the transmission dynamics of resistant strains and more accurate prediction of a future disease scenario. Adequate monitoring of drug resistance, especially MDR/XDR-TB in new patients and its transmission, molecular characterization of the drug-resistant strains, and analysis of patients' immune status and genetic susceptibility are also needed to address the problem of the fitness, virulence and transmissibility of drug-resistant *M. tuberculosis* strains.

Author details

Hum Nath Jnawali and Sungweon Ryoo*

*Address all correspondence to: scientist1@empal.com

Korean Institute of Tuberculosis, Osong Saengmyeong, Cheongwon-gun, Chungcheongbuk-do, Republic of Korea

References

[1] Espinal, M. A, Laszlo, A, Simonsen, L, Boulahbal, F, Kim, S. J, Reniero, A, Hoffner, S, Rieder, H. L, Binkin, N, Dye, C, Williams, R, & Raviglione, M. C. Global trends in resistance to antituberculosis drugs. The New England Journal of Medicine (2001). , 344(17), 1294-303.

[2] Masjedi, M. R, Farnia, P, Sorooch, S, Pooramiri, M. V, Mansoori, S. D, Zarifi, A. Z, Velayati, A. A, & Hoffner, S. Extensively drug resistant tuberculosis: 2 years of surveillance in Iran. Clinical Infectious Diseases (2006). , 43(7), 840-7.

[3] Eker, B, Ortmann, J, Migliori, G. B, Sotgiu, G, Muetterlein, R, Centis, R, Hoffmann, H, Kirsten, D, Schaberg, T, Ruesch-gerdes, S, & Lange, C. Multidrug- and extensively drug-resistant tuberculosis, Germany. Emerging Infectious Diseases (2008). , 14(11), 1700-6.

[4] Almeida Da Silva P. E, & Palomino J. C. Molecular basis and mechanisms of drug resistance in *Mycobacterium tuberculosis*: classical and new drugs. The Journal of Antimicrobial Chemotherapy 2011. , 66(7), 1417-30.

[5] Bernstein, J, Lott, W. A, Steinberg, B. A, & Yale, H. L. Chemotherapy of experimental tuberculosis. V. Isonicotinic acid hydrazide (nydrazid) and related compounds. American Review of Tuberculosis (1952). , 65(4), 357-64.

[6] Bardou, F, Raynaud, C, Ramos, C, Laneelle, M. A, & Laneelle, G. Mechanism of isoniazid uptake in *Mycobacterium tuberculosis*. Microbiology 1998. , 144(Pt 9), 2539–44.

[7] Zhang, Y, Heym, B, Allen, B, Young, D, & Cole, S. The catalase-peroxidase gene and isoniazid resistance of *Mycobacterium tuberculosis*. Nature (1992). , 358(6387), 591-3.

[8] Middlebrook, G. Isoniazid resistance and catalase activity of tubercle bacilli. American Review of Tuberculosis (1954). , 69(3), 471-2.

[9] Winder, F. Mode of Action of the Antimycobacterial Agents and Associated Aspects of the Molecular Biology of Mycobacteria. In: Ratledge C, Stanford J, eds. The Biology of Mycobacteria. Vol I. New York, NY, USA: Academic Press; (1982). , 354-438.

[10] Zhang, Y, & Telenti, A. Genetics of Drug Resistance in *Mycobacterium tuberculosis*. In Molecular Genetics of Mycobacteria. Hatful, G.F., and Jacobs, W.R., Jr (eds). Washington, DC: ASM Press; (2000). , 235-254.

[11] Banerjee, A, Dubnau, E, Quemard, A, Balasubramanian, V, Um, K. S, Wilson, T, Collins, D, & De Lisle, G. Jacobs WR Jr. *inhA*, a gene encoding a target for isoniazid and ethionamide in *Mycobacterium tuberculosis*. Science (1994). , 263(5144), 227-30.

[12] Hazbón, M. H, Brimacombe, M, Bobadilla del Valle, M, Cavatore, M, Guerrero, M. I, Varma-Basil, M, Billman-Jacobe, H, Lavender, C, Fyfe, J, García-García, L, León, C. I, Bose, M, Chaves, F, Murray, M, Eisenach, K. D, Sifuentes-Osornio, J, Cave, M. D, Ponce de León, A, & Alland, D. Population genetics study of isoniazid resistance mutations and evolution of multidrug-resistant *Mycobacterium tuberculosis*. Antimicrobial Agents and Chemotherapy (2006). , 50(8), 2640-9.

[13] Heym, B, Alzari, P M, Honore, N, & Cole, S. T. Missense mutations in the catalase-peroxidase gene, *kat*G, are associated with isoniazid resistance in *Mycobacterium tuberculosis*. Molecular Microbiology (1995). , 15(2), 235-45.

[14] Leung, E. T, Ho, P. L, Yuen, K. Y, Woo, W. L, Lam, T. H, Kao, R. Y, Seto, W. H, & Yam, W. C. Molecular characterization of isoniazid resistance in *Mycobacterium tuberculosis*: identification of a novel mutation in *inhA*. Antimicrobial Agents and Chemotherapy (2006). , 50(3), 1075-8.

[15] Rinder, H, Thomschke, A, Rüsch-gerdes, S, Bretzel, G, Feldmann, K, Rifai, M, & Löscher, T. Significance of *ahpC* promoter mutations for the prediction of isoniazid resistance in *Mycobacterium tuberculosis*. European Journal of Clinical Microbiology and Infectious Diseases (1998). , 17(7), 508-11.

[16] Sherman, D. R, Mdluli, K, Hickey, M. J, Arain, T. M, Morris, S. L, Barry, C. E 3rd, & Stover, C. K. Compensatory *ahpC* gene expression in isoniazid-resistant *Mycobacterium tuberculosis*. Science (1996). , 272(5268), 1641-3.

[17] Ramaswamy, S, & Musser, J. M. Molecular genetic basis of antimicrobial agent resistance in *Mycobacterium tuberculosis*: 1998 update. Tubercle and Lung Disease (1998). , 79(1), 3-29.

[18] Mitchison, D. A. Basic mechanisms of chemotherapy. Chest (1979). Suppl): , 771-81.

[19] Telenti, A, Imboden, P, Marchesi, F, Schmidheini, T, & Bodmer, T. Direct, automated detection of rifampin-resistant *Mycobacterium tuberculosis* by polymerase chain reaction and single-strand conformation polymorphism analysis. Antimicrobial Agents and Chemotherapy (1993). , 37(10), 2054-8.

[20] Somoskovi, A, Parsons, L. M, & Salfinger, M. The molecular basis of resistance to isoniazid, rifampin, and pyrazinamide in *Mycobacterium tuberculosis*. Respiratory Research (2001). , 2(3), 164-8.

[21] Caws, M, Duy, P. M, Tho, D. Q, Lan, N. T, Hoa, D. V, & Farrar, J. Mutations prevalent among rifampin and isoniazid-resistant *Mycobacterium tuberculosis* isolates from a hospital in Vietnam. Journal of Clinical Microbiology (2006). , 44(7), 2333-7.

[22] Heep, M, Rieger, U, Beck, D, & Lehn, N. Mutations in the beginning of the *rpoB* gene can induce resistance to rifamycins in both Helicobacter pylori and *Mycobacterium tuberculosis*. Antimicrobial Agents and Chemotherapy (2000). , 44(4), 1075-7.

[23] Mitchison, D. A. The action of antituberculosis drugs in short-course chemotherapy. Tubercle (1985). , 66(3), 219-25.

[24] Konno, K, Feldmann, F. M, & Mcdermott, W. Pyrazinamide susceptibility and amidase activity of tubercle bacilli. The American Review of Respiratory Disease (1967). , 95(3), 461-9.

[25] Mcdermott, W, & Tompsett, R. Activation of pyrazinamide and nicotinamide in acidic environment in vitro. American Review of Tuberculosis (1954). , 70(4), 748-54.

[26] Zhang, Y, & Mitchison, D. The curious characteristics of pyrazinamide: a review. The International Journal of Tuberculosis and Lung Disease (2003). , 7(1), 6-21.

[27] Scorpio, A, & Zhang, Y. Mutations in *pncA*, a gene encoding pyrazinamidase/nicotinamidase, cause resistance to the antituberculous drug pyrazinamide in tubercle bacillus. Nature Medicine (1996). , 2(6), 662-7.

[28] Cheng, S. J, Thibert, L, Sanchez, T, Heifets, L, & Zhang, Y. *pncA* mutations as a major mechanism of pyrazinamide resistance in *Mycobacterium tuberculosis*: spread of a

mono-resistant strain in Quebec, Canada. Antimicrobial Agents and Chemotherapy (2000). , 44(3), 528-32.

[29] Lemaitre, N, Sougakoff, W, Truffot-pernot, C, & Jarlier, V. Characterization of new mutations in pyrazinamide-resistant strains of Mycobacterium tuberculosis and identification of conserved regions important for the catalytic activity of the pyrazinamidase PncA. Antimicrobial Agents and Chemotherapy (1999). , 43(7), 1761-3.

[30] Ando, H, Mitarai, S, Kondo, Y, Suetake, T, Sekiguchi, J. I, Kato, S, Mori, T, & Kirikae, T. Pyrazinamide resistance in multidrug-resistant Mycobacterium tuberculosis isolates in Japan. Clinical Microbiology and Infection (2010). , 16(8), 1164-8.

[31] Juréen, P, Werngren, J, Toro, J. C, & Hoffner, S. Pyrazinamide resistance and pncA gene mutations in Mycobacterium tuberculosis. Antimicrobial Agents and Chemotherapy (2008). , 52(5), 1852-4.

[32] Suzuki, Y, Suzuki, A, Tamaru, A, Katsukawa, C, & Oda, H. Rapid detection of pyrazinamide-resistant Mycobacterium tuberculosis by a PCR-based in vitro system. Journal of Clinical Microbiology (2002). , 40(2), 501-7.

[33] Park, S. K, Lee, J. Y, Chang, Lee, M. K, Son, H. C, Kim, C. M, Jang, H. J, Park, H. K, & Jeong, S. H. pncA mutations in clinical Mycobacterium tuberculosis isolates from Korea. BMC Infectious Diseases (2001). , 1, 4.

[34] Scorpio, A, Lindholm-levy, P, Heifets, L, Gilman, R, Siddiqi, S, Cynamon, M, & Zhang, Y. Characterization of pncA mutations in pyrazinamide-resistant Mycobacterium tuberculosis. Antimicrobial Agents and Chemotherapy (1997). , 41(3), 540-3.

[35] Louw, G. E, Warren, R. M, Donald, P. R, Murray, M. B, Bosman, M, Van Helden, P. D, Young, D. B, & Victor, T. C. Frequency and implications of pyrazinamide resistance in managing previously treated tuberculosis patients. The International Journal of Tuberculosis and Lung Disease (2006). , 10(7), 802-7.

[36] American Thoracic Society, CDC, Infectious Diseases Society of America. Treatment of tuberculosis. MMWR Recommendations and Reports (2003)., 52(RR-11), 1–77.

[37] Takayama, K, & Kilburn, J. Inhibition of synthesis of arabinogalactan by ethambutol in Mycobacterium smegmatis. Antimicrobial Agents and Chemotherapy (1989). , 33(9), 1493-9.

[38] Wolucka, B. A, Mcneil, M. R, De Hoffmann, E, Chojnacki, T, & Brennan, P. J. Recognition of the lipid intermediate for arabinogalactan/arabinomannan biosynthesis and its relation to the mode of action of ethambutol on mycobacteria. The Journal of Biological Chemistry (1994). , 269(37), 23328-35.

[39] Zhang, Y, & Yew, W. W. Mechanisms of drug resistance in Mycobacterium tuberculosis. The International Journal of Tuberculosis and Lung Disease (2009). , 13(11), 1320-30.

[40] Telenti, A, Philipp, W. J, Sreevatsan, S, Bernasconi, C, Stockbauer, K. E, Wieles, B, & Musser, J. M. Jacobs WR Jr. The *emb* operon, a unique gene cluster of *Mycobacterium tuberculosis* involved in resistance to ethambutol. Nature Medicine (1997). , 3(5), 567-70.

[41] Belanger, A. E, Besra, G. S, Ford, M. E, Mikusová, K, Belisle, J. T, Brennan, P. J, & Inamine, J. M. The *embAB* genes of *Mycobacterium avium* encode an arabinosyl transferase involved in cell wall arabinan biosynthesis that is the target for the antimycobacterial drug ethambutol. Proceedings of the National Academy of Sciences of the United States of America (1996). , 93(21), 11919-24.

[42] Ramaswamy, S. V, Amin, A. G, Göksel, S, Stager, C. E, Dou, S. J, El Sahly, H, Moghazeh, S. L, Kreiswirth, B. N, & Musser, J. M. Molecular genetic analysis of nucleotide polymorphisms associated with ethambutol resistance in human isolates of *Mycobacterium tuberculosis*. Antimicrobial Agents and Chemotherapy (2000). , 44(2), 326-36.

[43] Sreevatsan, S, Stockbauer, K. E, Pan, X, Kreiswirth, B. N, & Moghazeh, S. L. Jacobs WR Jr, Telenti A, Musser JM. Ethambutol resistance in *Mycobacterium tuberculosis*: critical role of *embB* mutations. Antimicrobial Agents and Chemotherapy (1997). , 41(8), 1677-81.

[44] Sreevatsan, S, Stockbauer, K. E, Pan, X, Kreiswirth, B. N, Moghazeh, S. L, Jacobs, W. R Jr, Telenti, A, & Musser, J. M. Ethambutol resistance in *Mycobacterium tuberculosis*: critical role of *embB* mutations. Antimicrobial Agents and Chemotherapy (1997). , 41(8), 1677–81.

[45] Alcaide, F, Pfyffer, G. E, & Telenti, A. Role of *embB* in natural and acquired resistance to ethambutol in mycobacteria. Antimicrobial Agents and Chemotherapy (1997). , 41(10), 2270-3.

[46] Lee, A. S, Othman, S. N, Ho, Y. M, & Wong, S. Y. Novel mutations within the *embB* gene in ethambutol-susceptible clinical isolates of *Mycobacterium tuberculosis*. Antimicrobial Agents and Chemotherapy (2004). , 48(11), 4447-9.

[47] Mokrousov, I, Otten, T, Vyshnevskiy, B, & Narvskaya, O. Detection of *embB306* mutations in ethambutol-susceptible clinical isolates of *Mycobacterium tuberculosis* from Northwestern Russia: implications for genotypic resistance testing. Journal of Clinical Microbiology (2002). , 40(10), 3810-3.

[48] Safi, H, Fleischmann, R. D, Peterson, S. N, Jones, M. B, Jarrahi, B, & Alland, D. Allelic exchange and mutant selection demonstrate that common clinical *embCAB* gene mutations only modestly increase resistance to ethambutol in *Mycobacterium tuberculosis*. Antimicrobial Agents and Chemotherapy (2010). , 54(1), 103-8.

[49] Perdigão, J, Macedo, R, Ribeiro, A, Brum, L, & Portugal, I. Genetic characterisation of the ethambutol resistance-determining region in *Mycobacterium tuberculosis*: prevalence and significance of *embB306* mutations. International Journal of Antimicrobial Agents (2009). , 33(4), 334-8.

[50] British Medical Research CouncilStreptomycin treatment of pulmonary tuberculosis. A Medical Research Council Investigation. BMJ (1948). , 2, 769-82.

[51] British Medical Research Council. Streptomycin treatment of pulmonary tuberculosis. A Medical Research Council Investigation. BMJ (1948). , 2, 769-82.

[52] Gale, E. F, Cundliffe, E, Reynolds, P. E, Richmond, M. H, & Waring, M. J. The molecular basis of antibiotic action. John Wiley and Sons, Inc., New York. (1981).

[53] Douglass, J, & Steyn, L. M. A ribosomal gene mutation in streptomycin-resistant *Mycobacterium tuberculosis* isolates. The Journal of Infectious Diseases (1993). , 167(6), 1505-6.

[54] Finken, M, Kirschner, P, Meier, A, Wrede, A, & Böttger, E. C. Molecular basis of streptomycin resistance in *Mycobacterium tuberculosis*: alterations of the ribosomal protein S12 gene and point mutations within a functional 16S ribosomal RNA pseudoknot. Molecular Microbiology (1993). , 9(6), 1239-46.

[55] Funatsu, G, & Wittman, H. G. Ribosomal proteins. XXXIII. Location of amino-acid replacements in protein S12 isolated from *Escherichia coli* mutants resistant to streptomycin. Journal of Molecular Microbiology (1972). , 68(3), 547-50.

[56] Honore, N, & Cole, S. T. Streptomycin resistance in mycobacteria. Antimicrobial Agents and Chemotherapy (1994). , 38(2), 238-22.

[57] Nair, J, Rouse, D. A, Bai, G. H, & Morris, S. L. The *rpsL* gene and streptomycin resistance in single and multiple drug-resistant strains of *Mycobacterium tuberculosis*. Molecular Microbiology (1993). , 10(3), 521-7.

[58] Noller, H. F. Structure of ribosomal RNA. Annual Review of Biochemistry (1984). , 53, 119-62.

[59] De Stasio, E. A, Moazed, D, Noller, H. F, & Dahlberg, A. E. Mutations in 16S ribosomal RNA disrupt antibiotic-RNA interactions. The EMBO Journal (1989). , 8(4), 1213-6.

[60] Cooksey, R. C, Morlock, G. P, Mcqueen, A, Glickman, S. E, & Crawford, J. T. Characterization of streptomycin resistance mechanisms among *Mycobacterium tuberculosis* isolates from patients in New York City. Antimicrobial Agents and Chemotherapy (1996). , 40(5), 1186-8.

[61] Okamoto, S, Tamaru, A, Nakajima, C, Nishimura, K, Tanaka, Y, Tokuyama, S, Suzuki, Y, & Ochi, K. Loss of a conserved 7-methylguanosine modification in 16S rRNA confers low-level streptomycin resistance in bacteria. Molecular Microbiology (2007). , 63(4), 1096-106.

[62] Spies, F. S. da Silva PE, Ribeiro MO, Rossetti ML, Zaha A. Identification of mutations related to streptomycin resistance in clinical isolates of *Mycobacterium tuberculosis* and

possible involvement of efflux mechanism. Antimicrobial Agents and Chemotherapy (2008). , 52(8), 2947-9.

[63] Spies, F. S, da Silva, P. E, Ribeiro, M. O, Rossetti, M. L, & Zaha, A. Identification of mutations related to streptomycin resistance in clinical isolates of *Mycobacterium tuberculosis* and possible involvement of efflux mechanism. Antimicrobial Agents and Chemotherapy (2008). , 52(8), 2947-9.

[64] Bartlett, J. G, Dowell, S. F, Mandell, L. A, File Jr, T. M, Musher, D. M, & Fine, M. J. Practice guidelines for the management of community-acquired pneumonia in adults. Infectious Diseases Society of America. Clinical Infectious Diseases (2000). , 31(2), 347-82.

[65] Wang, J. Y, Hsueh, P. R, Jan, I. S, Lee, L. N, Liaw, Y. S, Yang, P. C, & Luh, K. T. Empirical treatment with a fluoroquinolone delays the treatment for tuberculosis and is associated with a poor prognosis in endemic areas. Thorax (2006). , 61(10), 903-8.

[66] Ginsburg, A. S, Grosset, J. H, & Bishai, W. R. Fluoroquinolones, tuberculosis, and resistance. The Lancet of Infectious Diseases (2003). , 3(7), 432-42.

[67] Chang, K. C, & Yew, W. W. Chan RCY. Rapid assays for fluoroquinolone resistance in *Mycobacterium tuberculosis*: a systematic review and meta-analysis. The Journal of Antimicrobial Chemotherapy (2010). , 65(8), 1551-61.

[68] Hillemann, D, Rusch-gerdes, S, & Richter, E. Feasibility of the GenoType MTBDRsl assay for fluoroquinolone, amikacin-capreomycin and ethambutol resistance testing of *Mycobacterium tuberculosis* strains and clinical specimens. Journal of Clinical Microbiology (2009). , 47(6), 1767-72.

[69] Takiff, H. E, Salazar, L, Guerrero, C, Philipp, W, Huang, W. M, Kreiswirth, B, & Cole, S. T. Jacobs WR Jr, Telenti A. Cloning and nucleotide sequence of *Mycobacterium tuberculosis gyrA* and *gyrB* genes and detection of quinolone resistance mutations. Antimicrobial Agents and Chemotherapy (1994). , 38(4), 773-80.

[70] Alangaden, G. J, Manavathu, E. K, Vakulenko, S. B, Zvonok, N. M, & Lerner, S. A. Characterization of fluoroquinolone-resistant mutant strains of *Mycobacterium tuberculosis* selected in the laboratory and isolated from patients. Antimicrobial Agents and Chemotherapy (1995). , 39(8), 1700-3.

[71] Cheng, A. F, Yew, W. W, Chan, E. W, Chin, M. L, Hui, M. M, & Chan, R. C. Multiplex PCR amplimer conformation analysis for rapid detection of *gyrA* mutations in fluoroquinolone-resistant *Mycobacterium tuberculosis* clinical isolates. Antimicrobial Agents and Chemotherapy (2004). , 48(2), 596-601.

[72] Pitaksajjakul, P, Wongwit, W, Punprasit, W, Eampokalap, B, Peacock, S, & Ramasoota, P. Mutations in the *gyrA* and *gyrB* genes of fluoroquinolone-resistant *Mycobacterium tuberculosis* from TB patients in Thailand. The Southeast Asian Journal of Tropical Medicine and Public Health (2005). Suppl 4): 228-37.

[73] Lee, A. S, Tang, L. L, Lim, I. H, & Wong, S. Y. Characterization of pyrazinamide and ofloxacin resistance among drug resistant *Mycobacterium tuberculosis* isolates from Singapore. International Journal of Infectious Diseases (2002). , 6(1), 48-51.

[74] Sun, Z, Zhang, J, Zhang, X, Wang, S, Zhang, Y, & Li, C. Comparison of *gyrA* gene mutations between laboratory-selected ofloxacin-resistant *Mycobacterium tuberculosis* strains and clinical isolates. International Journal of Antimicrobial Agents (2008). , 31(2), 115-21.

[75] Musser, J. M. Antimicrobial agent resistance in mycobacteria: molecular genetic insights. Clinical Microbiology Reviews (1995). , 8(4), 496-514.

[76] Matrat, S, Veziris, N, Mayer, C, Jarlier, V, Truffot-pernot, C, Camuset, J, Bouvet, E, Cambau, E, & Aubry, A. Functional analysis of DNA gyrase mutant enzymes carrying mutations at position 88 in the A subunit found in clinical strains of *Mycobacterium tuberculosis* resistant to fluoroquinolones. Antimicrobial Agents and Chemotherapy (2006). , 50(12), 4170-3.

[77] Kocagöz, T, Hackbarth, C. J, Unsal, I, Rosenberg, E. Y, Nikaido, H, & Chambers, H. F. Gyrase mutations in laboratory selected, fluoroquinolone-resistant mutants of *Mycobacterium tuberculosis* H37Ra. Antimicrobial Agents and Chemotherapy (1996). , 40(8), 1768-74.

[78] Alangaden, G. J, Kreiswirth, B. N, Aouad, A, Khetarpal, M, Igno, F. R, Moghazeh, S. L, Manavathu, E. K, & Lerner, S. A. Mechanisms of resistance to amikacin and kanamycin in *Mycobacterium tuberculosis*. Antimicrobial Agents and Chemotherapy (1998). , 42(5), 1295-7.

[79] Jugheli, L, Bzekalava, N, De Rijk, P, Fissette, K, Portaels, F, & Rigouts, L. High level of cross-resistance between kanamycin, amikacin, and capreomycin among *Mycobacterium tuberculosis* isolates from Georgia and a close relation with mutations in the *rrs* gene. Antimicrobial Agents and Chemotherapy (2009). , 53(12), 5064-8.

[80] Maus, C. E, Plikaytis, B. B, & Shinnick, T. M. Molecular analysis of cross-resistance to capreomycin, kanamycin, amikacin, and viomycin in *Mycobacterium tuberculosis*. Antimicrobial Agents and Chemotherapy (2005). , 49(8), 3192-7.

[81] Johansen, S. K, Maus, C. E, Plikaytis, B. B, & Douthwaite, S. Capreomycin binds across the ribosome subunit interface using tlyA-encoded 2'-O-methylations in 16S and 23S rRNAs. Molecular Cell (2006). , 23(2), 173-82.

[82] World Health Organization (WHO)Policy Guidance on Drug-Susceptibility Testing (DST) of Second-Line Antituberculosis Drugs. Report (WHO/HTM/TB/2008.392): 1-20. WHO, Geneva, Switzerland. (2008).

[83] Migliori, G. B, Lange, C, Centis, R, Sotgiu, G, Mütterlein, R, Hoffmann, H, Kliiman, K, De Iaco, G, Lauria, F. N, Richardson, M. D, & Spanevello, A. Cirillo DM; TBNET Study Group. Resistance to second-line injectables and treatment outcomes in multi

drug-resistant and extensively drug-resistant tuberculosis cases. The European Respiratory Journal (2008). , 31(6), 1155-9.

[84] Engström, A, Perskvist, N, Werngren, J, Hoffner, S. E, & Juréen, P. Comparison of clinical isolates and in vitro selected mutants reveals that *tlyA* is not a sensitive genetic marker for capreomycin resistance in *Mycobacterium tuberculosis*. The Journal of Antimicrobial Chemotherapy (2011). , 66(6), 1247-54.

[85] Via, L. E, Cho, S. N, Hwang, S, Bang, H, Park, S. K, Kang, H. S, Jeon, D, Min, S. Y, Oh, T, Kim, Y, Kim, Y. M, Rajan, V, Wong, S. Y, Shamputa, I. C, Carroll, M, Goldfeder, L, Lee, S. A, Holland, S. M, Eum, S, Lee, H, & Barry, C. E. rd. Polymorphisms associated with resistance and cross-resistance to aminoglycosides and capreomycin in *Mycobacterium tuberculosis* isolates from South Korean patients with drug-resistant tuberculosis. Journal of Clinical Microbiology (2010). , 48(2), 402-11.

[86] Via, L. E, Cho, S. N, Hwang, S, Bang, H, Park, S. K, Kang, H. S, Jeon, D, Min, S. Y, Oh, T, Kim, Y, Kim, Y. M, Rajan, V, Wong, S. Y, Shamputa, I. C, Carroll, M, Goldfeder, L, Lee, S. A, Holland, S. M, Eum, S, Lee, H, & Barry, C. E. 3rd. Polymorphisms associated with resistance and cross-resistance to aminoglycosides and capreomycin in *Mycobacterium tuberculosis* isolates from South Korean patients with drug-resistant tuberculosis. Journal of Clinical Microbiology (2010). , 48(2), 402-11.

[87] Zaunbrecher, M. A. Sikes RD Jr, Metchock B, Shinnick TM, Posey JE. Over-expression of the chromosomally encoded aminoglycoside acetyltransferase *eis* confers kanamycin resistance in *Mycobacterium tuberculosis*. Proceedings of the National Academy of Sciences of the United States of America (2009). , 106(47), 20004-9.

[88] Zaunbrecher, M. A, Sikes, R. D Jr, Metchock, B, Shinnick, T. M, & Posey, J. E. Over-expression of the chromosomally encoded aminoglycoside acetyltransferase *eis* confers kanamycin resistance in *Mycobacterium tuberculosis*. Proceedings of the National Academy of Sciences of the United States of America (2009). , 106(47), 20004-9.

[89] Stanley, R. E, Blaha, G, Grodzicki, R. L, Strickler, M. D, & Steitz, T. A. The structures of the anti-tuberculosis antibiotics viomycin and capreomycin bound to the 70S ribosome. Nature Structural and Molecular Biology (2010). , 17(3), 289-93.

[90] Debarber, A. E, Mdluli, K, Bosman, M, Bekker, L. G, & Barry, C. E. rd. Ethionamide activation and sensitivity in multidrug-resistant *Mycobacterium tuberculosis*. Proceedings of the National Academy of Sciences of the United States of America (2000). , 97(17), 9677-82.

[91] DeBarber, A. E, Mdluli, K, Bosman, M, Bekker, L. G, & Barry, C. E 3rd. Ethionamide activation and sensitivity in multidrug-resistant *Mycobacterium tuberculosis*. Proceedings of the National Academy of Sciences of the United States of America (2000). , 97(17), 9677-82.

[92] Banerjee, A, Dubnau, E, Quemard, A, Balasubramanian, V, Um, K. S, Wilson, T, Collins, D, & De Lisle, G. Jacobs WR Jr. *inhA*, a gene encoding a target for isoniazid and ethionamide in *Mycobacterium tuberculosis*. Science (1994)., 263(5144), 227-30.

[93] Zhang, Y, Heym, B, Allen, B, Young, D, & Cole, S. The catalase/peroxidase gene and isoniazid resistance of *Mycobacterium tuberculosis*. Nature (1992)., 358(6387), 591-3.

[94] Rengarajan, J, Sassetti, C. M, Naroditskaya, V, Sloutsky, A, Bloom, B. R, & Rubin, E. J. The folate pathway is a target for resistance to the drug *para*-aminosalicylic acid (PAS) in mycobacteria. Molecular Microbiology (2004)., 53(1), 275–82.

[95] Leung, K. L, Yip, C. W, Yeung, Y. L, Wong, K. L, Chan, W. Y, Chan, M. Y, & Kam, K. M. Usefulness of resistant gene markers for predicting treatment outcome on second-line anti-tuberculosis drugs. Journal of Applied Microbiology (2010)., 109(6), 2087–94.

[96] WHO. Guidelines of the programmatic management of drug-resistant tuberculosis. http://whqlibdoc.who.int/publications/2006/9241546956_eng.pdf (accessed July 30, 2010).

[97] WHO. Guidelines for the programmatic management of drug-resistant tuberculosis. http://whqlibdoc.who.int/publications/2008/9789241547581_eng.pdf (accessed July 30, 2010).

[98] Caminero, J. A. Treatment of multidrug-resistant tuberculosis: evidence and controversies. The International Journal of Tuberculosis and Lung Disease 2006., 10(8), 829–37.

Chapter 9

Laboratory Diagnosis of Tuberculosis - Latest Diagnostic Tools

Gunes Senol

Additional information is available at the end of the chapter

1. Introduction

Early diagnosis of tuberculosis and drug resistance improves survival and by identifying infectious cases promotes contact tracing, implementation of institutional cross-infection procedures, and other public-health actions. There have been many advances in methodology for tuberculosis diagnosis [1-3].

For every stages of diagnosis, there are new approaches. New tests are available by level of laboratory and phase of application.

2. Microscoby

Microscopy has been a diagnostic tool for TB for over a century, and still currently the most rapid diagnostic method. Standard light microscopy (LM) and fluorescent microscopy (FM) are common methods. The recent development of light emitting diodes (LED), with the appropriate fluorescent light output for FM and low power consumption, has led to the development of simple, robust LED FM microscopes, requiring minimal mains or battery power and no dark room requirement. The WHO has recommended rolling it out as an alternative to LMs in resource-limited settings, based on studies that have shown comparable performance of LM and standard FM systems [4,5].

3. Culture and drug resistance testing

3.1. Phenotypic methods

Significant effort has been invested into further development of simple, alternative phenotypic methods such as the nitrate reductase assay (NRA), thin-layer agar (TLA), colour test (Color Test), the microscopic observation drug susceptibility assay (MODS), the colorimetric redox indicator (CRI) method and phage-based assays, most of which can be set up directly on specimens [6,7,8]. These methods can detect MTB and resistance to INH and RMP. While MODS, NRA and CRI have been endorsed by the WHO, current evidence was considered to be insufficient for recommending the use of TLA or phage-based assays [8].

MODS is an extensively validated method that has almost perfect agreement with conventional DST for INH, RMP and MDR-TB (100%, 97% and 99%). The results are available within a median of 7 days; the method is cheap, non-commercial and works well on all types of primary specimens as well as on isolates. However, it requires relatively long, detailed staff training. [6,7,9,10]

TLA recently demonstrated a good performance of the MDR-/XDR-TB colour test for the identification of MTB complex and detection of resistance to INH, RMP and ciprofloxacin in cultures [11].

3.2. Genotypic methods

Molecular techniques are aimed at the nucleic acid of the mycobacterium as the analyte. Ribosomal rRNA is useful genetic target for the identification of organisms, since it often contains spesific sequences and is present in the cells and media in high quantity due to the growth of the mycobacteria. There are various applications of molecular tecniques for the detection and identification of MTB.

PCR is the common format of nucleic acid amplification tests (NAAT); other methodologies include ligase chain reaction, strain displacement amplification, loop-mediated isothermal amplifi cation (LAMP) and transcription mediated amplification. More recently, real-time (RT) PCR technologies based on fluorescent- probe detection or melting-curve analysis have been developed [12-16].

These molecular techniques also aimed detecting resistance genes. Example includes; DNA probe and DNA sequencing of MTB gene such as catalase (katG) or RNA polymerase (rpoB). Mutations in these genes have been associated with resistance to isoniazid and rifampicin respectively. The using of molecular primers in real- time PCR reaction can differentiate between the presence of the wild- type sequence and mutated sequence associated with drug resistance. Molecular tests are rapid (within few hours), highly sensitive and specific, but expensive, requires expertise and may not differentiate active infection as DNA from a dead organism during antibiotic treatment can be detected and amplified by PCR [17]. Genotypic methods are not routinely used in the mycobacterium laboratory; they are essentially for research purposes [18,19].

Line-probe assays and XPERT MTB/RIF: Line probe assays (LPAs) are actual molecular tests. Three main LPAs for the rapid diagnosis of TB and/or rapid detection of RMP resistance and MDR-/XDR-TB are currently available on the market: INNO-LiPA Rif. TB (Innogenetics, Belgium), GenoType®MTBDR/MTBDRplus and Geno-Type® MTBDRsl (both Hain Lifescience, Germany). These assays are based on the targeted amplification (PCR) of specific fragments of the MTB genome, followed by hybridisation of PCR products to oligonucleotide probes immobilised on membranes. INNO-LiPA Rif TB detects only RMP resistance, GenoType MTBDR/MTBDRplus detects both RMP and INH resistance, and GenoType MTBDRsldetects resistance to flouroquinolons, injectable second-line drugs and ethambutol. These tests are designed for detection the MTB isolates in respiratory specimens. Xpert® MTB/RIF (Cepheid Inc, USA) is a fully automated RT-PCR based assay for the detection of TB bacteria and resistance to RMP in direct clinical specimens [20].

4. Lysis-centrifugation blood culture system

The recovery of mycobacterium from peripheral blood and bone marrow samples may be improved by lyses- centrifugation blood culture method. In this method, blood is put into a tube containing an anticoagulant and an agent to effect rupture of both erythrocytes and neutrophils. Following centrifugation of the tube, the sediment is inoculated into the appropriate culture media. This method has increased both the yield and shortened the time of recovery of mycobacteria from blood cultures [21].

5. Phage Amplification Technique (PAT)

This is a bacteriophage based test to detect MTB in sputum. Non-pathogenic mycobacteria (sensor cells) were used for control bacteria in the test. The phage replicate, infect and lyses the sensor cells leaving zones of clearing (holes) in the agar. The areas of clearing indicates that the patient sputum contain viable MTB. It is fast with a turnaround time of 2 days. It is cheap, requires few equipments, sensitive (detection as low as 100 tubercles per ml of sputum). It can be adapted for sensitivity testing. Limitations are applicability to sputum specimen only and technically demanding [22].

6. Immunological methods

Immunodiagnostic tests can provide indirect evidence current or past infections of MTB. Exception of tuberculin skin test, immunodiagnostic tests are of limited application due to cross reactivity and poor sensitivity.

6.1. Detection of antibodies

Although the detection of antibodies against MTB in the blood is a relatively simple and costeffective method, recent meta-analyses and systematic reviews concluded that commercial serological tests provided inconsistent results [23,24]. As the overall test performance and data quality of these assays were poor, the WHO currently recommends against their use for the diagnosis of pulmonary and extrapulmonary TB.

Antibodies against lipoarabinomannans, A60, 38Kd and 16 Kd are mostly studied [25].

6.2. Detection of antigens

Lipoarabinomannan (LAM) was identified as a promising target for antigen detection for TB diagnosis due to its temperature stability and could be detected in urine. LAM-based assays are currently being developed by a number of commercial companies, and preliminary results indicate their potential applicability in the rapid diagnosis of TB by detecting LAM in a variety of body fluids, including urine [26]. LAM-based assays are included in the WHO TB diagnosis re-tooling programme [27] and forma part of a Foundation for Innovative New Diagnostics (FIND) funded TB Project [19,28].

MTB antigen detection provides direct evidence of TB. Such as LAM, 65Kd, 14 Kd antigens were widely used. It is very quick and easy to perform. Main limitation is low sensitivity (detect high levels of antibody). It does not rule out TB in patients with poor antibody response as in HIV and malnutrition and not specific due to cross reactivity with other species of mycobacteria in the environment [26].

7. Interferon-Gamma Release Assays (IGRA)

Because of the difficulties with the tuberculin test interpretation, the interferon-gamma assay test was developed. Two available formats of the interferon-gamma release assays are; the Quantiferon-TB Gold and T Spot-TB test. The IGRA assay is based on the ability of the MTB antigens, which includes the Early Secretory Antigen Target 6 (ESAT-6) and Culture Filtrate Protein 10 (CFP-10) to stimulate host production of interferon –gamma. These antigens are not present in NTM or in BCG vaccine, so, these tests can distinguish latent TB infection from BCG immunization and NTM infections. Requiring a single visit to draw a blood sample and result available within 24 hours are main advantages. It does not boost immune response measured by subsequent tests which can happen with tuberculin skin test. It does not cause to readers bias as in tuberculin skin test and not affected by prior BCG vaccination. Blood must be processed within 12 hours while leukocytes are still viable. There are limited data for sensitivity of IGRAs in children younger 17 years of age and immunocompromised patients e.g. HIV/AIDS, diabetics, treatment with immunosuppressive drugs [29].

8. The future of TB diagnostics

The rapid technological evolution in the laboratory diagnosis of TB, especially in the application of molecular biology h as diminished the time required for identification and susceptibility testing. Continuous effort endeavor for increasing reproducibility, improvment of performance and cost containment. WHO founded an organisation (FIND-Foundation for Innovative New Diagnostics) for researching fast, relible and inexpensive tests as given Table 1 [28].

	Concept phase	Feasibility phase	Devolapment phase	Evaluation phase	Demonstration phase	Implementation phase
Reference laboratory level	-	-	-	-	-	Liquid culture & DST Rapid speciation Line probe assay (1st line drugs)
Disrtict/peripheral level	-	Rapid colorimetric DST	-	Line probe assay /2nd line drugs)	LAMP TB	LED florecence microscopy Xpert MTB/RIF
Community level	LFI sensitivity increase	Antibody detection Antigen detection	Beta lactamase detection	-	-	-

LFI sensitivity increase: Alternative quantitative fluorescence (LFI) sensitivity increase

Table 1. WHO projects for TB diagnostic tests. LAMP TB: Loop mediated isothermal amplification (LAMP) for TB

9. Assays being developed/evaluated

Another new approach to diagnosis of TB is biosensing technologies. Variety of portable, rapid, and sensitive biosensors with immediate "on-the-spot" interpretation have been developed for MTB detection based on different biological elements recognition systems and basic signal transducer principles. Combination of nanotechnology and biosensing technology has very promising.

Transrenal DNA detection provides a challenging new target for molecular TB diagnosis. No commercial assays are currently available, largely due to the difficulties in the development of TB detection/read-out assays.

Combined high-resolution melting (HRM) curve analysis using a closed-tube RT-PCR is potentially an ideal screening method with a positive predictive value (PPV) of 100% and negative predictive value (NPV) of at least 99.9%, for screening large specimen numbers in any TB laboratory.

New amplification methodologies and refinements of 'molecular beacon' approaches, such as linear-after-the exponential PCR, offer future improvements, particularly in drug resistance analysis [30-32].

MTB urease is a bacterial virulence factor. Isotopcally labelled urea as substrate, Urea tracer has detected in exaled breath using portable infrared spectrofotometer. Signal correleted with bacterial load. [33]

A biophotonic detection platform has been developed that utilizes reporter enzyme fluorescence to detect β-lactamase produced by MTB. This innovative new technology is now being adapted for point of care (POC) use [28]

10. Conclusions and further work

This is an exciting time for new TB diagnostics. This is in part a reflection of the funding and application of good science, a clear understanding of unmet needs, a commercial sector that is considering new approaches to a global market, and the complexity of and limited progress in new drug and vaccine development, which has encouraged more academic and industrial partners to participate in diagnostic development.

Overall, the technology for the diagnosis of TB and RMP resistance in pulmonary specimens is well advanced, with high specificity and increasingly high sensitivity. Rapid, high-specificity molecular assays for TB identification and drug resistance cannot replace the standard diagnostic methods, such as microbiology, clinical and radiological assessments, and conventional DST for active TB in pulmonary (particularly sputum smear-negative) and extra-pulmonary TB specimens. Implementation of all of these tools in routine laboratory practice requires the implementation of appropriate quality assurance systems.

The performance of molecular tools of extra-pulmonary specimens varies and should be considered separately for each specifi c specimen type. Evidence for the use of these assays to identify TB and detect drug resistance in TB-HIV co-infected individuals is limited. There is a need for designed studies among children, including HIV-positive children. There also remains a need to increase the sensitivity of TB detection among all patients, but especially among immunocompromised patients and children [20].

Author details

Gunes Senol

Infectious Diseases and Clinical Microbiology, Izmir Chest Diseases and Chest Surgery Training Hospital, Izmir, Turkey

References

[1] Dinnes J, Deeks J, Kunst H, Gibson A, Cummins E, Waugh N, et al. A systematic review of rapid diagnostic tests for the detection of tuberculosis infection. Health Technol Assess 2007; 11:1-196.

[2] Lange C, Mori T. Advances in the diagnosis of tuberculosis. Respirology 2010; 15:220-40.

[3] Wallis RS, Pai M, Menzies D, Doherty TM, Walzl G, Perkins MD, et al. Biomarkers and diagnostics for tuberculosis: progress, needs, and translation into practice. Lancet 2010; 375:1920-37.

[4] Minion J, Pai M, Ramsay A, Menzies D, Greenaway C. Comparison of LED and conventional fluorescence microscopy for detection of acid-fast bacilli in a low-incidence setting. PLoS One 2011; 6: e22495

[5] Trusov A, Bumgarner R, Valijev R, et al. Comparison of L umin™ LED fl uorescent attachment, fluorescent microscopy and Ziehl-Neelsen for AFB diagnosis. Int J Tuberc Lung Dis 2009; 13: 836–41.

[6] Bwanga F, Hoffner S, Haile M, Joloba M L. Direct susceptibility testing for multidrug-resistant tuberculosis: a meta-analysis. BMC Infect Dis 2009; 9: 67.

[7] Balabanova Y, Drobniewski F, Nikolayevskyy V, et al. An integrated approach to rapid diagnosis of tuberculosis and multidrug resistance using liquid culture and molecular methods in Russia. PLoS One 2009; 4: e7129.

[8] World Health Organization. Non-commercial culture and drug susceptibility testing methods for screening patients at risk for multidrug-resistant tuberculosis: policy statement. WHO/HTM/TB/2011.9 Geneva, Switzerland: WHO, 2011. http://whqlibdoc. who.int/publications/2011/9789241501620_eng.pdf Accessed February 2012.

[9] Minion J, Leung E, Menzies D, Pai M. Microscopic-observation drug susceptibility and thin layer agar assays for the detection of drug resistant tuberculosis: a systematic review and metaanalysis. Lancet Infect Dis 2010; 10: 688–98.

[10] Leung E, Minion J, Benedetti A, Pai M, Menzies D. Microcolony culture techniques for tuberculosis diagnosis: a systematic review. Int J Tuberc Lung Dis 2012; 16: 16–23, i–iii.

[11] Toit K, Mitchell S, Balabanova Y, Evans C, et al. The colour test for drug susceptibility testing of Mycobacterium tuberculosis strains. Int J Tuberc Lung Dis 2012;16: 1113-8.

[12] Ling D I, Flores L L, Riley L W, Pai M. Commercial nucleic acid amplifi cation tests for diagnosis of pulmonary tuberculosis in respiratory specimens: meta-analysis and meta-regression. PLoS One 2008; 3: e1536.

[13] Nagdev K J, Kashyap R S, Parida M M, et al. Loop-mediated isothermal amplifi cati-on for rapid and reliable diagnosis of tuberculous meningitis. J Clin Microbiol 2011; 49: 1861–5.

[14] Boehme C C, Nabeta P, Hillemann D, et al. Rapid molecular detection of tuberculosis and rifampin resistance. N Engl J Med 2010; 363: 1005–15.

[15] Boehme C C, Nicol M P, Nabeta P, et al. Feasibility, diagnostic accuracy, and effec-tiveness of decentralised use of the Xpert MTB/RIF test for diagnosis of tuberculosis and multidrug resistance: a multicentre implementation study. Lancet 2011;377: 1495–505.

[16] Pietzka A T, Indra A, Stoger A, et al. Rapid identifi cation ofmultidrug-resistant My-cobacterium tuberculosis isolates by rpoB gene scanning using high-resolution melting curve PCR analysis. J Antimicrob Chemother 2009; 63: 1121–7.

[17] Dinnes J, Deek J, Kurnst H, et al. A Systemic Review of Rapid Diagnostic Test for the Detection of Tuberculosis Infection, Health Technol Assess 2007; 11:1-314.

[18] Somoskovi A, Song Q et al. Use of molecular methods to identify the Mycobacterium tuberculosis complex and other mycobacteria species and to detect rifampicin resist-ance in Mycobacterium tuberculosis complex isolates following growth detection with BACTEC MGIT 960 SYSTEM. J Clin Microbiol 2003; 41:2822-6.

[19] Lin S-Y, Probert W, Desmond E. Rapid detection of isoniazid and rifampicin muta-tions in Mycobacterium tuberculosis complex from cultures or smear positive sputa by use of molecular beacon. J Clin Microbial. 2004; 42:4204-8.

[20] Drobniewski F, Nikolayevsky V, Balabanova Y, Bang D, Papaventsis D. Diagnosis of tuberculosis and drug resistance: what can new tools bring us? Int J Tuberc Lung Dis 16:860-70.

[21] Gill VJ, Park CH, Stock F, et al. Use of Lysis-Centrifugation (Isolator) and radiometric (BACTEC) Blood Culture Systems for the Detection of Mycobacteria. J Clin Microbiol 1985; 22:543-6

[22] Washinton W, Stephen A, William J et al. Koneman's Colour Atlas and Textbook of Diagnostic Microbiology; 6th Ed. Lippincott Publishing. 2006; Chapter 19:1066-117

[23] World Health Organization. Commercial serodiagnostic tests for diagnosis of tuber-culosis: policy statement. WHO/HTM/TB/2011.5. Geneva, Switzerland: WHO, 2011.

[24] Steingart K R, Flores L L, Dendukuri N, et al. Commercial serological tests for the di-agnosis of active pulmonary and extra-pulmonary tuberculosis: an updated system-atic review and meta-analysis. PLoS Med 2011; 8: e1001062.

[25] Kunnath-Velayudhan S, Salamon H, Wang H Y, et al. Dynamic antibody responses to the Mycobacterium tuberculosis proteome. Proc Natl Acad Sci USA 2010; 107: 14703–8.

[26] Patel V B, Singh R, Connolly C, et al. Comparison of a clinical prediction rule and a LAM antigen-detection assay for the rapid diagnosis of TBM in a high HIV prevalence setting. PLoS One 2010; 5: e15664

[27] World Health Organization. New technologies for tuberculosis control: a framework for their adoption, introduction andimplementation. WHO/HTM/STB/2007.40. Geneva, Switzerland: WHO, 2007

[28] http://www.finddiagnostics.org/programs/tb/find_activities/index.html

[29] Menzies D, Pai M, Comstock G. Meta analysis: New Tests for the Diagnosis of Latent Tuberculosis Infection: Areas of Uncertainty and Recommendation for Research. Ann Intern Med 2007; 146:340-54.

[30] Green C, Huggett J F, Talbot E, Mwaba P, Reither K, Zumla A I. Rapid diagnosis of tuberculosis through the detection of mycobacterial DNA in urine by nucleic acid amplifi cation methods. Lancet Infect Dis 2009; 9: 505–11.

[31] Chen X, Kong F, Wang Q, Li C, Zhang J, Gilbert G L. Rapid detection of isoniazid, rifampin and ofl oxacin resistance in *Mycobacterium tuberculosis* clinical isolates using high-resolution melting analysis. J Clin Microbiol 2011; 49: 3450–7.

[32] Casali N, Broda A, Rice J, et al. A novel single-tube PCR assay for rapid identification of MDR-TB. London, UK: 22nd European Congress of Clinical Microbiology and Infectious Diseases, 1– 4 April 2012. [Abstract P1919]

[33] Maiga M, Abaza A, Bishai WR. Current tuberculosis diagnostic tools and role ofurease breath test. Ind J Med Res 2012;135: 731-6.

Chapter 10

Diagnostic Evaluation of Tuberculosis

Mochammad Hatta and A. R. Sultan

Additional information is available at the end of the chapter

1. Introduction

Tuberculosis is still one of the leading causes of death by infectious diseases with 2 million deaths per year and 9.2 million new cases of tuberculosis disease annually [1-3]. Besides, more than 2 milliard people are infected with latent tuberculosis infection (LTBI) [1-3]. Despite continuous effort in the prevention, monitoring and treatment of tuberculosis, the disease remains a major health problem in many countries [4-6], particularly in developing countries like Indonesia [7]. National tuberculosis programs and other programs conducted by foreign organizations still fail to eliminate the transmission and incidence of tuberculosis. Transmission is even on the rise in developing countries despite the availability of effective therapies for tuberculosis, whereas the spread and the incidence of tuberculosis in Europe and North America are under control. Several reasons may be responsible for this failure, such us the difficulty of providing adequate anti-tuberculosis medication in many developing countries due to cost issues, the emergence of multi-drug resistant (MDR) strains of *M. tuberculosis*, and the dramatically high co-incidence of tuberculosis in HIV-infected patients [2, 7]. Another important issue is delay of diagnosis due to the lack of a proper method to identify tuberculosis agents [1, 8].

Smear is the cheapest and most widely available detection method for *M. tuberculosis*. In this technique, the diagnosis of tuberculosis is based on identification of acid-fast bacilli (AFB) in a patient's sputum [9, 10]. Many staining techniques are available for AFB smear, the most common one of which is the modified Ziehl-Neelsen stain. Unfortunately, the sensitivity and the specificity of those techniques are low due to difficulty in the identification and differentiation of the various species of *M. tuberculosis* [10]. Two studies found that the AFB smear was positive in only half of patients with subsequent culture positive for *M. tuberculosis* [9, 10]. Another worldwide available detection method is the conventional culture method on

Lowenstein-Jensen (LJ) medium. This method is the gold standard in the identification of M. *tuberculosis* and still serves as the reference method due to its high sensitivity (89%) and specificity (98%) [4, 7, 9, 10]. However, this technique requires equipments or materials that are often unavailable in resource-poor settings. In addition, this technique is time consuming; the results only can be obtained after 6–12 weeks. In addition, the incidence of other bacterial contamination on culture tends to be high [7, 11]. Even a modern culture method such as the BACTEC MGIT 960 culture system, which uses the modified Middlebrook 7H9 broth and a fluorescent signaling system, allows for earlier detection of growth, but still takes at least 10 days to give any result [9].

The goal of tuberculosis control programs is to identify and to cure as many cases as possible; therefore the critical role of early diagnosis is obvious [11]. Under-diagnosis may lead to further spread of the disease because undiagnosed patients can spread the disease unnoticeably [11]. Accurate and early diagnosis is the first important step to effective management. Several new methods for the identification of tuberculosis are available, which including serologic tests and also various molecular methods developed as a result of major advances in understanding the genetic aspects of tuberculosis [8, 9, 11]. Those detection methods can be grouped into two types First, by detection of mycobacteria or its components directly; second by measurement of immunologic responses to mycobacterium infection [9]. In this chapter we present a short review of some these promising detection methods used in the laboratory to identify tuberculosis.

2. Direct detection methods

The genus mycobacterium consists of almost 100 different species, which all appear similar on AFB staining and culture [7, 10, 12]. Many of these can be isolated from humans, although many also can be found in the environment including in animals. It is not easy, however, to distinguish between pathogen and saprophyte species. Each mycobacterium isolate must be evaluated individually regarding its potential to cause a disease; therefore identification of mycobactera is a lengthy and tedious effort. Since the introduction of nucleic acid amplification assays as diagnostic tool for mycobacteria identification, several probes/gene amplification systems for tuberculosis have been developed for rapid and specific identification of M. *tuberculosis* and other mycobacteria [12, 13]. These techniques allow for the confirmation of identity of isolates, direct detection of gene sequences from the clinical specimens and also for molecular detection of drug resistance [12]. Many previous publications have shown the sensitivity and specificity of several molecular detection assays such as BDProbeTec ET, (Becton Dickinson), COBAS AMPLICOR (Roche), Amplified M. *tuberculosis* Direct Test AMTDT (Gen Probe, USA) for identification of mycobacteria[9].

The use of nucleic-acid probe identification systems was a one step ahead in the rapid identification of mycobacterium species of M. *tuberculosis* complex, M. *avium* complex, M.

avium, M. intracellulare, M. kansasii, and *M. gordonae* and also other nontuberculous mycobacteria (NTM) in culture because the result can be obtained after 2 hours [10, 12]. But the sensitivity and specificity of this probe technology will only approximate 100% if there are more than 100 *mycobacteria* present in the sample, except for *M. kansasii* (87%) [12]. Thus, these probes are not sensitive enough to be used directly in clinical specimens like sputum. Also, it still needs to be confirmed by other conventional detection methods such as biochemical test and molecular tests to able to identify the species identity within the *M. tuberculosis* complex, such as for *M. microti, M. bovis, M. bovis of* BCG,, *M. canettii,* and *M. africanum* [10]. There has been extensive research to design an identification system for ribosomal RNA/DNA fingerprinting and for development of probes that targeting specific rRNA, ribosomal DNA, spacer and flanking sequences of various types of mycobacterium species including *M. tuberculosis, M. leprae, M. avium, M. gardonae,* etc [12, 13]. Those rRNA targeting probes are 10-100 fold more sensitive than DNA targeting. However, since the lowest detection limit is still around 100 organisms. it still needs more evaluation before it can be applied to clinical specimens [12].

Several techniques based on polymerase chain reaction (PCR) and isothermal amplification assay have been developed [7-10, 12]. Various researchers have described the rapid detection of *M. tuberculosis* by PCR, and many have reported a high sensitivity in detecting *M. tuberculosis* in clinical samples by means of DNA amplifications [7, 14]. Such techniques involve amplification of specific gene regions followed by hybridization with species specific primers, and also frequently followed by sequencing and or restriction fragment length polymorphism (RFLP) analysis [12]. RFLP is still most widely used in clinical microbiology laboratories due to its simplicity and lower costs than PCR Sequencing [12]. Multiplex PCR has been used to detect *M. tuberculosis* complex bacteria and other mycobacterium. This technique is based on the amplification of the most widely used specific insertion sequences IS6110 and 16S [7-9]. Based on our experience, multiplex PCR has sensitivity up to 81.62% with negative predictive value up to 79.51% [7]. Nevertheless, taking into account the "simple and economical" issue this technique is probably not suited for most of the countries with a high tuberculosis burden [11]. Other rapid molecular amplification detection method which is being used in our laboratory is multiplex PCR-reverse cross blot hybridization, which can be modified to identify multiple species of mycobacteria at one time by using a specific probe for each species. Compared to the culture and microscopic method, this technique had a sensitivity of 86.03%, negative predictive value of 82.41% and it can be applied to detect NTM [7]. The multiplex PCR reverse cross blot hybridization technique is more complicated than conventional multiplex PCR; but it can detect considerably more NTM species such as *M. avium, M. intracellulare, M. kansasii, M. fortuitum, M. chelonae, M. genavense and M. smegmatis* (Fig. 1) [7].

In term of accuracy and duration time that it needs to get a result, Raman spectroscopy is one of the most promising techniques. This vibrational spectroscopy-based detection method can detect and differentiate various molecular compositions of microorganism [15-18] and therefore is suitable to identify the species and strains of microorganism. Buijtels et al., demonstrated that Raman spectroscopy differentiated between *M. tuberculosis* with NTM with accuracy up to 100% and with 92.5% correct species identification. This technique is also are much faster; results can be obtained within 3 hours since positive automated cultured system is obtained [18]. In view of the importance of early diagnosis to prevent further spread of tuberculosis in the community, this time efficiency is the most significant contribution of Raman spectroscopy.

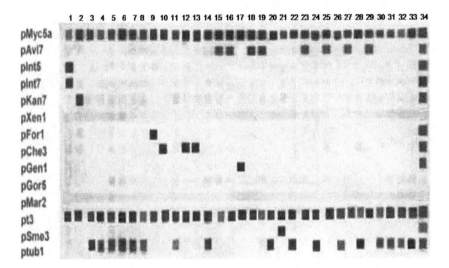

Figure 1. Multiplex PCR reverse cross blot hybridization assay is able to detect various species of mycobacteria simultaneously. Each column (Col) represents certain species of mycobacteria; Col 1, *M. intracellulare*; Col 2, *M. kansasii* ; Col 3-8, 11, 14, 20, 22, 24, 26, 28, 30-33, *M. tuberculosis*; Col 9, *M. fortuitum*; Col 10, 12, 13, *M. chelonae*; Col 15, 16, 18, 19, 23, 25, 27, 29, *M. avium*; Col 17, *M. genavense*; Col 21, *M. smegmatis* ; 34, pool PCR product of mycobacteria. [7]

3. Indirect detection methods

Even those remarkable molecular detection methods are not yet up to the mark when it comes to in the identification of tuberculosis, particularly latent tuberculosis infection (LTBI). Approximately 2 milliard people are silent tuberculosis patients, i.e. they have been infected by *M. tuberculosis* but show no tuberculosis symptoms [1, 2]. LTBI has been defined by evidence of a cellular immune response to *M. tuberculosis* derived antigens. It may be the result of incomplete elimination of *M. tuberculosis* by the host's adaptive immune system, resulting in asymptomatic infection with almost undetectable bacilli [2]. Thus, the diagnosis of LTBI currently depends on detecting the host's immune response to the infection [2]. Affected individuals have little risk of progression from LTBI to active tuberculosis, but any disruption of their cellular immunity – such as in HIV co-infection cases – can considerably increase this risk [2]. Currently, the diagnosis of LTBI is commonly made with the tuberculosis skin test (TST), which is based on the delayed hypersensitivity to purified protein derivative (PPD). Unfortunately, patients sensitized to environmental nontuberculous mycobacteria or patients vaccinated with the bacillus Calmette–Guérin (BCG) vaccine may have a false positive result. On the other hand, a false negative result may occur in immunosuppressed patients and also in children [2]. This immunologic response is often not conclusive as antibodies and delayed type hypersensitivity response persist long after infection or after the diseases has disappeared [12]

Interferon Gamma Release Assays (IGRAs) have been introduced in the clinical setting for the diagnosis of LTBI [19-21]. These more specific whole-blood tests are based on the principle of measuring host interferon-y (IFN-y) released by T-cells specific to *M. tuberculosis* as a marker. IFN-y is stimulated by *early secretory antigen target 6* (ESAT-6) and *culture filtrate protein 10* (CFP-10). These are not present in the BCG or in the most of the NTM [2]. There are two types of IGRAs: The enzyme-linked immunospot assay (ELISpot)-based IGRA, where individual IFN-y producing T-cells responding to *M. tuberculosis* antigens stimulation are counted [22], and the QuantiFERON-TB Gold In-Tube test, an ELISA-based IGRA where the IFN-y produced by those T-cells is measured after stimulation with *M. tuberculosis* antigens [2]. Pai et al. showed that the sensitivity of the ELISpot and ELISA-based approach was around 90% and 70%, respectively, and that the specificity of both was 93% [2, 20]. As there is still no gold standard for the diagnosis of LTBI, these assays potentially may serve as routine diagnosis test other than TST to identify people with LTBI [2].

Cytokine-based detection methods could be useful not only in the detection of LTBI cases but also of active tuberculosis cases. However, considering the high number of LTBI in the community, a single cytokine identification method such as IGRAs is not sufficient to detect active tuberculosis. For this reason the identification of multiple tuberculosis biomarkers-cytokines seems to be a promising strategy. Several studies have shown the potential usefulness of TNA-a, IL-2, IP-10, MIG along with IF-g simultaneously [23-26]. Using a multiplex microbead-based assay, Wang et al. showed significant differences in expression of these cytokines/chemokines between active tuberculosis patients and healthy controls. Regarding active pulmonary tuberculosis the sensitivity of IFN-y, IP-10 and MIG was 75.3% and the specificity was 89.7%. They also demonstrated the potential usefulness of this multiplex microbead-based assay for the detection of new tuberculosis cases by documenting a sensitivity of 96.3% [23].

Untill now, smear and culture methods are still the gold standard to detect mycobacteria. Based on our experience, combination of conventional and advanced detection methods would greatly improve the sensitivity and specificity of the assays. Detection of the *mycobacteria* species are quite difficult with culture, therefore we using multiplex PCR as the first confirmation assay to detect the species while it also as confirmation test for negative results from either smear or culture assay. Hence, to overcome the limitation of multiplex PCR in species detection, multiplex PCR- reverse cross blot hybridization assay would further expand the range of *mycobacteria* species detection (Fig. 2).

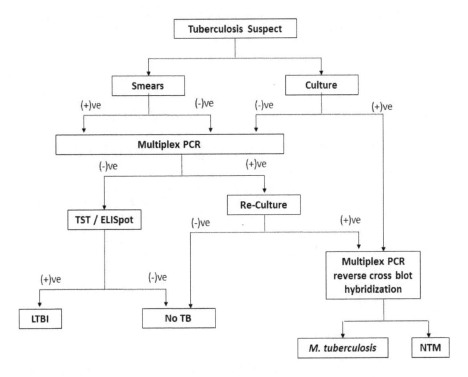

Figure 2. Microbiologic diagnosis of tuberculosis. Multiplex PCR are used to confirm smears results and negative result of culture assay. Patients with negative multiplex PCR result would be proceed for ELISpot or Tuberculin skin test (TST) to detect latent tuberculosis (LTBI), while specimen from patient with positive culture result would get final confirmation by Multiplex PCR reverse cross blot hybridization assay to further detect the mycobacterium species

4. Conclusion

Conventional methods for the diagnosis of tuberculosis, such as the smear and culture methods have some limitations, particularly the low specificity and sensitivity as well as the time-consuming nature. Now these limitations have been overcome in some novel and rapid detection methods. Various gene amplification techniques have demonstrated their usefulness in the identification of mycobacteria and its various species. The rapid detection of *M. tuberculosis* by probes, PCR or other molecular techniques and some newest serologic assays offer good opportunities to improve the diagnosis and therapy of tuberculosis [2, 7-9, 12, 13].

However despite the availability of diagnostic tools for laboratory identification of tuberculosis at high sensitivity and specificity, the "simple and economically" aspect of those new methods is still a matter of consideration. The question is whether they can be used in simple clinical settings and whether they are economically affordable for developing countries, in most of which tuberculosis is still rampant [11].

Summary

Tuberculosis still remains a major health problem in many developing countries, despite continuous long-standing vaccination and surveillance programs, and worldwide availability of effective anti-tuberculosis drugs. Early detection is of major importance in the control of tuberculosis. The emergence of multidrug resistant *Mycobacterium tuberculosis* and the association of HIV with tuberculosis outbreaks in community both illustrate that rapid diagnosis is essential. Therefore, a fast and reliable diagnosis of tuberculosis would greatly improve the control of the tuberculosis. Regrettably, current conventional laboratory diagnostic methods of tuberculosis are still time-consuming. The rapid development of novel diagnostic methods for the identification of mycobacteria and its species bring new hope, however, for the diagnosis and management this infectious disease. Meanwhile those techniques still seem to clash with simplicity and economically affordable issues.

Author details

Mochammad Hatta and A. R. Sultan

Departments of Medical Microbiology, Molecular Biology and Immunology Laboratory, Faculty of Medicine, Hasanuddin University, Makassar, Indonesia

References

[1] Jain, S. K, Lamichhane, G, Nimmagadda, S, Pomper, M. G, & Bishai, W. R. Antibiotic treatment of tuberculosis: old problem, new solution. Microbe (2008).

[2] Connell, D. W, Berry, M, & Cooke, G. Kon OM: Update on tuberculosis: TB in the early 21st century. Eur Respir Rev (2011).

[3] Nhlema Simwaka B. Benson T, Salaniponi FM, Theobald SJ, Squire SB, Kemp JR: Developing a socio-economic measure to monitor access to tuberculosis services in urban Lilongwe, Malawi. Int J Tuberc Lung Dis (2007).

[4] Golub, J. E, Mohan, C. I, & Comstock, G. W. Chaisson RE: Active case finding of tuberculosis: historical perspective and future prospects. Int J Tuberc Lung Dis (2005).

[5] Caminero JA: Multidrug-resistant tuberculosis: epidemiologyrisk factors and case finding. Int J Tuberc Lung Dis (2010).

[6] Jassal, M. S. Bishai WR: Epidemiology and challenges to the elimination of global tuberculosis. Clin Infect Dis (2010). Suppl 3:S, 156-164.

[7] Hatta, M, Sultan, A. R, & Tandirogang, N. Masjudi, Yadi: Detection and identification of mycobacteria in sputum from suspected tuberculosis patients. BMC Res Notes (2010).

[8] Raza, S. T, Ali, G, Hasan, S, & Mahdi, F. Molecular diagnosis of tuberculosis: a new primer design. Iranian Journal of clinical infectious diseases (2009).

[9] Yam WC: Recent advadces in rapid laboratory diagnosis of tuberculosis. The Hongkong Medical Diary (2006).

[10] Hale, Y. M, & Pfyffer, G. E. Salfinger M: Laboratory diagnosis of mycobacterial infections: new tools and lessons learned. Clin Infect Dis (2001).

[11] Walker D: Economic analysis of tuberculosis diagnostic tests in disease control: how can it be modelled and what additional information is needed? Int J Tuberc Lung Dis (2001).

[12] Katoch VM: Advances in Molecular Diagnosis of Tuberculosis. MJAFI (2003).

[13] Kaminski, D. A. Hardy DJ: Selective utilization of DNA probes for identification of Mycobacterium species on the basis of cord formation in primary BACTEC 12B cultures. J Clin Microbiol (1995).

[14] Kox, L. F, Noordhoek, G. T, Kunakorn, M, Mulder, S, & Sterrenburg, M. Kolk AH: Microwell hybridization assay for detection of PCR products from Mycobacterium tuberculosis complex and the recombinant Mycobacterium smegmatis strain 1008 used as an internal control. J Clin Microbiol (1996).

[15] Ibelings, M. S, Maquelin, K, Endtz, H. P, & Bruining, H. A. Puppels GJ: Rapid identification of Candida spp. in peritonitis patients by Raman spectroscopy. Clin Microbiol Infect (2005).

[16] Kirschner, P. Bottger EC: Species identification of mycobacteria using rDNA sequencing. Methods Mol Biol (1998).

[17] Maquelin, K, Dijkshoorn, L, & Van Der Reijden, T. J. Puppels GJ: Rapid epidemiological analysis of Acinetobacter strains by Raman spectroscopy. J Microbiol Methods (2006).

[18] Buijtels, P. C, Willemse-erix, H. F, Petit, P. L, Endtz, H. P, Puppels, G. J, Verbrugh, H. A, Van Belkum, A, & Van Soolingen, D. Maquelin K: Rapid identification of mycobacteria by Raman spectroscopy. J Clin Microbiol (2008).

[19] Ewer, K, Deeks, J, Alvarez, L, Bryant, G, Waller, S, Andersen, P, & Monk, P. Lalvani A: Comparison of T-cell-based assay with tuberculin skin test for diagnosis of Mycobacterium tuberculosis infection in a school tuberculosis outbreak. Lancet (2003).

[20] Pai, M, & Zwerling, A. Menzies D: Systematic review: T-cell-based assays for the diagnosis of latent tuberculosis infection: an update. Ann Intern Med (2008).

[21] Lalvani, A. Pareek M: Interferon gamma release assays: principles and practice. En-
ferm Infecc Microbiol Clin (2010).

[22] Lalvani A: Spotting latent infection: the path to better tuberculosis controlThorax
(2003).

[23] Wang, X, Jiang, J, Cao, Z, Yang, B, & Zhang, J. Cheng X: Diagnostic performance of
multiplex cytokine and chemokine assay for tuberculosis. Tuberculosis (Edinb)
(2012).

[24] Harari, A, Rozot, V, Enders, F. B, Perreau, M, Stalder, J. M, Nicod, L. P, Cavassini, M,
Calandra, T, Blanchet, C. L, Jaton, K, et al. Dominant TNF-alpha+ Mycobacterium tuberculosis-specific CD4+ T cell responses discriminate between latent infection and
active disease. Nat Med (2011).

[25] Krummel, B, Strassburg, A, Ernst, M, Reiling, N, Eker, B, Rath, H, Hoerster, R, Wap-
pler, W, Glaewe, A, Schoellhorn, V, et al. Potential role for IL-2 ELISpot in differenti-
ating recent and remote infection in tuberculosis contact tracing. PLoS One (2010).
e11670.

[26] Ruhwald, M, Dominguez, J, Latorre, I, Losi, M, Richeldi, L, Pasticci, M. B, Mazzolla,
R, Goletti, D, Butera, O, Bruchfeld, J, et al. A multicentre evaluation of the accuracy
and performance of IP-10 for the diagnosis of infection with M. tuberculosis. Tuberculosis (Edinb) (2011).

Multi-Drug Resistant Tuberculosis

Chapter 11

Management of Drug-Resistant TB

Zakaria Hmama

Additional information is available at the end of the chapter

1. Introduction

Although major progress has been made to reduce global incidence of drug-susceptible tuberculosis (TB), the emergence of multidrug-resistant (MDR) and extensively drug-resistant (XDR) TB over the past decade presents an unprecedented public health challenge to which countries of concern are responding far too slowly. Indeed, a recent WHO TB surveillance report indicates the highest global level of drug-resistance ever recorded, which affected disproportionately developing countries with an estimated 440,000 MDR-TB cases worldwide resulting in 150,000 deaths in 2009 [1]. Even more troubling is being the recent emergence of new strains of totally drug-resistant *M. tuberculosis* (Mtb), currently occurring in densely populated cities such as Teheran (Iran) [2] and Mumbai (India) [3]. Given that an untreated TB patient can infect up to 15 contacts in a year in overcrowded areas [4], it is highly likely that totally drug-resistant TB will continues spreading and one would worry that TB will again become an incurable disease.

While part of the increase in drug resistance can be attributed to difficulty in treating patients who are double infected with HIV, which represent about 13% of total TB cases [5], detailed field studies revealed that the emergence drug-resistant TB is clearly a direct consequence of misdiagnosis and mismanagement of drug susceptible TB, which result in only a fraction of TB patients getting correct diagnosis and appropriate therapy ([6,7] and Fig.1). In other words, "Resistance is man-made, caused by exposure to the wrong treatment, the wrong regimen, the wrong treatment duration" says TB expert Giovanni Miglio [8]. Therefore, a comprehensive approach to ensure rapid detection, proper treatment and public health measures needs to be applied globally to cure TB patients and prevent further transmission of the disease. This chapter discusses various challenges facing the management of drug resistant TB and presents the efforts of WHO and its partners for the development of strategies and guidelines for optimal TB control.

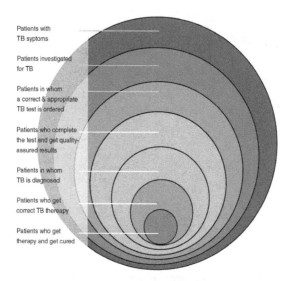

Patients with
TB syptoms

Patients investigated
for TB

Patients in whom
a correct & appropriate
TB test is ordered

Patients who complete
the test and get quality-
assured results

Patients in whom
TB is diagnosed

Patients who get
correct TB therapy

Patients who get
therapy and get cured

Figure 1. Misdiagnosis and mismanagement can result in only fraction of TB patients getting correct diagnosis, appropriate therapy, and positive outcomes. Reprinted from Ref. 9 with permission from Dr. Madhukar Pai.

2. Standard treatment for drug-susceptible TB

Symptoms associated with active TB are generally defined as loss of weight and energy, poor appetite, fever, a productive cough, and night sweats. Although highly suggestive of TB, such symptoms might easily be assigned to another disease. Therefore accurate diagnosis is important before initiating drug therapy. The current standard laboratory test consists on the analysis of 3 sputum specimens for acid-fast bacilli smears and culture, with nucleic acid amplification performed on at least 1 specimen [10].

In 1994, the WHO introduced the DOTS (Directly Observed Treatment, Short-course) as a major plan to control TB globally [11]. The DOTS strategy focuses on five main points of action: 1) government commitment to control TB, 2) diagnosis based on sputum-smear microscopy tests done on patients with TB symptoms, 3) direct observation short-course chemotherapy treatments, 4) a continuous supply of drugs, and 5) standardized reporting and recording of cases and treatment outcomes [11]. The standard short course (SSC) treatment recommended by WHO [12] consists of 2 months of intensive phase of daily oral administration of isoniazid (INH), rifampicin (RMP), pyrazinamide (PZA) and ethambutol (EMB) followed by 4 months continuous phase of daily INH and RMP alone.

INH is only active against growing tubercle bacilli [13]. RMP is active against both growing and stationary phase bacilli with low metabolic activity and is associated with high sterilizing activity *in vivo* [14]. PZA plays a unique role in shortening TB treatment from the previous 12 months to 6 months because it kills the persistent Mtb population in the lung [15]. EMB is active against growing Mtb but has no effect on dormant bacilli. The combination of drugs acting at different stages of the Mtb life cycle during SSC therapy has been successful in TB treatment in most endemic countries when patients adhere to a fairly strict daily regimen. SSC therapy causes minor or no side effects and is affordable, costing less than $40 for a full course of treatment. Side effects, if they occur, are manageable and usually do not result in the interruption of the treatment.

Aproximately 90% of people infected with Mtb develop an efficient immune response that successfully contains the infection but unfortunately without killing all the bacteria. Surviving bacteria persist in the lung as non-replicative (i.e. dormant) organisms [16]. In this stage of latent TB infection (LTBI), people do not exhibit TB symptoms and cannot pass the infection on to other individuals. However, in weakened immune system conditions (old age, HIV infection or therapeutic immunosupression), dormant bacteria revert into dividing organisms leading to TB reactivation [16].

LTBI is highly suspected in individuals previously exposed to those with known active TB, which would include people in hospitals, homeless shelters and prisons, or people having recently traveled to countries where TB is highly endemic. The stage of clinical latency is of surpassing importance for TB control as most cases of active TB arise from the vast reservoir of the latently infected population [17]. In fact, it estimated that the infection reactivates and cause active TB in approximately 5 to 10% of latently infected persons [18].

Purified protein derivative (PPD) skin test (also known as the Mantoux test) is the major diagnostic tool used to identify LTBI patients. A positive skin reaction to the PPD test reflects a local cellular immune response, which is interpreted as recent or remote exposure to the TB bacterium. However, despite its usefulness and simplicity, the PPD test have a low predictive value since false-positive reactions can occur as a result of previous BCG vaccination or sensitization to environmental mycobacteria [19,20,21]. In fact, the skin test uses a crude mix of Mtb antigens shared among many mycobacterial species. As a replacement for the PPD test, new interferon-gamma release assays (IGRAs) have been recently developed and shown to be more accurate for LTB diagnosis [22]. IGRAs measure *ex-vivo* production of IFN-gamma by circulating T cells in whole blood in response to more specific Mtb antigens such as ESAT6, CFP10 and TB7.7.

Although LTBI is symptom-free and non contagious, many countries have adopted its treatment in order to reduce the risk of infection progression to active TB and the spread of the disease to the general population. Six to 9 month treatment with INH alone was proven to be effective and safe [10]. Unfortunately, if LTBI results from exposure to a person with MDR- or TB XDR-TB, preventive treatment options are very limited or may not be possible. In both active and latent TB cases, it is crucial that health care providers make every effort to ensure that infected persons complete the entire course of treatment. They must explain clearly the benefit of the treatment and also possible side effects (or drug interactions). Additionally, They should identify potential barriers to the course of treatment, which will help to establish an efficient plan to ensure adherence.

Understanding the mechanisms of TB latency is crucial to development of better control strategies. Infection with Mtb occurs initially in alveolar macrophage, in which the bacteria replicate and induce cytokines that initiate the inflammatory response in the lungs, leading ultimately to the formation of granuloma [23]. Granuloma is defined as an immune structure consisting of connective tissue, lymphocytes and activated macrophages, which has a central necrotic core containing extracellular bacteria. Within the granuloma the bacterium is exposed to multiple stresses that include, among others, hypoxic, nutrient limiting, oxidative, nitrosative and acidic conditions [24,25], which trigger a genetic program controlled by the transcription factor DosR [25]. The later regulates the development of a quiescent physiological state, which maintains viability of non-dividing bacteria for extended periods of time. The granuloma contains the infection and prevents its spread to other organs [26]. However, dormant bacteria are capable of reactivation controlled by Rpf (resuscitation promoting factor) genes, which is associated with reversal of the non-replicating state into a metabolically active growing and dividing bacteria [27]. Thus, life-long immunity is not gained by a first episode of active TB disease and the disease may develop again at a later stage, either through relapse with the same strain or reinfection with a new strain.

Deciphering the molecular basis of dormancy and reactivation is therefore necessary for developing more efficient TB therapies. Adjuncts of agents that would block transitions between active growth, dormancy, and resuscitation or kill effectively dormant bacteria can significantly enhance the efficacy of current treatments for latent infection. Such agents would also shorten the treatment duration of active TB.

3. Molecular basis of Mtb resistance to SSC drugs

The frequency of spontaneous mutations that confer resistance to an individual TB drugs *in vitro* are well known and vary from 1 in 10^5 (EMB) to 1 in 10^{10} (RMP) [28].

Resistance to INH: INH is a drug precursor that is activated by Mtb catalase-peroxidase enzyme (KatG) to generate a range of highly reactive species [29]. Active INH targets essentially enoylacyl carrier protein reductase (InhA enzyme), which is involved in mycolic acid synthesis [29]. Resistance to INH occurs more frequently than for most anti-TB drugs, at a frequency of 1 in 10^6 bacilli *in vitro* [13]. Clinical isolates of INH-resistant Mtb often lose catalase and peroxidase activities due to KatG S315T mutation [30]. Resistance to INH can also occur through mutations in the promoter region of *inhA*, causing overexpression of InhA, or by mutations at the InhA active site, lowering InhA affinity for INH [31]. *katG* mutation can be associated with *inhA* mutations, leading to higher levels of INH resistance [32].

Resistance to RMP: RMP interferes with RNA synthesis by binding to the β subunit of mycobacterial RNA polymerase, which is encoded by *rpoB*. Mtb resistance to RMP occurs at a frequency of 10^{-7} to 10^{-8} as a result of mutations in *rpoB*. Mutations at positions 531, 526 and 516 in *rpoB* are among the most frequent (96%) in RMP-resistant strains [33].

Resistance to PZA: PZA requires conversion to its active form, pyrazinoic acid (POA), by the pyrazinamidase/nicotinamidase enzyme encoded by Mtb *pncA*, which then permeates through the membrane, disrupts bacterial membrane potential and affects membrane transport [34]. PZA resistance is linked to defective pyrazinamidase/nicotinamidase activity, which results from mutations that might occur at different regions (3-17, 61-85 and 132-142) of *pncA* [34]. While most PZA-resistant strains (72–97%) have *pncA* mutations, some do not have *pncA* mutations but rather express defective pyrazinamidase/nicotinamidase activity [13], which suggests possible mutations in a putative *pncA* regulatory gene, yet to be identified.

Resistance to EMB: Arabinosyl transferase, encoded by *embB*, an enzyme involved in the synthesis of cell wall arabinogalactan, has been proposed as the target of EMB in Mtb [35]. Mutation to EMB resistance occurs at a frequency of 10^{-5} [13]. The *embB* codon 306 mutation account for only 68% EMB resistant strains [36], suggesting that there may be other mechanisms of EMB resistance. Therefore, further studies are needed to identify potential new mechanisms of EMB resistance.

Because the mutations described above are unlinked, the probability of developing bacillary resistance to 4 drugs used simultaneously is unlikely. Clinical drug-resistant TB is definitely the result of genetic mutation amplification through mismanagement of the TB disease. This includes intermittent therapy due to irregular drug supply, inappropriate drug prescriptions and most importantly poor patient adherence to treatment [37]. Sequential accumulation of mutations in different genes involved in individual drug resistance results in the emergence of multiple drug resistance.

4. Diagnosis of multidrug resistant tuberculosis

Conventional culturing of the etiologic agent combined with drug susceptibility testing (DST) is the 'gold standard' for diagnosing drug resistant TB in order to initiate adequate treatment. However, this approach is rarely used because it requires 3 to 4 months to produce results. Indeed, only 7% of all MDR-TB cases are detected globally [1]. Hence, the deficiency in tools for rapid DST is associated with inadequate treatment regimens, which tragically increase transmission and spread of drug resistant TB, especially in HIV-infected individuals [38]. This alarming situation stimulated the development of a great number of rapid culture- and molecular-based methods that are currently being evaluated in TB diagnosis laboratories. The Nitrate Reductase Assay (NRA) is based on detection of nitrate reduction into nitrite by Mtb organisms capable of growth in the presence of the test antibiotic [39]. Whereas the Microscopic Observation of Drug Susceptibility (MODS) uses inverted microscope to detect the formation of cord-like structure by Mtb isolates resistant to the test drug [40]. The commercial Mycobacterium Growth Indicator Tube 960 (MGIT 960) is a drug-containing culture system based on the fluorescence detection of resistant bacteria [41]. The Genotype MTBDR*plus* is a molecular line-probe assay that detects simultaneously mutations in the rpoB gene that confers resistance to RMP as well as mutations in the katG gene and the inhA promoter, which are associated with resistance to INH [42]. The Alamar blue and resazurin assays are liquid-based colorimetric tests [43]; a color change in wells containing drug-exposed bacteria reflects resistance. The MTT assay relays on the ability of drug-resistant (viable) bacteria to cleave the tetrazolium rings of MTT, which produces a violet-purple color [44]. Many of these assays gave excellent detection of MDR-TB, within a significantly shorter time frame when compared to conventional culturing methods (Table 1).

The effective implementation of these rapid diagnostic tests for TB and drug resistance will increase the proportion of patients promptly placed on appropriate therapy, and therefore will improve substantially management and control of TB disease globally. However a major limitation to the use of these rapid tests is their affordability and the availability of equipped laboratories in resource-constrained countries, which unfortunately tend to have the highest burden of MDR-TB cases. Thus, global initiatives are needed to make new diagnostics accessible to low-income countries.

	MTBDRplus	MODS	NRA	AB	Resazurin	MTT	MGIT 960	LJPM
Average time to results, days	2	7	7	8	8	8	9	30
Results within 8 days, %	100	90	77	87	87	74	42	-
Results within 10 days, %	100	100	100	100	97	87	81	-

MODS = microscopic observation drug susceptibility; NRA = nitrate reductase assay; AB =Alamar Bbue ; MTT = 3-[4,5-dimethyl- thiazol-2-yl)-2,5-diphenyltetrazolium bromide; MGIT = Mycobacterium Growth Indicator Tube; LJPM = Löwenstein-Jensen proportion method.

Table 1. Time to results and percentage of results obtained within 8 and 10 days. Reprinted from Ref. 45 with permission of the International Union Against Tuberculosis and Lung Disease. Copyright © The Union.

5. Treatment of drug-resistant TB

The emergence of MDR- and XDR-TB has shattered the initial optimism that DOTS based programmes would progressively eliminate TB. MDR TB is defined as resistance to at least the two most potent first-line TB drugs—ie, INH and RMP [46,47]. XDR TB strains are resistant to INH or RMP, any fluoroquinolone, and at least one of three second-line injectable drugs—ie, capreomycin, kanamycin, and amikacin [46,47]. In order to control the spread of drug resistant TB, the WHO extended the DOTS programme in 1998 to include the treatment of MDR-TB (called "DOTS-Plus") [48]. Implementation of DOTS-Plus requires the capacity to perform drug-susceptibility testing and the availability of second-line agents, in addition to all the requirements for DOTS. Clinical pilot experiences from the past few years showed that high cure rates of drug resistant TB are achieved in settings where DOTS-Plus has been established [49-51].

Resistance to INH is the most common form of TB drug resistance reported, either in isolation or in combination with other drugs [13]. INH monoresistant TB is relatively easy to treat with SCC treatment. Up to 98% cure and less than 5% relapse can be achieved when all four drugs

INH, RMP, PZA and EMB are used during the 6-month treatment period [52]. RMP-resistant TB often carries a much more ominous prognosis, as the outcome of SCC treatment is poor in terms of both disease status at the end of the treatment and relapse [13]. Moreover, RMP monoresistance in Mtb is rare and usually reflects resistance to INH as well, i.e., MDR-TB [53]. In fact, SCC cures less than 60% of MDR-TB, with a recurrence rate of about 28% among patient with apparent success [38,54].

The current recommendation for individualized treatment regimens is a combination of at least four drugs to which the Mtb isolate is likely to be susceptible [55]. Drugs are chosen with a stepwise selection process through 5 groups of TB drugs (Table 2) on the basis of efficacy and safety [55]. More than 5 drugs can be used if the sensitivity to a given drug is unclear or if the regimen contains few bactericidal drugs. The duration of the intensive phase of treatment (when an injectable drug is given) should be at least 6 months (or 4 months after culture conversion). The continuation phase (without the injectable drug) should last until 18 months after culture conversion [55].

Although the effectiveness and feasibility of MDR-TB management in resource-limited settings have been demonstrated, less than 2% of all estimated MDR-TB patients currently receive appropriate treatment [5]. Thus, the growing MDR-TB epidemic globally requires moving beyond the pilot project stage in order to scale up DOTS-plus based TB management as a routine component of national TB control programmes. However, there are potential difficulties with implementing DOTS-Plus in low-income countries as it can absorb a large part of resources dedicated to existing DOTS programmes, and subsequently decrease the overall standard of care [56]. Note that the emergence of drug resistant TB in these countries is actually the result of limited resources to implement the simple DOTS programme.

A major barrier to the management of drug resistant TB in low-income countries is the prohibitive price of second-line drugs. Therefore in an attempt to address this issue, in 2000, the WHO and its partners established the Green Light Committee (GLC) initiative to facilitate access to quality-assured second-line TB drugs at reduced prices [57,58]. Evaluation of the first GLC-endorsed pilot projects of MDR-TB management in five resource-limited countries showed treatment success rates of 59%–83% [59]. During 2012, the number of patients with MDR-TB approved for treatment by the GLC Committee was only 42,033 with 13,000 actually starting treatment. It is clear that these numbers remain small compared to the estimated annual incidence (440,000 cases) of MDR-TB [1]. Therefore, substantial funding through public-private partnerships is desperately needed to scale up the availability of second line drugs.

Other than the price of second-line drugs, frequent adverse events and the long duration of the regimen further compromise adherence to TB treatment, even in the most advanced industrialized countries. These drawbacks have resulted in resurgence in research efforts during last decade to develop new TB drugs. In recent years, a number of new drug candidates with novel modes of action and excellent activity against Mtb have entered clinical trials [60]. OPC-67683 (nitro-dihydro-imidazooxazole) and diarylquinoline TMC207 are the most promising of these new drugs since both are highly active against drug-resistant and susceptible Mtb strains and possess excellent sterilizing activity [61]. These and other drugs under

TB drug group	Daily dose
Group one: first-line oral TB drugs (use all possible drugs)	
Isoniazid	5 mg/kg
Rifampicin	10 mg/kg
Ethambutol	15–25 mg/kg
Pyrazinamide	30 mg/kg
Group two: fluoroquinolones (use only one, because they share genetic targets)	
Ofloxacin	15 mg/kg
Levofloxacin	15 mg/kg
Moxifloxacin	7.5–10 mg/kg
Group three: injectable TB drugs (use only one, because they share very similar genetic targets)	
Streptomycin	15 mg/kg
Kanamycin	15 mg/kg
Amikacin	15 mg/kg
Capreomycin	15 mg/kg
Group four: less-effective second-line TB drugs (use all possible drugs if necessary)	
Ethionamide/Prothionamide	15 mg/kg
Cycloserine/Terizidone	15 mg/kg
P-aminosalicylic acid (acid salt)	150 mg/kg
Group five: less-effective drugs or drugs on which clinical data are sparse (use all necessary drugs if there are less ily than four from the other groups)	
Clofazimine	100 mg
Amoxicillin with clavulanate (every 12 h)	875/125 mg
Linezolid	600 mg
Imipenem (every 6 h)	500–1000 mg
Clarithromycin (every 12 h)	500 mg
High-dose isoniazid	10–15 mg/kg
Thioacetazone	150 mg

Table 2. Categories of TB drugs. Reprinted from Ref. 55 with permission of the International Union Against Tuberculosis and Lung Disease. Copyright © The Union

development give hope that a safe and effective TB regimen of shorter duration will be available within the next few years.

6. Adverse drug reactions to second line TB drugs

The treatment of MDR-TB is a challenging issue due to the adverse events associated with long-term exposure (18 to 24 months) to second line drugs, all in great contrast to the short treatment period of drug sensitive TB. Adverse events significantly influence treatment outcome and patient compliance, leading to acquisition of more resistance and spread of drug-resistant strains. Initial evidence of the prevalence of adverse events associated with the use of second-line drugs was deducted from observation of patients enrolled in five DOTS-Plus sites: Estonia, Latvia, Peru, the Philippines and the Russian Federation. The data collected from these sites showed that among 818 patients enrolled on MDR-TB 30% required removal of suspected drugs from the regimen due to adverse events [62] and Table 3.

Adverse events can be distinguished as major or minor and may not be consistently found among all patients treated for MDR-TB [39]. The major adverse events associated with second line drugs include auditory toxicity (ototoxicity) and neurologic side effects [63].

Ototoxicity causes damage to the outer hair cells in the cochlea and vestibular labyrinth leading to permanent hearing loss. Ototoxic hearing loss is common in patients treated with amino-glycosides (Streptomycin, Kanamycin and Amikacin). A prospective cohort study of the incidence of ototoxicity in MDR-TB individuals (with normal hearing) showed that 57% of aminoglycoside-treated patients developed high-frequency of hearing loss [64]. The same study showed that HIV-positive patients (70%) were more likely to develop hearing loss than HIV-negative patients (42%). Susceptibility to hearing loss increases further in patients bearing mutations in mitochondrial genes [65]. Numerous mutations linked to susceptibility to ototoxicity have been identified in the mitochondrial MT-RNR1 gene that encodes the human 12S rRNA ribosomal subunit. In particular, the A1555G mutation causes increased binding of aminoglycosides to the 12S rRNA ribosomal subunit [66], which results in the disruption of mitochondrial protein synthesis and death of the cell. In this regard, a recent study in South Africa detected A1555G mutation in a significant proportion of the population (0.9% of Black and 1.1% of Afrikaner), indicative of high proportion of individuals genetically predisposed to developing aminoglycoside-induced hearing loss. It is unfortunate that the widespread and poorly controlled use of aminoglycosides will lead to many individuals suffering from permanent deafness. Auditory monitoring should be an integral part of the care programme of MDR-TB patients, particularly in countries where aminoglycosides are still commonly used. In addition, identification of patients who are genetically predisposed will significantly reduce the risk of developing ototoxicity.

Patients with neurologic side effects (depression, psychosis and suicidal tendencies) have less favorable outcome and increased risk of death. Cycloserine is the most significant TB drug associated with central nervous system (CNS) toxicity. Cycloserine is used as second line drug in TB treatment based of its structural analogy to D-alanine. Cycloserine competitively inhibits two necessary enzymes (alanine racemase and alanine ligase) that incorporate alanine into an alanyl-alanine dipeptide, an essential component of the mycobacterial cell wall [67]. Early studies revealed that neurological and psychiatric manifestations are present in as many as 33% of patients treated with cycloserine [68]. The principal side effects associated with cycloserine therapy are convulsions, exacerbations of bipolar states and multiple neurological symptoms including excitation, dizziness, headaches, insomnia and anxiety [69]. Cycloserine-mediated neurologic side effects are exacerbated even more when used in combination with isoniazid [70]. These variable psychotropic responses are related to cycloserine action as an

Adverse event*	Suspected agent(s)†	Affected n (%)
Nausea/vomiting	PAS, TM, FQ	268 (32.8)
Diarrhoea	PAS, TM	173 (21.1)
Arthralgia	FQ, TM, CS, AG	134 (16.4)
Dizziness/vertigo	CS, CM, AG, FQ	117 (14.3)
Hearing disturbances	CM, TM, AG	98 (12.0)
Headache	CS, FQ	96 (11.7)
Sleep disturbances	CS, FQ	95 (11.6)
Electrolyte disturbances	CM, TM	94 (11.5)
Abdominal pain	PAS, TM	88 (10.8)
Anorexia	PAS, TM	75 (9.2)
Gastritis	TM, PAS	70 (8.6)
Peripheral neuropathy	TM, AG, CS	65 (7.9)
Depression	CS	51 (6.2)
Tinnitus	CM, CS, AG	42 (5.1)
Allergic reaction	FQ	42 (5.1)
Rash	FQ, PAS	38 (4.6)
Visual disturbances	CS, TM	36 (4.4)
Seizures	CS	33 (4.0)
Hypothyroidism	TM, PAS	29 (3.5)
Psychosis	CS	28 (3.4)
Hepatitis	TM	18 (2.2)
Renal failure/nephrotoxicity	AG, CM	9 (1.2)

Table 3. Frequency of adverse events and suspected agents among 818 patients receiving MDR-TB treatment. PAS: para-aminosalicyclic acid; TM: thioamides; FQ: fluoroquinolones; CS: cycloserine; AG: aminoglycosides; CM: capreomycin.. Reprinted from Ref. 62 with permission of the International Union Against Tuberculosis and Lung Disease. Copyright © The Union.

agonist of the neuronal NMDA (N-methyl-D-aspartate) receptor for glutamate [71], which is a major excitatory neurotransmitter in the mammalian CNS [72]. The most dramatic effect of cycloserine reported so far is the suicide of 2 patients during the postoperative antibiotic treatment course following pulmonary resection [73]. Because of its neurological toxicities, cycloserine was prevented very early from being part of first line TB drugs but was recently reintroduced as one of the cornerstones of treatment for MDR- and XDR-TB [46]. Although co-administration of pyridoxine (vitamin B6) with cycloserine can reduce partially the neurological side effects, the later should be prescribed after psychiatric evaluation for patients with apparent convulsions and agitation [55]. Some clinicians favor terizidone (two cycloserine molecules combined) as they found the side effects associated with it are less severe and more manageable [55]. However, given the little evidence demonstrating safety and efficacy of terizidone, it should be used with caution in TB patients intolerant to cycloserine.

Although adverse events associated with second-line drugs are a major obstacle in the management of MDR-TB, compared with first line treatment, DOTS-Plus programmes have achieved cure rates of greater than 70% even in resource-poor settings [74,75]. In general, the main adverse effects of anti-TB drugs occur during the first two to three weeks of treatment. If they are recognized in time and managed properly, high rates of treatment completion and cure can be achieved. Proper monitoring should include patient education, clinical examination and appropriate laboratory tests. Special training for staff on the various adverse events associated with second line drugs is essential for successful management. In particular, staff should consider altering dosages when appropriate, supplementary drugs to treat adverse events and replacement of drugs when toxicity cannot be managed.

7. Management approaches for the contacts of MDR TB patients

MDR-TB and XDR-TB cases are currently on the increase and it is expected that the number of their contacts will also increase, especially in densely populated area. Therefore, identification and proper management of these contacts are major components of drug resistant TB containment. In this regard, WHO recommend the identification of all close contacts of MDR-TB cases through contact tracing and their evaluation for TB infection.

A contact is defined as an individual who has a risk of acquiring TB because it has been exposed to Mtb by sharing air space with a person with infectious TB (the source case). The index case (a person with suspected or confirmed TB disease) is defined as the initial case of TB for a contact investigation [76]. He is not necessarily identical with the source case [76]. Many guidance documents focus on the source case and not the index case, as it is the source case who will have exposed the contacts, not necessarily the index case. Close contacts are those people sharing common habitation rooms with the source case. This can also include individuals with evidence of prolonged and frequent exposure to a source case in the workplace, school, prison, hospital ward, or social settings [77]. Contact tracing is defined as the systematic finding of contacts of patients with infectious TB disease [77]. The tracing helps identifying individuals who are particularly at high risk, such as individuals with HIV infection, young children and elderly.

The management of contacts of drug-resistant TB patients, in term of preventive chemoprophylaxis, remains a complex issue with a significant ethical dimension. In case of drug-susceptible TB, the provision of preventive INH therapy to suspect LTBI individuals is effective at reducing the risk of developing disease among infected contacts [10]. In theory, such a preventive approach should also work for LTBI individuals exposed to MDR and XDR Mtb strains. Unfortunately, health care providers cannot predict with certainty the susceptibility pattern of a contact's isolate from the source case's isolate. Indeed, many divergent drug susceptibility test profiles in source-contact pairs have been reported [78,79], due either to infection of the contact by another source case or to infection before the source case acquires resistance. Such a scenario likely occurs in high-burden TB areas where different drug resistant strains may circulate in homes, schools, and work places. Therefore, the lack of effective drugs with acceptable adverse-event profile in an otherwise healthy individual is a prominent barrier to the treatment of drug resistant TB contacts. Indeed, if, to some extent, the occurrence of toxicity is accepted by MDR-TB patients (since the alternative is high risk of death), convincing healthy contacts to cope with adverse-events during preventive therapy in is fundamentally different.

Given the lack of clear evidence in support of preventive therapy, the WHO does not recommend universal use of second-line drugs for chemoprophylaxis in MDR-TB contacts. Current guidance for the management of drug resistant TB contacts are largely based on expert opinions, which do not reject nor support provision of preventive therapy with the currently available drugs. In this context a guidance document presenting the most up-to-date evidence and expert opinion regarding the management of contacts of MDR- and XDR-TB patients has been recently proposed (March 2012) by the European Centre for Disease Prevention and Control (ECDC) [76]. Box 1 summarizes key recommendations provided by ECDC document.

Which factors should be evaluated to decide whether to provide preventive therapy to MDR TB contacts considered to have LTBI?

When evaluating an MDR TB contact and deciding between the two options (to provide preventive therapy and/or careful clinical observation and information), an overall individual risk assessment should be conducted, taking into consideration the following: the MDR TB contact's risk for progression to TB disease; the drug susceptibility pattern of the source case of infection; and the contact's risk for adverse drug events if initiating preventive therapy.

Are there any specific risk groups to whom special attention should be paid?

Children below the age of five years and immunocompromised persons in close contact with MDR TB patients and considered to have LTBI are at particular risk of progressing to TB disease. These risk groups might benefit from preventive therapy. The preventive therapy may be interrupted if, based on further examination, infection is found to be unlikely.

Persons over five years of age in close contact with MDR TB patients and considered to have LTBI could also be considered for preventive therapy if the individual risk assessment indicates this course of action.

If the decision is made to put an individual on preventive therapy, the selection of the drugs should be based on: the drug susceptibility pattern of the source case's likely infecting strain;

local patterns of drug resistance;

the potential adverse events in individual patients, taking into account age and other risk factors;

the selection of single or multiple drugs and the duration of treatment will depend on the availability of drugs with bactericidal activity for the particular infecting strain; alternatively, the decision can follow national guidelines.

Which arrangements should be in place if preventive therapy is considered?

If preventive therapy is considered by the expert physician or other healthcare provider, national legislation should ensure that the treatment costs for the patient are covered.

If preventive therapy is considered to be relevant for a particular individual, careful clinical monitoring and follow-up is essential for the detection of drug-adverse events and signs of TB disease if the preventive therapy is not effective.

Specific opinions for XDR TB contacts

As the currently available treatment options are very limited for XDR TB, it is likely that the risks of preventive therapy outweigh the benefits for contacts of XDR TB patients. Thus, the option to inform and observe the contacts will be preferable, given the currently available drugs and evidence.

How should health authorities conduct follow-ups for MDR TB and XDR TB contacts suspected to have LTBI?

All MDR TB and XDR TB contacts considered to have LTBI who, after a comprehensive individual risk assessment, are not given preventive therapy should be followed-up by careful clinical observation.

Follow-ups should be performed according to existing national guidelines.

All persons in contact with MDR TB or XDR TB (after exclusion of TB disease) should be informed about the risks and symptoms, carefully observed, and provided with easy access to a specialized TB clinic in case of symptoms between assessments. No specific time period for follow-up or periodicity of clinical assessments is recommended, but regular systematic, clinical observation is essential for the early detection of TB disease.

Individuals repeatedly in contact with infectious MDR TB or XDR TB cases (e.g. healthcare workers) should be re-examined periodically.

Box 1. ECDC expert opinions regarding preventive therapy of MDR- and XDR-TB contacts.

Studies conducted so far on the benefits and adverse events of preventive therapy are not conclusive in term of optimal treatment and duration for preventive treatment of MDR-TB contacts [80]. Therefore, well-designed randomized clinical trials for preventive therapy are urgently needed in settings where MDR-TB therapy and a strong national programme infrastructure are already in place. Further research is also needed to define the most effective contact-tracing procedures for contacts and the most effective follow-up procedures in healthcare workers constantly exposed to drug resistant TB. In addition, specific management approaches need to be established for children below the age of five years, children with HIV infection, immunocompromised individuals, pregnant women, and the elderly. Finally, whether MDR Mtb strains are more or less infectious and/or transmissible than drug-suscep-tible strains need to be clarified.

8. Compliance issues from patients and health care providers

The treatment for MDR-TB is long and complex and relies on a handful of antibiotics with uncertain efficacy. The WHO has launched an 8-point plan to ensure optimal management of XDR-TB patients with currently available drugs (Box 2). However, guidelines do not always translate easily into real world practice. In addition to directly observed treatment, what support can be offered to convince a patient to continue painful treatment? And how should patients who have exhausted all treatment options with existing second-line drugs be cared for?

1. Strengthen quality of basic TB and HIV/AIDS control
2. Scale up programmatic management of MDR-TB and XDR-TB
3. Strengthen laboratory services
4. Expand MDR-TB and XDR-TB surveillance
5. Develop and implement infection control measures
6. Strengthen advocacy, communication and social mobilization
7. Pursue resource mobilization at all levels
8. Promote research and development of new tools

Box 2. WHO 8-point plan

In many cases, MDR-TB treatment results in poor compliance with subsequent development of further drug resistance (i.e. XDR-TB), which leaves infected patients, namely HIV positive individuals, virtually untreatable using currently available drugs. The WHO defines a defaulter as being off drugs for more than 8 weeks after completing at least one month of treatment [81]. It is an operational definition to guide physicians in the decision of using a retreatment or second line regimen if the patient comes back to the health facility after defaulting. However it is imperative that health providers understand predictive factors for treatment default so that they can implement additional measures to target the population at risk. In this context, a recent review (2010) assessed TB treatment compliance and the factors predictive for poor adherence based on the analysis of 4 studies performed in Sub-Saharan Africa in the last 10 years [82]. The review revealed a high proportion of patients defaulting, which varied between 11.3% and 29.6%. Defaulting appears to be associated with many factors such as distance from the hospital, not being on the first course of TB medications, lack of repeated smears, drug-associated side effects, transportation difficulties, absence of family support and poor knowledge about TB disease and its treatment. Thus it is unfortunate that health care institutions continue to blame vulnerable and powerless patients who are unable, for this multitude of reasons, to comply with the treatment. Since distance from health care centers is a major factor, national programmes should at least consider making drugs more widely available, by either providing TB treatment in smaller health centers, or organizing mobile TB clinics, especially in rural areas.

It is time to admit that TB disease is not a 'patient problem' by default but rather a social and community responsibility that requires close cooperation and collaboration at all levels of the health care system. Forcing a patient to continue an ineffective, toxic regimen that results in uncertain outcome also raises an ethical issue yet to be resolved. Ereqat and colleagues reported a recent case of a MDR-TB patient who withdrew from treatment after 2 years while still sputum-positive [83]. Due to persistent efforts to force compliance, the patient disappeared carrying with him the potential to infect all people with whom he has contact. The authors suggest consulting with legal practitioners about the legality of enforced treatment and how patients who refuse or interrupt treatment can be managed to protect them and their potential contacts. It is obvious that in the absence of alternative treatment, this approach might end up with a response to TB without medication (i.e incarceration). For this type of recalcitrant patients, other TB specialists [84,85] propose directing efforts towards exploring possible regimens with better chances of cure and securing an appropriate living environment. Indeed, the threat of incarceration will just encourage patients to disappear and propagate the disease. Providing supportive accommodation with access to counseling and palliative care, when required, should reduce the risk of transmission to others [84]. Overall, until newer drugs become available, management that balances the risk of disease spread with individual human rights is likely to be more humane and less costly to health services compared with involuntary detention [85]. In this context, Upshur and Colleagues propose a list of additional considerations to the management of drug resistant TB as moral correlates to the current WHO 8-point plan (Box 3).

A paramount issue in TB management is that in many countries with limited resources most of the healthcare is provided by the private sector where the number of qualified medical personnel to prevent and treat drug resistant TB remains very limited. In this regard, the World Medical Association (WMA, http://www.wma.net) revealed that many doctors are no longer being taught to diagnose and treat TB. Thus, private physicians make frequent errors in dealing

---

1. Adherence research

2. Building the evidence-base for infection control practices

3. Supporting communities

4. Enhancing public health response while addressing the social determinants of health

5. Embracing palliative care

6. Advocacy for research

Box 3. Additional considerations to the WHO 8-point plan

with TB cases. They prescribe too few drugs or the wrong drugs, give inadequate doses of drugs, or prescribe an inadequate duration of treatment [86]. The standardized method of determining cure is based on bacteriologic laboratory testing for the growth of Mtb on culture media. However many health care providers rely on clinical observation to determine treatment outcome [87], either because of shortages in equipment and adequate infrastructure or because they trust their own observation above test results. Such mismanagement is a major cause of acquired drug resistance and treatment failure. On the other hand, on many occasions lung cancer was misdiagnosed and treated as sputum negative TB, a medical error due to high TB prevalence and radiological similarities [88].

It is therefore important that healthcare personnel at the forefront in the fight against TB acquire appropriate and state-of-the art training on TB management. In this regards, the WMA launched in its website a new online refresher course for care providers in many languages. The course provides basic clinical care information for TB including the latest diagnostics, treatment and information about multidrug-resistant TB. It also provides information on how to ensure patient adherence and infection control and includes many aspects of TB care and management. Dr. Julia Seyer, medical adviser at the WMA, said: 'When we started an online MDR-TB training course in 2006, we discovered that many physicians were missing the most basic knowledge about normal TB'.

In summary, both the lack of patient adherence to treatment and deficiencies in programme managements are compromising the effectiveness of MDR TB treatment and the interaction of these two issues raises further the barrier to achieving efficient TB control. From the various opinions on the issue of non-compliance it can be concluded that:

- Addressing therapy-related adverse events should contribute positively in improving patient's compliance. Therefore, potential adverse effects must be carefully evaluated when designing the therapy plan. Alternative plans should be discussed with the patients to minimize the possibility of therapeutic barriers.

- Healthcare system quality is significantly related to compliance. Long waiting times and unhappy experiences during clinic visits are frequent complains from TB patients. A healthcare system that considers patient satisfaction would enhance patient adherence to TB treatment.

- Compliance is also affected by the characteristics of TB disease. While non-adherence is not a major issue when treating short duration infections, this is not the case for TB, a chronic disease by definition. Therefore, special effort should be made to explain the nature of the disease with a particular focus on the asymptomatic stage of TB.

- Healthcare expenditures are a very important factor that affects compliance. TB patients often feel that the cost of long-term treatment would be a financial burden, which definitely threatens therapy compliance. Therefore, health care personnel should discuss the patient's resources and help identifying sources that might provide financial assistance to low-income patients.

Overall providing care centered on patient needs and expectations is a key component for the success of TB control programmes.

9. Programmatic management of drug resistant TB

Policies, strategies, protocols and guidelines for TB management are well explained and articulated on the paper. However, their implementation in resource-limited sittings remains challenging due to weak case finding strategies, unclear patient tracing mechanisms (especially defaulters), a lack of MDR-TB rapid diagnostic tools, absence of childhood TB case finding approaches and inadequate patient support services. Furthermore, specialized drug resistant TB services are limited to locations that often exclude many patients living in remote areas from receiving adequate health care. Recording systems, mainly paper-based, are time consuming for health care providers, and therefore reduces time for quality care. Addressing these many challenges requires collaboration from different components of national TB control programmes. These components include case detection, treatment, prevention, surveillance, and adequate monitoring/evaluation of the programme's performance. Such objectives are the backbone of DOTS-Plus management programme introduced by the WHO in 1998 [48]. Many DOTS-plus pilot projects provided evidence base for this strategy in the management of drug resistant TB [59,89,90]. Based on the success of pilot projects, the WHO issued in 2006 guidelines for what is now called programmatic management of drug-resistant TB (PMDT), which were recently updated with extra focus on the detection and treatment of drug-resistant TB in resources limited settings [91]. Priority topics identified in the new WHO document are:

- Case-finding through use of rapid molecular tests; investigation of contacts and other high-risk groups;

- Regimens for MDR-TB and their duration in HIV-positive and HIV-negative patients;

- Monitoring during treatment;

- Models of care.

PMDT is currently highly supported by funding for MDR-TB treatment, which has dramatically increased in the past few years. Multi-billion dollar funds are now available through governments and donors, including the Global Fund to Fight AIDS, Tuberculosis and Malaria, UNITAID and the GLC committee [90]. Such fund was essential to demonstrate the feasibility and effectiveness of PMDT in many resource-limited settings, where it is needed most [92].

The current status of MDR-TB epidemic requires urgent moving of PMDT beyond this pilot project stage in order to respond to the call of Stop TB for the treatment of 1.6 million MDR-TB patients in the near future [93].

Although the last WHO document on TB control provides comprehensive guidelines for good PMDT, The WHO recognizes that many crucial management issues remain to be addressed. Thus, during the development of the recent PMDT document, a review published in 2008 [92] revealed some important gaps in knowledge that need to be addressed in order to optimize PMDT:

• Lack of high quality evidence from randomized controlled trials for optimizing treatment regimens in patients with MDR-TB, including the best combination of drugs and treatment duration;

• Very limited information about treatment and management of pediatric MDR-TB;

• Identification of the most effective chemoprophylaxis for contacts of MDR-TB cases;

• The therapy for symptomatic relief from adverse reactions linked to second-line TB drugs.

It is also important to note that social stigma and discrimination are still major obstacles for access to TB care services in many countries [94,95]. Similarly, financial issues and geographical accessibility is also a barrier for the continuation of treatment [96,97]. Misconceptions about TB are highly prevalent, which discourages seeking help in time or encourage those with TB to seek help from traditional healers [98]. Therefore national TB programmes must also include specific strategies to combat these issues in order to optimize the implementation of good PMDT.

Diversity in the epidemiology of MDR-TB poses a challenge for its management in various settings [99]. Ideally, TB management approaches need to be adapted to each particular setting. However it is possible to build a minimal package that could be adapted to specific countries wishing to implement proper TB management approaches. Accordingly, in 2003 a Stop TB Working Group on DOTS-Plus for MDR-TB identified key research questions to be answered in order to scale up the management of all forms of drug-resistant TB and to maximize its public health impact [99]. The working group felt that evidence is needed to address the following questions:

• How can regimens be selected (either at the programme or at the individual patient level) based on standardized and reproducible DST that adequately reflects *in vivo* responsiveness to treatment?

• How can setting specific treatment strategies be optimized with respect to effectiveness, complexity (dosing, eligibility, duration, and monitoring of outcome and side effects), safety, adherence, and affordability?

• What is the minimum infrastructure needed to scale-up PMDT, in terms of:

    ○ laboratory and treatment provision

    ○ efficient and equitable patient selection

    ○ prevention of transmission to other patients and health care workers

- How should infected contacts of DR-TB patients be managed?

Ensuring that these research questions are addressed is the responsibility of all parties involved in the management of MDR-TB. If adequately addressed, they will generate a solid evidence-base to support existing WHO guidelines.

The integration of PMDT into existing TB control programmes beyond the limited pilot project phase has become a critical emergency in order to respond to the increasing spread of MDR/XDR-TB worldwide. However, analysis of current WHO strategies by many experts in the field of TB management [100] suggest that successful PMDT will still require:

- New and improved tools for drug resistance testing;

- Clinical trials to test the efficacy and effectiveness of simplified and shorter second-line treatment regimens as well as of candidate second-line drugs;

- New and improved strategies for identifying patients with drug-resistant disease, promoting treatment adherence, and improving infection control;

- Better epidemiological data to explain geographic variations in occurrence of drug resistance and to identify the greatest contributors to development of drug resistance in specific settings;

- Clinical trials to test the efficacy and effectiveness of new regimens for prophylactic treatment of contacts of patients with DR-TB.

10. Patient centered care approach

Acquiring adequate care for TB is becoming increasingly complex and costly when patients are infected with drug resistant Mtb. This problem is further amplified when patient access to health care centers is limited and adequate patient-clinician relationships are absent. To address this issue Stop TB included patient centered approach as one of its important underlying principles. It insists on respect for patients right as individuals and as partners in TB care and control. Therefore what are usually characterized as 'patient problems' need to be reconfigured into solidarity with patients and programmatic challenges. Patient-centeredness can be traced back to the adoption of the right to health as part of the International Human right declaration in 1948 [101], but it is only in the 1990s, as result of the community reaction to the AIDS epidemic, that its importance has been perceived. Since then, the rise in prevalence of all forms of TB in HIV individuals has become one of the major stimulating factors for implementation of patient-centered approaches in TB care.

Promoting patient-centered case management involves assessing each TB patient's needs and identifying a treatment plan that ensures the completion of therapy. Policies and guidelines for patient-centered approaches are currently widely distributed. Unfortunately, their application in the field is progressing very slowly. Applying a patient-centered approach takes time and requires effort at many levels. It is a new way of thinking, teaching, providing care, prevention and communication [102]. Therefore, many countries will continue to experience substantial difficulties in treating drug resistant TB patients at high risk of defaulting.

A systematic review of factors that contribute to non-adherence [103] indicate that many social and economic barriers prevent patients from successfully completing their treatment. A wide range of interacting factors impact on the patient behavior, which is subject to changes during the course of treatment. According to Doctor Without Borders [104], one of the major challenges faced by drug resistant TB patients is the long and arduous treatment period, which can involve large numbers of tablets each day, as well as injectables, both expensive and not always easily available or accessible. Low-income patients living in remote area often struggle to reach specialized TB clinics, in particular when the harsh winter weather affect severely the country's road network and compromises the transportation system. Therefore, in the absence of efficient patient-centered approaches, it is almost impossible to convince patients to continue this forceful effort every day for up to two years.

In the Russian Federation, the proportion of MDR-TB patients defaulting from treatment has increased from 12% in 2001 to almost 30% in 2004 [105], despite the expansion of the DOTS programme to include the treatment of drug resistant TB in 2000. This failure to control drug resistant TB was mainly attributed to the absence of patient-centered strategies adapted to many risk factors for non-adherence such as poverty, unemployment, homelessness, alcoholism, drug abuse and mental illness, to name a few [105]. In response to the alarming proportion of defaulters, a novel patient-centered TB treatment delivery programme (Sputnik) was introduced in Tomsk City [106]. Sputnik care providers accompanied patients through treatment by remaining responsible for patients from the time of enrollment in the programme until the end of treatment (Box 4). The programme paid a particular attention to care giving. In addition to clinical preparation, nurses received a comprehensive training on how to care for patients facing a myriad of biosocial challenges. Indeed, a review of the emotional support that nurses provide to patients living with MTR-TB [107] concluded that nursing of TB patients could be improved with an integrated approach where the nurses are responsible for treating not only the patient, but also ambient factors that affect health, such as family and community.

A high nurse-to patient ratio (2:15),

More staff time per patient to facilitate bonding and defaulter searching

Provision of portable phones to nurses, which increases flexibility

Easier access to specialists

Expanded social and psychological support, which included clothing and assistance with procuring documentation required to access social services

---

Box 4. Sputnik programme package

The application of the Sputnik programme led to a mean adherence of 79.0% and a cure rate of 71.1%, indicating that adapted patient-centered approaches contributed significantly to improving TB patient adherence.

In 1998, the Centers for Disease Control and Prevention (CDC) and the Institute of Medicine of the National Academy of Sciences conducted a study to determine if TB eradication in the United State was feasible. The resulting report *"Ending Neglect: The Elimination of Tuberculosis in the United States"* concluded that TB elimination would require "aggressive and decisive action beyond what was in effect." One of the top objectives of the new CDC plan is to ensure that patient-centered case management and monitoring of treatment outcomes are the standard of care for all TB patients [108]. In particular, the CDC guidelines recommend all patients with active TB must be tested for HIV infection and that all patients double infected with Mtb and HIV infection must be appropriately and adequately treated. To ensure adherence to treatment, the CDC recommend the inclusion of multiple enablers (e.g., transportation vouchers and housing for the homeless) and incentives that will motivate the patient (e.g., food coupons), and other treatment enhancers such as alternative treatment delivery sites, and strategies to overcome social and cultural barriers.

Addressing social and economic barriers definitely increases patient access to adequate TB care. However, health education would also strengthen patient-centered approaches. Understanding an illness and how it affects ones life, as well as available treatment options, are necessary for a patient and community to take an active role in TB management. With input from community health professionals from several countries, a literacy tool kit "Within Our Reach: A TB Literacy Toolkit" was developed in 2009 for health educators, outreach workers, counselors, and supervisors who provide services to TB patients [109] and (Box 5).

Increasing knowledge about TB, the link between TB and HIV, TB treatment, and TB transmission

Raising awareness that TB is a serious but treatable disease

Giving patients confidence that they can complete TB treatment and be cured

Educating caregivers and families about how to support TB patients

Reducing stigma attached to TB and HIV

Box 5. Supporting objectives of the TB Literacy Toolkit

The tools are designed to educate TB and HIV patients, their caregivers, and their communities about TB and what it takes to complete a full course of TB treatment. The kit developers suggest that individual sessions should be conducted with flipcharts between the health provider and patient, and videos should be played in a waiting area or during community education events.

Patient-centeredness has become a central approach towards realizing universal access for all patients to efficient TB care. However scaling up this approach is progressing slowly in high TB-burden countries and is mainly challenged by the socio-economic determinants of knowledge and attitudes about TB among health care providers and the general population. Therefore optimal patient-centeredness approach requires collaborative efforts between all organizations serving TB patients to ensure that health care providers, policy makers, community leaders and the public are knowledgeable about TB disease.

11. Drug resistant TB infection (tansmission) in the community and hospitals

TB is a highly contagious disease, acquired mainly through inhalation of airborne aerosols. Infection can occur by inhaling as few as 5-10 living bacteria. People with active TB infection spread the bacterium not only by coughing and sneezing but also by spitting, speaking, singing or laughing. The infectiousness of a TB patient is directly related to the number of droplet nuclei carrying Mtb that are expelled into the air. These droplets rapidly evaporated to form tiny particle nuclei, which could remain airborne for several days [110]. Given this mode of propagation, a person with active TB can spread the germs to up to 15 people in a year, if left untreated [4]. Therefore the process of TB spread also needs to be controlled in order to successfully combat the TB epidemic. In this regards, Nardell recommend the term "transmission control of TB" instead of "infection control of TB", since a third of the world's population is already infected with TB, a situation that appear to be stationary [111].

Because MDR strains carry mutations in major metabolic activities, in particular INH resistant strains lacking catalase activity [112], some researchers have suggested that they may be less virulent and less transmissible [113]. Contrasting with this hypothesis, the epidemic that occurred in New York City in the 1990s [114,115], which affected mainly HIV-infected persons, proved that MDR strains are highly virulent and transmissible. Current data on MDR TB prevalence in Africa, Eastern Europe and Asia [116] provides further evidence of this phenomenon. Drug resistant TB can be transmitted in virtually any setting but healthcare settings, correctional institutions and homeless shelters have an increased risk of transmission. The level of drug resistance TB in hospital settings varies according to local TB prevalence. For instance an university hospitals in Paris (France), reported MDR rates of respectively 1.2% among TB cases [117], while in university hospitals in Manila (Philippine), this figure was an alarming 53.5% [118].

It is generally thought that the emergence of drug-resistant TB (usually termed acquired) occurs in settings where patients fail to adhere to proper treatment regimens or receive inadequate treatment. It is difficult to assign the current magnitude of the epidemic to acquired resistance alone. Another mechanism for the perpetuation of resistance, which has largely been neglected in the development of TB control programmes, is the direct transmission of drug-resistant strains (called primary or transmitted resistance) [119]. In the 2006 XDR-TB outbreak in KwaZulu-Natal (South Africa), 52 of 53 people who contracted the disease (all of them HIV infected) died within weeks [120]. This outbreak received international attention because 85 percent of infected patients had genetically similar XDR strain, indicating that resistance was likely transmitted rather than acquired. Consistent with these findings, a study conducted in Tomsk (Siberia) –a setting where HIV infection is not widespread and effective TB treatment is available– to identify factors leading to increases in MDR-TB cases [121], revealed that a patient was six times more likely to develop MDR-TB if hospitalized for drug-susceptible TB than if not hospitalized. These results strongly suggest that nosocomial transmission of TB rather than resistance (acquired predominantly by nonadherence) is increasingly responsible for the rising MDR TB case rates in Russia and probably in many other places.

Worthy of note is that nosocomial transmission of TB is a risk not only to inpatients but also health care workers (HCWs). In fact, early studies revealed transmission of MDR-TB from patient to patient and from patient to HCWs [122]. A systematic review by Joshi and colleagues [123] demonstrated that TB is a significant occupational problem among HCWs in many low- and middle-income countries and that most health care facilities in these sittings lack resources to prevent nosocomial transmission of TB. HIV-infected HCWs have a particularly high risk of TB, which may be fatal if the disease is caused by a drug-resistant strain [124]. Indeed, dramatic nosocomial outbreaks of MDR TB occurred the late 1980s, largely in HIV infected HCWs, and caused many deaths [110]. This situation increased the concern of HCWs about the safety of working in institutions with a large numbers of admissions for active TB. Indeed, it is estimated that 1% to 10% of HCWs are infected annually in hospitals with more than 200 admissions per year for TB [110]. The risk of TB transmission to HCWs is particularly high in certain areas of the hospital, such as emergency rooms and units that admit patients with active TB [125].

A review of several reports of TB outbreaks with transmission to HCWs in industrialized countries revealed that many factors contribute to nosocomial transmission, such as delayed diagnosis, poor ventilation with positive pressure in isolation rooms, aerosolization of bacilli through mechanical ventilation, bronchoscopy and dressing change [110]. There was also strong evidence that technicians involved in cough-inducing procedures, histologic preparations and autopsies are at high risk, even in institutions caring for few patients with TB [126]. These outbreaks revealed many deficiencies in the knowledge of TB and its transmission as well as strategies used to control the disease. Therefore, various health authorities have implemented effective control programmes based on the early detection of TB and the prompt isolation and treatment of persons with TB in addition to introducing strong measures to prevent nosocomial transmissions of TB. For instance, the US Centers for Disease Control (CDC) [127] recommended the following levels of controls: **1. Administrative controls,** which reduce risk of exposure. **2. Environmental controls,** which prevent spread and reduce concentration of droplet nuclei. **3. Respiratory-protection controls,** which further reduce risk of exposure in special areas and circumstances. (Box 6).

Implementation of a full hierarchy of these measures lead to a significant reduction in nosocomial transmission of TB in the United States [128]. Whereas the extent of the epidemics in low and middle income countries is still attributed, in large part, to ineffective transmission control strategies. In these countries, double infection with TB and HIV has further accelerated the transmission of drug resistant TB and increased the spread of HIV. Such a dramatic situation blocks the efforts of both the Stop TB Partnership and anti-retroviral therapy programmes. It is regrettable that many health care institutions continue to house HIV positive individuals with patients who have drug-resistant TB, thus leading to nosocomial transmission with subsequent community transmission. In this regards, health authorities in Haiti implemented an effective community-based transmission control programme with a baseline triage and separation strategy [111]. Patients are admitted to either the general medical ward, a TB pavilion, or very basic isolation rooms based on smear results and HIV status (Fig. 2).

Administrative Controls
• Assign responsibility for TB infection control • Conduct TB risk assessment • Develop and institute a written TB infection-control plan • Ensure the timely availability of recommended laboratory processing, testing, and reporting of results • Implement effective work practices for the management of patients with suspected or confirmed TB disease • Ensure proper cleaning and sterilization or disinfection of potentially contaminated equipment • Train and educate health-care workers • Test and evaluate health-care workers for TB infection and disease • Apply epidemiology-based prevention principles • Use posters and signs demonstrating and advising respiratory hygiene and cough etiquette • Coordinate efforts with the local or state health department.

Environmental Controls
Reduce concentration of infectious droplet nuclei through the following technologies: • Ventilation technologies (Natural ventilation and Mechanical ventilation) • High efficiency particulate air filtration • Ultraviolet germicidal irradiation

Respiratory Protection Controls
• Implement a respiratory-protection programme • Train health-care workers on respiratory protection • Educate patients on respiratory hygiene and the importance of covering their cough • Test HCWs for mask fit and functionality

Box 6. TB Infection-Control Programme: Level of Controls

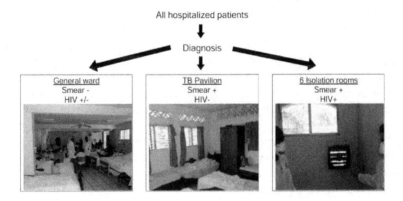

Figure 2. Community-based TB treatment triage strategy in Haiti. The general medical ward has natural ventilation and UV air disinfection. The TB ward has natural ventilation with fenestrated brick and more UV fixtures to disinfect the air than the general ward has. The six isolation rooms are off a common corridor, and each has a large exhaust fan built into the wall that draws air into the room from the corridor, as well as a UV fixture. Reprinted from Ref. 111 with permission of the International Union Against Tuberculosis and Lung Disease. Copyright © The Union

Although this simple baseline strategy is not sufficient, Nardell considers that its implementing in other resource-poor settings would contribute significantly to reduce the burden of TB epidemic [111].

12. Conclusion

Founded in 2001, the goal of The Stop TB Partnership for 2015 was to reduce the global burden of TB disease (deaths and prevalence) by 50% relative to 1990 levels. The reality of the global incidence of all forms of TB in 2012 indicates that this timetable is unrealistic. Despite billions of dollars already spent on TB control programs, less than 2% of drug resistant TB cases currently receive appropriate treatment in high burden countries allowing the disease to spread faster than the implementation of adequate management programs. This dramatic situation severely attenuates global efforts to control TB.

One of the major challenges now is to develop innovative approaches to expand the detection and treatment of drug resistant cases globally. To achieve this goal, substantial funding and development of extensive human resources is needed. Among the response priorities, the following are of paramount importance: 1) developing tools for rapid detection of drug resistance; 2) clinical trials to test simplified, safe and shorter second-line treatment regimens; 3) developing approaches to enhance treatment adherence; 4) clinical trials to test the efficacy of new prophylactic treatment regimens for contacts of patients; and finally 5) developing safe and more efficient second-line drugs.

However, even with increased detection and treatment of drug resistant TB, focusing on the care of TB and neglecting living conditions in low-income countries has little chance of completely reversing the burden of TB. The severity of the TB epidemic in the Western world during the 19th century was largely due to the low living standards prevalent among the poor during the industrial revolution. As living standards improved, TB mortality began to decrease long before any vaccinations or specific therapy was introduced. Reminiscent of the 19th century situation is the persistence of TB in poor and marginalized populations in most modern cities of the world. As the British historian Thomas Mc-Keown said in 1976, "the overall health of the population is less related to medical advances than to standards of living and nutrition" [101]. Thus the control and eventual eradication of the TB epidemic will need support and cooperation from multiple levels within the medical and scientific community, as well as all levels of government worldwide in order to address living standards and develop better drugs and therapeutic tools for the clinic.

Acknowledgements

This work was supported by operating grants from the Canadian Institutes of Health Research and BC Lung Association. The author is supported by scholar awards from the Michael Smith Foundation for Health Research, and the TB Vets Charitable Foundation. The author thanks Alice Lau and Jeffrey Helm for their editing help.

Author details

Zakaria Hmama

Division of Infectious diseases, Department of Medicine, University of British Columbia, BC, Canada

References

[1] WHO. Multidrug and extensively drug-resistant TB (M/XDR-TB): 2010 Global Report on Surveillance and Response. Available at: http://www.who.int/tb/publications/2010/978924599191/en/index.html

[2] Velayati AA, Masjedi MR, Farnia P, Tabarsi P, Ghanavi J, Ziazarifi AH, et al. Emergence of new forms of totally drug-resistant tuberculosis bacilli: super extensively drug-resistant tuberculosis or totally drug-resistant strains in iran. Chest 2009 Aug; 136(2):420-425.

[3] Udwadia ZF, Amale RA, Ajbani KK, Rodrigues C. Totally drug-resistant tuberculosis in India. Clin Infect Dis 2012 Feb 15;54(4):579-581.

[4] WHO. Tuberculosis Fact sheet N°104. 2012. Available at: http://www.who.int/mediacentre/factsheets/fs104/en/

[5] WHO report 2008. Global tuberculosis control - surveillance, planning, financing. Available at: http://www.who.int/tb/publications/global_report/2008/summary/en/index.html

[6] Jain A, Dixit P. Multidrug-resistant to extensively drug resistant tuberculosis: what is next? J Biosci 2008 Nov;33(4):605-616.

[7] Jain A, Mondal R. Extensively drug-resistant tuberculosis: current challenges and threats. FEMS Immunol Med Microbiol 2008 Jul;53(2):145-150.

[8] Migliori GB, De Iaco G, Besozzi G, Centis R, Cirillo DM. First tuberculosis cases in Italy resistant to all tested drugs. Euro Surveill 2007 May 17;12(5):E070517.1.

[9] Bhargava A, Pinto L, Pai M. Mismanagement of tuberculosis in India: Causes, consequences, and the way forward. Hypothesis 2011;9:e7.

[10] Sia IG, Wieland ML. Current concepts in the management of tuberculosis. Mayo Clin Proc 2011 Apr;86(4):348-361.

[11] Elzinga G, Raviglione MC, Maher D. Scale up: meeting targets in global tuberculosis control. Lancet 2004 Mar 6;363(9411):814-819.

[12] Treatment of Tuberculosis Guidelines, 4th edition. 2010. Available at: http://whqlib-doc.who.int/publications/2010/9789241547833_eng.pdf

[13] Zhang Y, Yew WW. Mechanisms of drug resistance in Mycobacterium tuberculosis. Int J Tuberc Lung Dis 2009 Nov;13(11):1320-1330.

[14] Mitchison DA. The action of antituberculosis drugs in short-course chemotherapy. Tubercle 1985 Sep;66(3):219-225.

[15] Wade MM, Zhang Y. Anaerobic incubation conditions enhance pyrazinamide activity against Mycobacterium tuberculosis. J Med Microbiol 2004 Aug;53(Pt 8):769-773.

[16] Kaufmann SH, McMichael AJ. Annulling a dangerous liaison: vaccination strategies against AIDS and tuberculosis. Nat Med 2005 04;11(4):S33-S44.

[17] Ernst JD. The immunological life cycle of tuberculosis. Nat Rev Immunol 2012 Jul 13;12(8):581-591.

[18] Selwyn PA, Hartel D, Lewis VA, Schoenbaum EE, Vermund SH, Klein RS, et al. A prospective study of the risk of tuberculosis among intravenous drug users with human immunodeficiency virus infection. N Engl J Med 1989 Mar 2;320(9):545-550.

[19] Rangaka MX, Wilkinson KA, Glynn JR, Ling D, Menzies D, Mwansa-Kambafwile J, et al. Predictive value of interferon-gamma release assays for incident active tuberculosis: a systematic review and meta-analysis. Lancet Infect Dis 2012 Jan;12(1):45-55.

[20] Horowitz HW, Luciano BB, Kadel JR, Wormser GP. Tuberculin skin test conversion in hospital employees vaccinated with bacille Calmette-Guerin: recent Mycobacterium tuberculosis infection or booster effect? Am J Infect Control 1995 Jun;23(3): 181-187.

[21] Farhat M, Greenaway C, Pai M, Menzies D. False-positive tuberculin skin tests: what is the absolute effect of BCG and non-tuberculous mycobacteria? Int J Tuberc Lung Dis 2006 Nov;10(11):1192-1204.

[22] Long SS. Interferon-gamma release assay for evaluation of latent tuberculosis infection. J Pediatr 2012 Oct;161(4):A3.

[23] Gengenbacher M, Kaufmann SH. Mycobacterium tuberculosis: success through dormancy. FEMS Microbiol Rev 2012 May;36(3):514-532.

[24] Betts JC, Lukey PT, Robb LC, McAdam RA, Duncan K. Evaluation of a nutrient starvation model of Mycobacterium tuberculosis persistence by gene and protein expression profiling. Mol Microbiol 2002 Feb;43(3):717-731.

[25] Boon C, Dick T. How Mycobacterium tuberculosis goes to sleep: the dormancy survival regulator DosR a decade later. Future Microbiol 2012 Apr;7(4):513-518.

[26] Flynn JL, Chan J. Tuberculosis: latency and reactivation. Infect Immun 2001 Jul;69(7): 4195-4201.

[27] Chao MC, Rubin EJ. Letting sleeping dos lie: does dormancy play a role in tuberculosis? Annu Rev Microbiol 2010;64:293-311.

[28] David HL. Probability distribution of drug-resistant mutants in unselected populations of Mycobacterium tuberculosis. Appl Microbiol 1970 Nov;20(5):810-814.

[29] Zhang Y, Heym B, Allen B, Young D, Cole S. The catalase-peroxidase gene and isoniazid resistance of Mycobacterium tuberculosis. Nature 1992 Aug 13;358(6387):591-593.

[30] Hazbon MH, Brimacombe M, Bobadilla del Valle M, Cavatore M, Guerrero MI, Varma-Basil M, et al. Population genetics study of isoniazid resistance mutations and evolution of multidrug-resistant Mycobacterium tuberculosis. Antimicrob Agents Chemother 2006 Aug;50(8):2640-2649.

[31] Rozwarski DA, Grant GA, Barton DH, Jacobs WR,Jr, Sacchettini JC. Modification of the NADH of the isoniazid target (InhA) from Mycobacterium tuberculosis. Science 1998 Jan 2;279(5347):98-102.

[32] Heym B, Alzari PM, Honore N, Cole ST. Missense mutations in the catalase-peroxidase gene, katG, are associated with isoniazid resistance in Mycobacterium tuberculosis. Mol Microbiol 1995 Jan;15(2):235-245.

[33] Telenti A, Imboden P, Marchesi F, Lowrie D, Cole S, Colston MJ, et al. Detection of rifampicin-resistance mutations in Mycobacterium tuberculosis. Lancet 1993 Mar 13;341(8846):647-650.

[34] Scorpio A, Zhang Y. Mutations in pncA, a gene encoding pyrazinamidase/nicotinamidase, cause resistance to the antituberculous drug pyrazinamide in tubercle bacillus. Nat Med 1996 Jun;2(6):662-667.

[35] Telenti A, Philipp WJ, Sreevatsan S, Bernasconi C, Stockbauer KE, Wieles B, et al. The emb operon, a gene cluster of Mycobacterium tuberculosis involved in resistance to ethambutol. Nat Med 1997 May;3(5):567-570.

[36] Ramaswamy SV, Amin AG, Goksel S, Stager CE, Dou SJ, El Sahly H, et al. Molecular genetic analysis of nucleotide polymorphisms associated with ethambutol resistance in human isolates of Mycobacterium tuberculosis. Antimicrob Agents Chemother 2000 Feb;44(2):326-336.

[37] Vareldzis BP, Grosset J, de Kantor I, Crofton J, Laszlo A, Felten M, et al. Drug-resistant tuberculosis: laboratory issues. World Health Organization recommendations. Tuber Lung Dis 1994 Feb;75(1):1-7.

[38] Espinal MA, Kim SJ, Suarez PG, Kam KM, Khomenko AG, Migliori GB, et al. Standard short-course chemotherapy for drug-resistant tuberculosis: treatment outcomes in 6 countries. JAMA 2000 May 17;283(19):2537-2545.

[39] Furin JJ, Mitnick CD, Shin SS, Bayona J, Becerra MC, Singler JM, et al. Occurrence of serious adverse effects in patients receiving community-based therapy for multi-drug-resistant tuberculosis. Int J Tuberc Lung Dis 2001 Jul;5(7):648-655.

[40] Moore DA, Evans CA, Gilman RH, Caviedes L, Coronel J, Vivar A, et al. Microscopic-observation drug-susceptibility assay for the diagnosis of TB. N Engl J Med 2006 Oct 12;355(15):1539-1550.

[41] Reisner BS, Gatson AM, Woods GL. Evaluation of mycobacteria growth indicator tubes for susceptibility testing of Mycobacterium tuberculosis to isoniazid and rifampin. Diagn Microbiol Infect Dis 1995 Aug;22(4):325-329.

[42] Levine ML, Moskowitz GW, Dorf BS, Bank S. Pneumatic dilation in patients with achalasia with a modified Gruntzig dilator (Levine) under direct endoscopic control: results after 5 years. Am J Gastroenterol 1991 Nov;86(11):1581-1584.

[43] Martin A, Portaels F, Palomino JC. Colorimetric redox-indicator methods for the rapid detection of multidrug resistance in Mycobacterium tuberculosis: a systematic review and meta-analysis. J Antimicrob Chemother 2007 Feb;59(2):175-183.

[44] Montoro E, Lemus D, Echemendia M, Martin A, Portaels F, Palomino JC. Comparative evaluation of the nitrate reduction assay, the MTT test, and the resazurin microtitre assay for drug susceptibility testing of clinical isolates of Mycobacterium tuberculosis. J Antimicrob Chemother 2005 Apr;55(4):500-505.

[45] Bwanga F, Joloba ML, Haile M, Hoffner S. Evaluation of seven tests for the rapid detection of multidrug-resistant tuberculosis in Uganda. Int J Tuberc Lung Dis 2010 Jul; 14(7):890-895.

[46] Caminero JA, World Health Organization, American Thoracic Society, British Thoracic Society. Treatment of multidrug-resistant tuberculosis: evidence and controversies. Int J Tuberc Lung Dis 2006 Aug;10(8):829-837.

[47] Mitnick CD, Shin SS, Seung KJ, Rich ML, Atwood SS, Furin JJ, et al. Comprehensive treatment of extensively drug-resistant tuberculosis. N Engl J Med 2008 Aug 7;359(6): 563-574.

[48] Iseman MD. MDR-TB and the developing world--a problem no longer to be ignored: the WHO announces 'DOTS Plus' strategy. Int J Tuberc Lung Dis 1998 Nov;2(11):867.

[49] Tupasi TE, Gupta R, Quelapio MI, Orillaza RB, Mira NR, Mangubat NV, et al. Feasibility and cost-effectiveness of treating multidrug-resistant tuberculosis: a cohort study in the Philippines. PLoS Med 2006 Sep;3(9):e352.

[50] Tupasi TE, Quelapio MI, Orillaza RB, Alcantara C, Mira NR, Abeleda MR, et al. DOTS-Plus for multidrug-resistant tuberculosis in the Philippines: global assistance urgently needed. Tuberculosis (Edinb) 2003;83(1-3):52-58.

[51] Riekstina V, Leimane V, Holtz TH, Leimans J, Wells CD. Treatment outcome cohort analysis in an integrated DOTS and DOTS-Plus TB program in Latvia. Int J Tuberc Lung Dis 2007 May;11(5):585-587.

[52] Five-year follow-up of a controlled trial of five 6-month regimens of chemotherapy for pulmonary tuberculosis. Hong Kong Chest Service/British Medical Research Council. Am Rev Respir Dis 1987 Dec;136(6):1339-1342.

[53] O'Riordan P, Schwab U, Logan S, Cooke G, Wilkinson RJ, Davidson RN, et al. Rapid molecular detection of rifampicin resistance facilitates early diagnosis and treatment of multi-drug resistant tuberculosis: case control study. PLoS One 2008 Sep 9;3(9):e3173.

[54] Becerra MC, Freeman J, Bayona J, Shin SS, Kim JY, Furin JJ, et al. Using treatment failure under effective directly observed short-course chemotherapy programs to identify patients with multidrug-resistant tuberculosis. Int J Tuberc Lung Dis 2000 Feb;4(2):108-114.

[55] Caminero JA, Sotgiu G, Zumla A, Migliori GB. Best drug treatment for multidrug-resistant and extensively drug-resistant tuberculosis. Lancet Infect Dis 2010 Sep; 10(9):621-629.

[56] Sterling TR, Lehmann HP, Frieden TR. Impact of DOTS compared with DOTS-plus on multidrug resistant tuberculosis and tuberculosis deaths: decision analysis. BMJ 2003 Mar 15;326(7389):574.

[57] Gupta R, Cegielski JP, Espinal MA, Henkens M, Kim JY, Lambregts-Van Weezenbeek CS, et al. Increasing transparency in partnerships for health--introducing the Green Light Committee. Trop Med Int Health 2002 Nov;7(11):970-976.

[58] Gupta R, Kim JY, Espinal MA, Caudron JM, Pecoul B, Farmer PE, et al. Public health. Responding to market failures in tuberculosis control. Science 2001 Aug 10;293(5532): 1049-1051.

[59] Nathanson E, Lambregts-van Weezenbeek C, Rich ML, Gupta R, Bayona J, Blondal K, et al. Multidrug-resistant tuberculosis management in resource-limited settings. Emerg Infect Dis 2006 Sep;12(9):1389-1397.

[60] Grosset JH, Singer TG, Bishai WR. New drugs for the treatment of tuberculosis: hope and reality. Int J Tuberc Lung Dis 2012 Aug;16(8):1005-1014.

[61] Rivers EC, Mancera RL. New anti-tuberculosis drugs in clinical trials with novel mechanisms of action. Drug Discov Today 2008 Dec;13(23-24):1090-1098.

[62] Nathanson E, Gupta R, Huamani P, Leimane V, Pasechnikov AD, Tupasi TE, et al. Adverse events in the treatment of multidrug-resistant tuberculosis: results from the DOTS-Plus initiative. Int J Tuberc Lung Dis 2004 Nov;8(11):1382-1384.

[63] Baghaei P, Tabarsi P, Dorriz D, Marjani M, Shamaei M, Pooramiri MV, et al. Adverse effects of multidrug-resistant tuberculosis treatment with a standardized regimen: a report from Iran. Am J Ther 2011 Mar-Apr;18(2):e29-34.

[64] Harris T, Bardien S, Schaaf HS, Petersen L, De Jong G, Fagan JJ. Aminoglycoside-induced hearing loss in HIV-positive and HIV-negative multidrug-resistant tuberculosis patients. S Afr Med J 2012 May 8;102(6):363-366.

[65] Human H, Hagen CM, de Jong G, Harris T, Lombard D, Christiansen M, et al. Investigation of mitochondrial sequence variants associated with aminoglycoside-induced ototoxicity in South African TB patients on aminoglycosides. Biochem Biophys Res Commun 2010 Mar 19;393(4):751-756.

[66] Qian Y, Guan MX. Interaction of aminoglycosides with human mitochondrial 12S rRNA carrying the deafness-associated mutation. Antimicrob Agents Chemother 2009 Nov;53(11):4612-4618.

[67] Lambert MP, Neuhaus FC. Mechanism of d-Cycloserine Action: Alanine Racemase from Escherichia coli W1. J Bacteriol 1972 Jun;110(3):978-987.

[68] Helmy B. Side effects of cycloserine. Scand J Respir Dis Suppl 1970;71:220-225.

[69] Pasargiklian M, Biondi L. Neurologic and behavioural reactions of tuberculous patients treated with cycloserine. Scand J Respir Dis Suppl 1970;71:201-208.

[70] Villar TG. Personal experience with cycloserine in 206 patients with pulmonary tuberculosis. Scand J Respir Dis Suppl 1970;71:196-200.

[71] Wood PL, Emmett MR, Rao TS, Mick S, Cler J, Iyengar S. In vivo modulation of the N-methyl-D-aspartate receptor complex by D-serine: potentiation of ongoing neuronal activity as evidenced by increased cerebellar cyclic GMP. J Neurochem 1989 Sep; 53(3):979-981.

[72] Weinberg RJ. Glutamate: an excitatory neurotransmitter in the mammalian CNS. Brain Res Bull 1999 Nov-Dec;50(5-6):353-354.

[73] Esteves Pinto E. Suicide of two patients during the postoperative course after pulmonary resection: possible effect of cycloserine. Scand J Respir Dis Suppl 1970;71:256-258.

[74] Mitnick C, Bayona J, Palacios E, Shin S, Furin J, Alcantara F, et al. Community-based therapy for multidrug-resistant tuberculosis in Lima, Peru. N Engl J Med 2003 Jan 9;348(2):119-128.

[75] Leimane V, Riekstina V, Holtz TH, Zarovska E, Skripconoka V, Thorpe LE, et al. Clinical outcome of individualised treatment of multidrug-resistant tuberculosis in Latvia: a retrospective cohort study. Lancet 2005 Jan 22-28;365(9456):318-326.

[76] ECDC Guidance. Management of contacts of MDR TB and XDR TB patients. 2012. Available at: http://www.ecdc.europa.eu/en/publications/Publications/201203-Guidance-MDR-TB-contacts.pdf

[77] Duarte R, Neto M, Carvalho A, Barros H. Improving tuberculosis contact tracing: the role of evaluations in the home and workplace. Int J Tuberc Lung Dis 2012 Jan;16(1): 55-59.

[78] Kritski AL, Marques MJ, Rabahi MF, Vieira MA, Werneck-Barroso E, Carvalho CE, et al. Transmission of tuberculosis to close contacts of patients with multidrug-resistant tuberculosis. Am J Respir Crit Care Med 1996 Jan;153(1):331-335.

[79] Furin JJ, Becerra MC, Shin SS, Kim JY, Bayona J, Farmer PE. Effect of administering short-course, standardized regimens in individuals infected with drug-resistant Mycobacterium tuberculosis strains. Eur J Clin Microbiol Infect Dis 2000 Feb;19(2): 132-136.

[80] van der Werf MJ, Langendam MW, Sandgren A, Manissero D. Lack of evidence to support policy development for management of contacts of multidrug-resistant tuberculosis patients: two systematic reviews. Int J Tuberc Lung Dis 2012;16(3):288-296.

[81] TB Case Definitions. Revision May 2011. Available at: http://www.stoptb.org/wg/gli/assets/documents/TBcasedefinitions_20110506b.pdf

[82] Castelnuovo B. A review of compliance to anti tuberculosis treatment and risk factors for defaulting treatment in Sub Saharan Africa. Afr Health Sci 2010 Dec;10(4): 320-324.

[83] Ereqat S, Spigelman M, Bar-Gal GK, Ramlawi A, Abdeen Z. MDR tuberculosis and non-compliance with therapy. Lancet Infect Dis 2011 Sep;11(9):662.

[84] Cox H, Hughes J, Ford N, London L. MDR tuberculosis and non-compliance with therapy. Lancet Infect Dis 2012 Mar;12(3):178; author reply 178-9.

[85] Upshur R, Singh J, Ford N. Apocalypse or redemption: responding to extensively drug-resistant tuberculosis. Bull World Health Organ 2009 Jun;87(6):481-483.

[86] Rao SN, Mookerjee AL, Obasanjo OO, Chaisson RE. Errors in the treatment of tuberculosis in Baltimore. Chest 2000 Mar;117(3):734-737.

[87] Alexy ER, Podewils LJ, Mitnick CD, Becerra MC, Laserson KF, Bonilla C. Concordance of programmatic and laboratory-based multidrug-resistant tuberculosis treatment outcomes in Peru. Int J Tuberc Lung Dis 2012;16(3):364-369.

[88] Singh VK, Chandra S, Kumar S, Pangtey G, Mohan A, Guleria R. A common medical error: lung cancer misdiagnosed as sputum negative tuberculosis. Asian Pac J Cancer Prev 2009 Jul-Sep;10(3):335-338.

[89] Van Deun A, Salim MA, Das AP, Bastian I, Portaels F. Results of a standardised regimen for multidrug-resistant tuberculosis in Bangladesh. Int J Tuberc Lung Dis 2004 May;8(5):560-567.

[90] Mukherjee JS, Rich ML, Socci AR, Joseph JK, Viru FA, Shin SS, et al. Programmes and principles in treatment of multidrug-resistant tuberculosis. Lancet 2004 Feb 7;363(9407):474-481.

[91] WHO. Guidelines for the programmatic management of drug-resistant tuberculosis. 2011.   Available   at: http://whqlibdoc.who.int/publications/ 2011/9789241501583_eng.pdf.

[92] Cobelens FG, Heldal E, Kimerling ME, Mitnick CD, Podewils LJ, Ramachandran R, et al. Scaling up programmatic management of drug-resistant tuberculosis: a prioritized research agenda. PLoS Med 2008 Jul 8;5(7):e150.

[93] WHO. The Global MDR-TB & XDR-TB Response Plan 2007-2008. 2007. Available at: http://whqlibdoc.who.int/hq/2007/who_htm_tb_2007.387_eng.pdf.

[94] Shanks L, Masumbuko EW, Ngoy NM, Maneno M, Bartlett S, Thi SS, et al. Treatment of multidrug-resistant tuberculosis in a remote, conflict-affected area of the Democratic Republic of Congo. Int J Tuberc Lung Dis 2012 Aug;16(8):1066-1068.

[95] Daftary A, Padayatchi N. Social constraints to TB/HIV healthcare: Accounts from co-infected patients in South Africa. AIDS Care 2012 Dec;24(12):1480-1486.

[96] Mauch V, Woods N, Kirubi B, Kipruto H, Sitienei J, Klinkenberg E. Assessing access barriers to tuberculosis care with the tool to Estimate Patients' Costs: pilot results from two districts in Kenya. BMC Public Health 2011 Jan 18;11:43.

[97] Lin X, Chongsuvivatwong V, Geater A, Lijuan R. The effect of geographical distance on TB patient delays in a mountainous province of China. Int J Tuberc Lung Dis 2008 Mar;12(3):288-293.

[98] Ngang PN, Ntaganira J, Kalk A, Wolter S, Ecks S. Perceptions and beliefs about cough and tuberculosis and implications for TB control in rural Rwanda. Int J Tuberc Lung Dis 2007 Oct;11(10):1108-1113.

[99] Gupta R, Espinal M, Stop TB Working Group on DOTS-Plus for MDR-TB. A prioritised research agenda for DOTS-Plus for multidrug-resistant tuberculosis (MDR-TB). Int J Tuberc Lung Dis 2003 May;7(5):410-414.

[100] Zellmer E, Zhang Z, Greco D, Rhodes J, Cassel S, Lewis EJ. A homeodomain protein selectively expressed in noradrenergic tissue regulates transcription of neurotransmitter biosynthetic genes. J Neurosci 1995 Dec;15(12):8109-8120.

[101] Cueto M. The origins of primary health care and selective primary health care. Am J Public Health 2004 Nov;94(11):1864-1874.

[102] TB CTA. Patient Centered Approach Strategy. Available at: http://www.tbcare1.org/ publications/toolbox/tools/access/PCA_Booklet.pdf.

[103] Munro SA, Lewin SA, Smith HJ, Engel ME, Fretheim A, Volmink J. Patient adherence to tuberculosis treatment: a systematic review of qualitative research. PLoS Med 2007 Jul 24;4(7):e238.

[104] Doctors without borders. Tuberculosis, 2012. Available at: http://www.doctorswithoutborders.org/news/issue.cfm?id=2404.

[105] Jakubowiak WM, Bogorodskaya EM, Borisov SE, Danilova ID, Kourbatova EV. Risk factors associated with default among new pulmonary TB patients and social support in six Russian regions. Int J Tuberc Lung Dis 2007 Jan;11(1):46-53.

[106] Gelmanova IY, Taran DV, Mishustin SP, Golubkov AA, Solovyova AV, Keshavjee S. 'Sputnik': a programmatic approach to improve tuberculosis treatment adherence and outcome among defaulters. Int J Tuberc Lung Dis 2011 Oct;15(10):1373-1379.

[107] Chalco K, Wu DY, Mestanza L, Munoz M, Llaro K, Guerra D, et al. Nurses as providers of emotional support to patients with MDR-TB. Int Nurs Rev 2006 Dec;53(4): 253-260.

[108] US Centers for Disease Control. Tuberculosis (TB). 2012; Available at: http:// www.cdc.gov/tb/publications/reportsarticles/iom/iomresponse/goal1.h tm. Guidelines, 2012.

[109] C-Hub. Within Our Reach: A TB Literacy Toolkit, 2012. Available at: http:// www.fhi360.org/en/HIVAIDS/pub/res_TBLiteracy_Toolkit.htm.

[110] Menzies D, Fanning A, Yuan L, Fitzgerald M. Tuberculosis among health care workers. N Engl J Med 1995 Jan 12;332(2):92-98.

[111] Nardell E, Dharmadhikari A. Turning off the spigot: reducing drug-resistant tuberculosis transmission in resource-limited settings. Int J Tuberc Lung Dis 2010 Oct; 14(10):1233-1243.

[112] Wilson TM, de Lisle GW, Collins DM. Effect of inhA and katG on isoniazid resistance and virulence of Mycobacterium bovis. Mol Microbiol 1995 Mar;15(6):1009-1015.

[113] Ramaswamy S, Musser JM. Molecular genetic basis of antimicrobial agent resistance in Mycobacterium tuberculosis: 1998 update. Tuber Lung Dis 1998;79(1):3-29.

[114] US Centers for Disease Control. Transmission of multidrug-resistant tuberculosis among immunocompromised persons in a correctional system--New York, 1991. MMWR Morb Mortal Wkly Rep 1992 Jul 17;41(28):507-509.

[115] US Centers for Disease Control. Outbreak of multidrug-resistant tuberculosis at a hospital--New York City, 1991. MMWR Morb Mortal Wkly Rep 1993 Jun 11;42(22): 427, 433-4.

[116] Zignol M, van Gemert W, Falzon D, Sismanidis C, Glaziou P, Floyd K, et al. Surveil-
       lance of anti-tuberculosis drug resistance in the world: an updated analysis,
       2007-2010. Bull World Health Organ 2012 Feb 1;90(2):111-119D.

[117] Robert J, Trystram D, Truffot-Pernot C, Cambau E, Jarlier V, Grosset J. Twenty-five
       years of tuberculosis in a French university hospital: a laboratory perspective. Int J
       Tuberc Lung Dis 2000 Jun;4(6):504-512.

[118] Mendoza MT, Gonzaga AJ, Roa C, Velmonte MA, Jorge M, Montoya JC, et al. Nature
       of drug resistance and predictors of multidrug-resistant tuberculosis among patients
       seen at the Philippine General Hospital, Manila, Philippines. Int J Tuberc Lung Dis
       1997 Feb;1(1):59-63.

[119] Van Rie A, Warren R, Richardson M, Gie RP, Enarson DA, Beyers N, et al. Classifica-
       tion of drug-resistant tuberculosis in an epidemic area. Lancet 2000 Jul 1;356(9223):
       22-25.

[120] Gandhi NR, Moll A, Sturm AW, Pawinski R, Govender T, Lalloo U, et al. Extensively
       drug-resistant tuberculosis as a cause of death in patients co-infected with tuberculo-
       sis and HIV in a rural area of South Africa. Lancet 2006 Nov 4;368(9547):1575-1580.

[121] Gelmanova IY, Keshavjee S, Golubchikova VT, Berezina VI, Strelis AK, Yanova GV,
       et al. Barriers to successful tuberculosis treatment in Tomsk, Russian Federation:
       non-adherence, default and the acquisition of multidrug resistance. Bull World
       Health Organ 2007 Sep;85(9):703-711.

[122] Pearson ML, Jereb JA, Frieden TR, Crawford JT, Davis BJ, Dooley SW, et al. Nosoco-
       mial transmission of multidrug-resistant Mycobacterium tuberculosis. A risk to pa-
       tients and health care workers. Ann Intern Med 1992 Aug 1;117(3):191-196.

[123] Joshi R, Reingold AL, Menzies D, Pai M. Tuberculosis among health-care workers in
       low- and middle-income countries: a systematic review. PLoS Med 2006 Dec;
       3(12):e494.

[124] O'Donnell MR, Jarand J, Loveday M, Padayatchi N, Zelnick J, Werner L, et al. High
       incidence of hospital admissions with multidrug-resistant and extensively drug-re-
       sistant tuberculosis among South African health care workers. Ann Intern Med 2010
       Oct 19;153(8):516-522.

[125] Biscotto CR, Pedroso ER, Starling CE, Roth VR. Evaluation of N95 respirator use as a
       tuberculosis control measure in a resource-limited setting. Int J Tuberc Lung Dis 2005
       May;9(5):545-549.

[126] Kantor HS, Poblete R, Pusateri SL. Nosocomial transmission of tuberculosis from un-
       suspected disease. Am J Med 1988 May;84(5):833-838.

[127] US Centers for Disease Control. TB elimination. Infection control in health care sit-
       tings.   Available   at: http://www.cdc.gov/tb/publications/factsheets/prevention/
       ichcs.pdf.

[128] Maloney SA, Pearson ML, Gordon MT, Del Castillo R, Boyle JF, Jarvis WR. Efficacy of control measures in preventing nosocomial transmission of multidrug-resistant tuberculosis to patients and health care workers. Ann Intern Med 1995 Jan 15;122(2): 90-95.

Chapter 12

Drug-Resistant Tuberculosis – Diagnosis, Treatment, Management and Control: The Experience in Thailand

Attapon Cheepsattayakorn

Additional information is available at the end of the chapter

1. Introduction

Multidrug-resistant tuberculosis (MDR-TB) is defined as TB bacilli revealing resistance to at least isoniazid and rifampicin whereas extensively drug-resistant tuberculosis (XDR-TB) is TB bacilli that develops resistance to at least isoniazid and rifampicin as well as to any quinolone drug and at least one of the second-line anti-TB injectable drug : kanamycin, amikacin, or capreomycin. Report from the World Health Organization (WHO)/International Union Against Tuberculosis and Lung Disease (IUATLD) Global Project on Drug Resistance Surveillance revealed that the prevalence of the primary multidrug-resistant tuberculosis during 1996-1999 ranged between 0-14.1 % [1]. In 1994, the first WHO-IUATLD global anti-TB drug resistance surveillance was carried out in 35 countries and subsequently, the second, third and fourth surveillances occurred in 1996-1999, 1999-2002 and 2002-2007, respectively. The emergence of clinically significant MDR-TB was in the early 1990s. Reports of Primary Drug-Resistance Surveillance in Thailand during 1997-1998, 2001-2002, and 2005-2006 were 2.02 % [2], 0.93 % [3], and 1.65 % [4], respectively while the secondary drug-resistance in 2005-2006 revealed 34.54 % [4]. However, number of patients with MDR-TB demonstrated in 2008 Annual Report of the Bureau of Tuberculosis, Thailand were only 294 while the WHO' s estimated number of patients were 2,774 [5]. The prevalence of primary plus secondary MDR-TB among prisoners in Thailand in 2002-2003 was 5.3 % while the prevalence of primary MDR-TB was 5.9 % [6]. Report from the 10th Zonal Tuberculosis and Chest Disease Centre, Chiang Mai, Thailand, 10th office of Disease prevention and Control, Department of Disease Control, Ministry of Public Health, Thailand in 2011 revealed only 88 patients who registered with MDR-TB at hospitals in northern Thailand [7] while only 16.3 %, 18.6 % and 18.6 % of 43 patients with laboratory confirmation were cure, completeness of treatment, and dead, respectively in 2009 report [8]. Findings from the Bureau of Tuberculosis of Thailand ' s 2007-2009 Research

Project on Anti-tuberculosis Drug Resistance Surveillance in Thailand (Situation of Multidrug-Resistant Tuberculosis in Thailand : Fiscal Year 2007-2009) that studied in 126 hospitals countrywide showed 877 patients with laboratory-confirmed MDR-TB and 64 patients with laboratory-confirmed XDR-TB while 21.5 % were dead and 12.74 % of these MDR/XDR-TB patients had human immunodeficiency virus (HIV) infection /acquired immunodeficiency syndrome (AIDS) compared to 21.57% of probable or presumptive MDR-TB patients co-infected with HIV/AIDS [9]. Only 18.2% of the studied data sources came from TB registered book for MDR-TB patients and most of them came from the hospital medical registry [9]. A previous study by Scano F *et al.* revealed 52 of the 53 patients with XDR-TB died [10]. The median survival time from collection of specimen to death of these patients was 16 days [10]. The prevalence of XDR-TB among all MDR-TB patient was as the following : 10.3% in Germany and 14.3% in Italy (1993-2004) ; 1.5% in Asia, 15.4% in Republic of Korea, 13.6% in Russia, 0.6% in Africa and Middle East, 6.5% in industrialized countries, and 6.6% overall worldwide (2000-2004); 12% in Hong Kong (2004); 10.9% in Iran (2006); 7.3% in India; and 4% in France (2006) [11]. The WHO notified that Thailand possibly underreported of MDR/XDR-TB prevalence due to delaying of transportation of the specimens for anti-tuberculosis drug susceptibility testing to the specialized centres and processes of unstandardized data collecting of the country [9]. More than 400,000 new MDR-TB cases globally occur each year while approximately half of a million cases occurred in 2007 and accounted for more than 5% of the annually global cases of TB disease. The emerging of drug-resistant TB is a global health problem, although emphasis has been placed on several " hotspots " (higher than 3% of its prevalence) worldwide because of lacking of good global data reported to the WHO. The emergence of MDR-TB and XDR-TB is a real health threat to achieve TB elimination.

2. Epidemiology

Development of anti-tuberculosis drug resistance can occur due to *Mycobacterium tuberculosis* genetic factor, previous anti-tuberculosis treatment-related factors and many other factors [11]. The mechanism of drug-resistance is shown in Figure 1. There is a constant rate of spontaneous mutation of 0.0033 mutations/deoxyribonucleic acid (DNA) replication that is unique for a diverse spectrum of prokaryotic organisms [12]. The average rates of spontaneous mutation for rifampicin, isoniazid, pyrazinamide, streptomycin, and ethambutol are 2.25×10^{-10}, 2.56×10^{-8}, 1×10^{-3}, 2.95×10^{-8}, and 1.0×10^{-7}, respectively [13]. A previous study in India revealed 3.4% and 25% of primary and acquired MDR-TB, respectively [14] which were higher than the primary MDR-TB and acquired MDR-TB prevalence previously surveyed in Thailand [2,3,4]. Liu CH *et al.* reported their study in China which presented 19.4% of MDR-TB, 1.3% of XDR-TB, 19.8% of poly-resistant TB, and 47.1% of any anti-tuberculosis drug resistance [15]. A surveillance data in 2007 from the WHO demonstrated 4.8% of MDR-TB cases among new TB cases worldwide [16] compared to the study from MDR-TB surveillance in Thailand between 2007-2009 revealed the MDR-TB prevalence of 0-0.21% (average 0.08%) which was highest in the central part of Thailand [9]. The prevalence among patients with previously TB treatment from the same surveillance project was between 1.58-58.72% (average 8.49%, higher than the percentage of hotspot of MDR-TB prevalence set by the WHO (3%, an indicator for implementation of DOTS (Directly Observed Treatment, Short Course)-Plus programmes) which was also found highest in the central part of Thailand while the northern part of Thailand was the second [9]. This Thailand's serious MDR-TB situation needs urgently management such as implementation of DOTS-Plus programmes. In 2006, Gandhi NR *et al.* firstly reported of XDR-TB co-infected with HIV/AIDS which had been studied in Kwazulu Natal, South Africa (KZN) [11]. XDR-TB epidemic in South Africa appears to be the primary mechanism through the acquisition of 63-75% of XDR-TB cases [11] whereas the strain of *Mycobacterium tuberculosis* infected among a large number of XDR-TB cases in KZN was F15/LAM4/KZN [11]. Generally, individual who is infected with *Mycobacterium tuberculosis* has approximately 5-10% lifetime risk of developing TB disease, but in an individual with HIV-infection/AIDS the risk is 5-15% a year [11]. This can contribute HIV-infection/AIDS to facilitate the control of outbreaks of MDR-TB and XDR-TB, although it has contributed to outbreaks of drug-resistant TB [17]. The patients with MDR-TB and HIV/AIDS co-infection will have exceedingly high mortality [16]. Gandhi NR *et al.* recently reported their study on risk factors for mortality among MDR/XDR-TB patients with HIV/AIDS co-infection which revealed that 80% of XDR-TB patients died whereas 63% of MDR-TB patients were dead following the diagnosis [18]. The CD4-T cell count less than 50 cells/mm^3 was the strongest independent factor for mortality among both patient groups [18]. History of TB treatment is the most significant predictor of development of MDR-TB [19]. High prevalence of HIV/AIDS co-infection and inadequate resources for case detection and management have contributed to the emergence of untreatable XDR-TB [20]. Unfortunately, the presence of XDR-TB in non—HIV-infected patients with MDR-TB is independent poor prognostic factors [11]. Prevalence of XDR-TB is globally accounted for approximately 5.4% of MDR-TB prevalence [21]. Drug-resistant TB and drug-resistant gram-negative bacterial infection and disease are associated with the most serious health problems in developing countries [22]. Estimated 81,000 patients with MDR-TB (18.4% of the estimated MDR-TB patients worldwide in 2011) live in the 53 countries of the WHO European Region [23]. This European MDR-TB problem contributed to launching of a new WHO Regional Office for Europe Action Plan to fight MDR-TB to contain the spread of drug-resistant TB in the region by the end of 2015 [23]. The new action plan set the targets to be achieved by the end of 2015, are : 1) decreasing 20% of the proportion of MDR-TB cases among previously treated patients 2) diagnosis of at least 85% of the estimated MDR-TB cases and 3) treating successfully at least 75% of notified MDR-TB cases [23]. If this plan is fully implemented and expected, by 2015, to successfully treat 127,000 MDR-TB cases, and to prevent the emergence of 250,000 new MDR-TB cases and 13,000 new XDR-TB cases [23]. This would interrupt the transmission of MDR-TB and save 120,000 lives in this region [23].

3. Systematic management of MDR/XDR-TB

Diagnostic and treatment consultation networks for MDR/XDR-TB which set by the 10th Zonal Tuberculosis and Chest Disease Centre, Chiang Mai, 10th Office of Disease Prevention and Control, Department of Disease Control, Ministry of Public Health, Thailand beyond the year

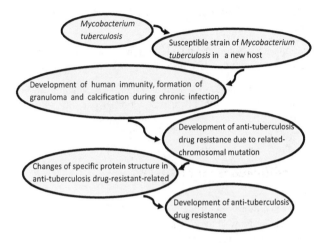

Figure 1. Mechanism of development of anti-tuberculosis drug resistance

2000 have been firstly initiated at tertiary care hospitals in northern Thailand. Data collecting on MDR/XDR-TB control has been tracked through the special project paper-based recording and reporting systems set by the 10th Zonal Tuberculosis and Chest Disease Centre which separated from the routine DOTS recording and reporting systems. Currently, a new computer programme has been developed by staff of this centre to efficiently record and report the MDR/XDR-TB data in the area of northern Thailand and attempt to gradually extend the use of this computer programme throughout the country.

4. Presumptive diagnosis of MDR-TB

The Thailand' s 2012 National Tuberculosis Management Guidelines [24] set the criteria for probable or suspected MDR-TB, are :

1. patients with history of TB retreatment, especially within 6 months after completeness of treatment or cure,

2. patients with interruption of 6 month-short course chemotherapy (2HRZE/4HR, H=iso-niazid, R=rifampicin, Z=pyrazinamide, E=ethambutol) and having continuously positive-sputum smear examinations after treatment interruption,

3. patients with history of multiple TB treatments, irregular anti-TB drug taking, and persistently positive-sputum smear examinations,

4. patients having positive-sputum smear examinations at the end of second and fifth months of the 6-month short course chemotherapy (2HRZE/4HR),

5. patients with evidence of HIV co-infection/AIDS before the 6-month short course chemo-
    therapy starting,

6. general TB patients with history of MDR-TB patient exposure, including health or medical
    personnel with TB disease who have history of MDR-TB patient exposure, and

7. other high-risk patients of MDR-TB, such as general TB patient with huge lung cavity,
    diabetic patients, prisoners with TB disease, and TB patients who live in the cross-
    borderline areas.

5. Laboratory investigations for MDR-TB

Several plans have been announced for the WHO Stop TB Department to collaborate with the
Foundation for Innovative New Diagnostics (FIND) to initiate and introduce rapid-culture
technology and new rapid drug-resistant tests in the southern African countries and the world
including the international standards for the second-line drug-susceptibility testing [11]. The
Thailand' s 2012 National Tuberculosis Management Guidelines [24] set the laboratory
investigations for MDR-TB which are direct acid-fast bacilli (AFB)-sputum smear examinations with sputum culture and drug susceptibility testing (DST). For reduction of the diagnosis
time for unrecognized drug-resistant TB, new rapid diagnostic technologies for drug resistance
from sputum smear or positive culture for smear-negative and extra-pulmonary TB must be
prioritized [10]. All TB control programmes in moderate- and high-MDR TB prevalent settings
should consider the promotion of culture and DST including implementation of use of
algorithms for the diagnosis of pulmonary and extra-pulmonary TB [10]. Rapid DST is
preferred to the conventional DST due to 1-2 days of resulting. Recently, the 2011 WHO
Guidelines recommends " Xpert MTB/RIF® " and line-probe assay which are new molecular
diagnostic technologies and can detect drug resistance to both isoniazid and rifampicin or only
rifampicin [24], but their disadvantage is inability to detect the resistance to every drugs used
in MDR-TB treatment for detecting probable XDR-TB, required expertise and expensive
technologies/equipments which limit their wider uses [25]. The conventional DST takes 1-3
months of the results that take markedly longer than the new molecular methods and is labor-
intensive [24]. Other alternative phenotypic methods based on the *Mycobacterium tuberculosis*
metabolism such as CO_2 (carbon dioxide) production, oxygen uptake, ATP (adenosine
triphosphate) bioluminescence, etc. have been experimented and demonstrated promising in
overcoming this obstacle of longer time resulting [25]. These methods also have impressive
sensitivity and specificity compared to the conventional DST [25]. Currently, molecular line
probe assays and automated liquid culture systems are recommended by the WHO as the gold
standard for the first-line and second-line DSTs. Liquid culture DST has been demonstrated
to have relatively good reliability and reproducibility for aminoglycosides, fluoroquinolones,
and polypeptides for detecting XDR-TB [26]. However, liquid culture DST for other second-
line drugs such as para-aminosalisylic acid, linezolid, clarithromycin, amoxicillin-clavulanate,
cycloserine, clofazimine, terizidone, ethionamide, and prothionamide is not recommended by
the WHO [26]. A recent study reported the use of spoligotyping and sequence 6110 restriction

fragment length polymorphism insertion analysis of genomic DNA which demonstrated that MDR-TB cases (74.0%) were more likely to be identified in clusters than anti-TB drug susceptible cases (33.6%) [27]. Xpert MTB/RIF assay recently has been introduced which meets the requirements of effective diagnosis of pulmonary TB as the following : allowing detection of both the *Mycobacterium tuberculosis* complex and resistance to the principal anti-TB drugs, especially rifampicin (RIF or R), availability on a global scale with standardized-easy use and robust diagnostic tools recently has been introduced [28]. This assay is a nucleic acid amplification test for detection of rifampicin resistance-associated mutations of the *rpoB* gene and *Mycobacterium tuberculosis* complex DNA in sputum [28]. It can be designed for use with other systems to automate and integrate sample processing, nucleic acid amplification, and detection of target sequences using reverse transcriptase polymerase chain reaction (PCR) and real-time PCR [28]. Between 2007-2009, the WHO has approved several drug-resistant TB diagnostic tests such as liquid culture (MGIT®, an automated liquid culture, developed by BD Diagnostic Systems, 2007) which has been used at the 10th Zonal Tuberculosis and Chest Disease Centre, Chiang Mai, Thailand, line-probe assays (INNO-Lipa®, line-probe assay that requires culture, developed by Innogenetics, 2008), noncommercial culture and drug susceptibility testing (Microscopic Observation Drug Susceptibility (MODS), developed by Academic Laboratories, 2009; Nitrate reductase assay, developed by Academic Laboratories, 2009; and Colorimetric drug susceptibility testing, developed by Academic Laboratories, 2009) [29]. GeneXpert MTB/ RIF®, a new automated nucleic acid amplification technique which was developed by Cepheid, The Foundation for Innovative New Diagnostics (FIND) and University of Medicine and Dentistry of New Jersey (UMDNJ) was reviewed by the WHO in 2011 [29] and currently has been recommended to measure the *Mycobacterium tuberculosis* DNA and the rifampicin-resistance sequence worldwide. This new technique has been set in Thailand at least 6 sets including the one set at the 10th Zonal Tuberculosis and Chest Disease Centre, Chiang Mai, Thailand in collaboration with the Unites States Centres for Disease Control and Prevention (US-CDC) for reference laboratories in Thailand. GeneXpert test's sensitivity is moderate at 67.2% in AFB-smear negative cases at one-time smear staining of the specimens, and increases to 80% when is performed three times [28]. This test provides the results within two hours and requires minimal training of the laboratory workers [29]. The limitations of the test are requirement of a consistent source of electricity that will limit its use outside of the settings where a regular electric power supply can be guaranteed, its expensive cost of the instrument, and cost per test cartridge [29]. Mishra B *et al*. used the automated BACTEC 460 TB system in study the emergence of drug-resistant TB at an urban tertiary care hospital in South India which revealed that 37.2% were MDR-TB isolates whereas 42% of the pulmonary *Mycobacterium tuberculosis* isolates and 20.4% of extra-pulmonary isolates were MDR [30]. Phenotypic and genotypic detections of anti-TB drug resistance are described as the following [31- 49]:

1. Phenotypic detection

1.1 Slide DST

This method has less equiptment, suitable for decentralization, 93% rifampicin susceptibility at 88% predictive value of resistance.

1.2 Mycobacteria Growth Indicator Tube (MGIT) Systems

This test has sensitivities of 100% for rifampicin, isoniazid, ethambutol and streptomycin, specificity of 100% for rifampicin, 97.7% for isoniazid, 98.0% for ethambutol and 89.8%% for streptomycin.

1.3 Microscopic observation broth-drug susceptibility assay (MODS)

This method has sensitivity of 72.7% and specificity of 99.7% for rifampicin, 72.6% and 97.9% for isoniazid, and 77.8% and 99.7% for MDR-TB.

1.4 Mycobacteriophage-based method

1.4.1 Commercial FASTPlaque assay (FASTPlaque TB test and FastPlaque TB-RIF™ (rifampicin DST) (Biotech Labs Ltd, Ipswich, UK))

This test has sensitivity and specificity of 31.2% and 94.9%, respectively in all anti-TB drug-susceptible and resistant TB patients, sensitivity and specificity of 33.3% and 93.9%, respectively in all anti-TB drug-susceptible and resistant TB patients with HIV-infection/AIDS.

1.4.2 Fluoromycobacteriophage assay (Figures 2, 3)

This method has 94% sensitivities for rifampicin and isoniazid and 98% sensitivity for streptomycin and specificities of 97% for isoniazid, 95% for rifampicin, and 98% for strepto-mycin (resazurin microplate technique), sensitivity of 94% for all three anti-TB drugs (rifam-picin, isoniazid, and streptomycin) (*EGFP*-phage technique) and specificities of 93% for rifampicin, 90% for isoniazid and 95% for streptomycin (*EGFP*-phage technique).

1.4.3 Luciferase reporter phage assay

This test has 100% sensitivity and 89-100% specificity for culture isolates.

1.5 Nitrate reductase assay

This method has sensitivity and specificity of 100% and 100% for rifampicin, 93% and 100% for isoniazid, 76% and 100% for streptomycin, and 55% and 99% for ethambutol, respectively.

1.6 Microcolony method (Thin-layer agar (TLA) method)

This test has sensitivities and specificities of 100% for both rifampicin and ofloxacin, and sensitivity of 100% and specificity of 98.7% for kanamycin, 100% overall accuracy for rifam-picin and isoniazid resistance.

1.7 Colorimetric redox indicator methods

This method has sensitivities of 100% for rifampicin, ofloxacin, kanamycin and capreomycin and 99.1% for isoniazid, specificity of 100% for rifampicin, isoniazid, ofloxacin and kanamycin, and 97.9% for capreomycin, overall accuracy of 98.4% for rifampicin, 96.6% for isoniazid, 96.7% for ofloxacin, 98.3% for kanamycin and 90% for capreomycin.

2. Genotypic detection (Nucleic Acid Amplification)

2.1 Line-probe assay (LPA)

2.1.1 INNO-LiPA Rif.TB® assay (Innogenetics, Ghent, Belgium)

This test has higher than 95% sensitivity and 100% specificity, sensitivity of 82.2% and specificity of 66.7% for MDR-TB detection.

2.1.2 GenoType® MTBDRplus kit (Hain Lifescience, Nehren, Germany)

This method has nearly 91% sensitivity for MDR-TB, possibly detects rifampicin and isoniazid resistance and confirms TB infection simultaneously.

2.1.3 Genotype MTBDRsl assay

This test has ethambutol, 89% sensitivity for ofloxacin, 87% sensitivity for capreomycin, 75% sensitivity for amikacin.

2.2 Real-time PCR

This technique has sensitivity of 89% and specificity of 99% (molecular beacons), overall sensitivity of 98-100% with 72% sensitivity in smear-negative specimens and specificity of 100% for Xpert MTB/RIF assay (Cepheid Xpert MTB/RIF®, Sunyvale, CA).

2.3 PCR sequencing

This technique has sensitivities of 96.7% for rifampicin-resistant isolates (*rpoB* gene), 64% for isoniazid-resistant isolates (*katG* gene) and 70% of ofloxacin-resistant isolates (*gyrA* gene) (PCR pyrosequencing).

2.4 DNA Microarrays (DNA biochip)

This technique has specificity of 97% and 95% for rifampicin, 91% and 60% for isoniazid, 96% and 67% for kanamycin, 93% and 73% for streptomycin, and 98% and 89% for ethambutol, respectively, simultaneous detection of multiple genetic sequences (oligonu-cleotide microarray).

Although genotypic methods have potentially fastest results, the massive cross-contamination is still the main risk. To prevent its, strict internal controls, special technique, and separation of working areas are required. The reproducibility of the results of the Xpert MTB/RIF assay under actual field conditions, the strength of the laboratories, and the manner and extent of its introduction are the impact of this new assay. The sources of error for genotypic methods are incomplete coverage of rifampicin-resistance gene-core region and mixtures (multiple mutations, wild-type strain/emerging mutant) and silent mutations. These sources of error may contribute to 1% false-resistant and 5% false-susceptible results [31].

Schematic representation of *phAE87* : *hsp60-EGFP* construction. Shuttle phasmid *phAE87* is a conditionally replicating derivative of phage TM4 in which the cosmid moiety is flanked by Pac I restriction sites. A plasmid derivative of *pYUB854* containing the *EGFP* gene (pMP14) was used to replace the cosmid in *phAE87* followed by lambda packaging and recovery in *E. coli*.

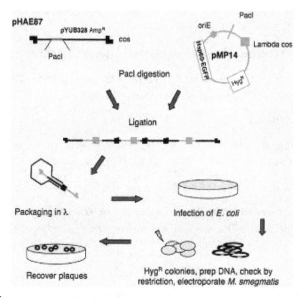

Source : Piuri M, Jacobs WR Jr, Hatfull GF. Fluoromycobacteriophages for rapid, specific, and sensitive antibiotic susceptibility testing of *Mycobacterium tuberculosis*. PLoS ONE 2009; 4(3) : e4870. doi: 10.1371/journal.pone.0004870

Figure 2. Fluoromycobacteriophages construction

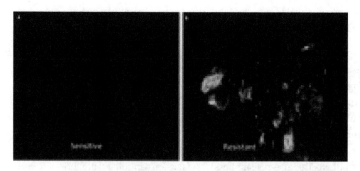

Source : Rondo'n L, Piuri M, Jacobs WR Jr, Waard Jde, Hatfull GF, Takiff HE. Evaluation of fluoromycobacteriophages for detecting drug resistance in *Mycobacterium tuberculosis*. J Clin Microbiol 2011; 49 (5) : 1838-1842.

Figure 3. A, B). Two strains of *Mycobacterium tuberculosis* were incubated separately in 7H9-OAD with 2 μg of rifampicin/ml for 24 hours, infected with the *EGFP*-phage, killed with paraformaldehyde, and then fixed on microscope slides. The images, obtained with a fluorescence microscope, show a susceptible-to-rifampicin strain (A) and a resistant-to-rifampicin strain (B).

6. Radiological features in patients with MDR/XDR-TB

A recent study in South Korea showed 100% of lung nodules, 60% of lung consolidation, and 47% of lung cavities that were mainly located in the upper and middle lung zones in XDR-TB patients whereas less frequent lung nodules and ground-glass opacity lesions were found in XDR-TB patients compared to the patients with anti-TB drug-susceptible pulmonary TB [50]. More frequent multiple lung cavities, lung nodules, and bronchial dilatation were found in both MDR-TB and XDR-TB patients compared to the patients with anti-TB drug-susceptible pulmonary TB [50]. There was no different radiological findings between MDR-TB and XDR-TB patients [50]. Another recent study in South Korea revealed that micronodules and tree-in-bud appearance were found in 100% of the pulmonary XDR-TB patients whereas lung consolidations, lung cavities, bronchiectasis, lobar consolidations were found in 85%, 85%, 80%, and 70%, respectively [51]. This study showed a significantly larger extent of tree-in-bud appearance and lung consolidations compared to the MDR-TB patients [51]. In childhood patients, chest radiological features at the time of diagnosis demonstrates lobar opacification, intrathoracic lymphadenopathy, particular hilar lymph nodes, and airway narrowing [52]. Chest radiological features of three patients with MDR-TB who attended the 10th Zonal Tuberculosis and Chest Disease Centre, Chiang Mai, Thailand are shown in the Figure 4 (A,B,C) which demonstrated a single cavity at the upper lung zone in two patients and no lung cavity in another one. These three patients possibly attended the 10th Zonal Tuberculosis and Chest Disease Centre, Chiang Mai, Thailand at the earlier stages compared to the above study results.

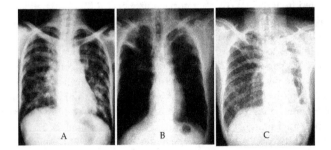

Figure 4. First-attendance chest radiological features of the three patients (A,B,C) with MDR-TB at the 10th Zonal Tuberculosis and Chest Disease Centre, Chiang Mai, Thailand A : Showing bilaterally diffuse lung infiltration with a cavity in the left upper lung zone, B : Showing fibrotic infiltration with surrounding new infiltration at the right upper lung zone with bilaterally diffuse emphysematous lung changes, C : Showing bilaterally diffuse infiltration with a cavity in the right upper lung zone with left pleural effusion.

7. Regimens used in treating patients with drug-resistant tuberculosis

A recent study on MDR-TB treatment revealed that use of later generation quinolones (moxifloxacin, gatifloxacin, sparfloxacin, levofloxacin), ofloxacin or ethionamide/prothionamide, use of four or more likely effective drugs in the initial intensive phase, and three or more likely effective drugs in the continuation phase was associated with the treatment success compared to the treatment failure or relapse [53]. The duration of initial phase up to 7.1-8.5 months and the total duration of treatment up to 18.6-21.5 months increased the chances of treatment success [53]. In 2011, the WHO recommended the regimens containing a fluoroquinolone, pyrazinamide, ethionamide (or prothionamide), para-aminosalicylic acid (or cycloserine), and a second-line injectable drug with more than 20 months of treatment duration [54]. Five MDR-TB control projects with used DST results and previous treatment history were conducted among 1,047 MDR-TB patients in 5 resource-limited settings with well-established DOTS programmes (Manila, Estonia, Latvia, Lima, and Tomsk) in 1999 for Lima and Manila, 2000 for Tomsk and Latvia, and 2001 for Estonia [55]. At least 4 drug (ethambutol, pyrazinamide, cycloserine, clofazimine, para-aminosalicylic acid, ethionamide, or prothionamide, augmentin, clarithromycin or thiacetazone) including an injectable drug (kanamycin, amikacin, capreomycin, or streptomycin) and a fluoroquinolone (ofloxacin, ciprofloxacin, or levofloxacin) were administered for the duration of treatment (18-24 months) except for the injectable drug, which was administered for a specified interval after the patient' s specimens were culture-negative [55]. Monthly sputum-AFB smear and culture were monitored [55]. Every 6-months (Manila and Lima) and 3-months chest radiographs (Tomsk, Latvia, and Estonia) were performed [55]. The treatment outcomes among new and previously treated MDR-TB patients revealed 74.8% and 68.3% cured patients, 2.5% and 0.3% completed treatment patients, 4.2% and 7.0% failed treatment patients, 3.4% and 14.2% dead patients, and 77.3% and 66.6% treatment success rates (cure rate + completed treatment rate), respectively [55]. The results showed worsen outcomes among previously treated patients. Report from the 10th Zonal Tuberculosis and Chest Disease Centre, Chiang Mai, Thailand, in 2011 which had been collected from the data of laboratory-confirmed 254 MDR-TB patients (72.8% of all probable MDR-TB cases) among 349 totally suspected-MDR-TB cases with 15.8% of HIV co-infection in northern Thailand between 2005-2010 gradually increased from 62.2% of probable MDR-TB cases in 2005 to 78.3% in 2010 and revealed 3.2% treatment-denial patients, 75.2% treatment-registered patients, 30.2% died before starting the second-line drug treatment regimens (pyrazinamide, ethambutol, ofloxacin, para-aminosalicylic acid administered for 18-24 months and one injectable drug (kanamycin, or amikacin) administered 5 days per week for the initial 6-month phase), 25.4% default-treatment patients (continuous interruption of treatment more than 2 months), 54.8% treatment success rate, and 22.2% unavailable-data patients [7]. Among 19 cases with pre-treatment death, 10 cases (52.63%) demonstrated HIV co-infection. Extra-pulmonary cases accounted for 2.4% of the laboratory-confirmed cases which was lower than percentage of susceptible extra-pulmonary TB cases in the same area [56]. Four cases with laboratory-confirmed MDR-TB emerged as XDR-TB during treatment [7]. A previous study on outcomes of a daily supervised-MDR-TB treatment regimen which consisted of initial phase of 6-9 months with kanamycin, ofloxacin, cycloserine, ethionamide, ethabutol, and pyrazinamide demonstrated that in cases of persistent culture positive at fourth month, the initial phase was extended for additional 3 months. Then ofloxacin, cycloserine, ethionamide, and ethambutol were continued for 18 months [57]. The results of the study revealed that 82% of cases demonstrated time to culture conversion at the second month or before. The culture conversion rates at third month and sixth month were 84% and 87%, respectively. The cure rate was 66%. At 24 months, 79% of the patients remained culture negative for more than 18 months. Adverse drug reactions were reported among 58% of cases and 2 failure cases emerged as XDR-TB during treatment [57]. A recent study on comparison between traditional hospital-based treatment-model of MDR-TB patient care and community-based model in rural areas of South Africa revealed that median times to starting the treatment and sputum smear conversion were shorter for community-based model (84 days versus 106.5 days and 59 days versus 92 days, respectively) [58]. Lack of sputum culture conversion at month 9 was a predictor of pulmonary MDR-TB treatment failure with 84% of sensitivity and 94% of specificity [59]. A recent study by Dheda K et al. demonstrated that the number of XDR-TB deaths was not significantly different compared between patients with and without HIV co-infection [60] whereas Well CD recently reported that lower cure rates and higher death rates were found in MDR-TB patients with HIV co-infection compared to the patients without HIV co-infection [61]. Survival of XDR-TB patients with HIV co-infection was associated with absence of biomarkers indicative of multiorgan dysfunction, less advanced stage of both diseases at time of diagnosis, and antiretrovirals provision [62]. Previous culture-proven MDR-TB, number of drug used in a MDR-TB treatment regimen, and treatment with moxifloxacin were independent predictors of death [60] while some previous reports showed that treatment success rates were poor (30-50%) in XDR-TB patients with HIV co-infection [63] and the MDR/XDR-TB prevalence was substantially precipitated by the HIV epidemic [64, 65]. In children with MDR-TB, the treatment guidelines are the same principles, using the same drugs as in adult patients with strict and prolonged supervision by expert pediatricians [66]. HIV co-infection are particular challenges and requires early starting of antiretroviral therapy with careful monitoring for drug-adverse side-effects [66]. Children with close contact with MDR-TB patients should be tested with tuberculin skin testing or interferon-gamma release assays, direct AFB-smear examinations, cultures, and DST and taking the chest radiological examinations [24]. Cases with close contact should be at least 2-year followed up [24]. If they are diagnosed MDR-TB, they must be treated with the empirical MDR-TB regimen [24]. Empirical MDR-TB treatment regimen is not recommended for MDR-TB chemoprophylaxis [24]. MDR-TB chemoprophylaxis for children with at least 2 second-line drugs for 6-12 months and reflecting the susceptibility profile of the source case' s isolate with daily supervision should be considered [52, 67]. The knowledge of mechanisms of the second-line drugs for children is necessary for ensuring the treatment adherence and long-term control of the disease.

A previous study on the second-line drug susceptibility among 40 MDR-TB strains in Turkey revealed mono-resistant to ethionamide 25%, amikacin 10.0%, kanamycin 2.5%, ofloxacin 2.5%, amikacin 0%, and clofazimine 0%, any resistant to ethionamide 37.5%, capreomycin 25.0%, kanamycin 5.0%, ofloxacin 5.0%, amikacin 5.0%, and clofazimine 2.5%, resistant to both ethionamide + capreomycin 5.0%, both capreomycin + clofazimine 2.5%, ofloxacin + ethionamide + capreomycin 2.5%, amikacin + ethionamide + capreomycin 2.5%, and kanamycin +

amikacin + ethionamide + capreomycin 2.5% [68]. Currently, the data of the second-line drug resistance are not available [9].

The Thailand' s 2012 National Tuberculosis Management Guidelines [24] recommends the guidelines for both pulmonary and extra-pulmonary MDR-TB treatment as the following flow diagram :

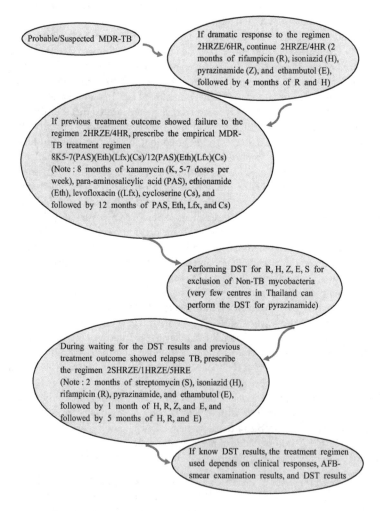

Figure 5. Flow Diagram of Management of Patient with Probable/Suspected MDR-TB

Currently, in Thailand, patients with persistent AFB-smear and/or culture positive after completeness of MDR-TB treatment will be prescribed isoniazid alone for lifelong while no

standardized treatment is recommended yet. Types of patients with MDR-TB, patient monitoring during MDR-TB treatment and assessment of sputum conversion, and classification of
treatment outcomes are shown in the Table 1, 2, and 3, respectively [24].

Type	Description
New case	patient who does not take any anti-TB drugs before or take any anti-TB drugs less than 1 month duration and the DST results show resistance to at least rifampicin and isoniazid
Relapse case	patient who cured of MDR-TB in the past and present or pre-treatment of relapse-MDR-TB DST results reveal MDR-TB
After default MDR-TB	patient who continuously interrupts the TB treatment more than 2 months and the DST results before treatment interruption demonstrates MDR-TB
After failure of the first- TB treatment	patient' s AFB examinations show positive results at the end of the fifth month and the DST results at the end of the second or fifth month reveal MDR-TB
After failure of retreatment	patient who treated with the retreatment regimen (2 months of streptomycin, rifampicin, isoniazid, pyrazinamide, and ethambutol, followed by 1 month of rifampicin, isoniazid, pyrazinamide, and ethambutol , and then followed by 5 months of isoniazid, pyrazinamide, and ethambutol for relapse cases) and the DST results at the end of third or fifth month demonstrate MDR-TB
Transfer in	patient who is referred from one setting to the other setting for further diagnosis, treatment, and management, transferred setting must report the outcome of treatment to the referred setting (first setting) for discharge registration as " transfer in "
Other	other patients who cannot be registered as the above 6 patient-registration types including patients who treated with empirical MDR-TB treatment regimen at the non-NTP settings (not registered as the above 6 patient-registration types)

Table 1. Registration of the patients with MDR-TB [24]

Patient monitoring during MDR-TB treatment	Assessment of sputum conversion
Direct AFB-smear examinations and cultures will be performed at month : 0, 1, 2, 3, 4, 5, 6, 7, 8, 10, 12, , 14, 16, 18, and 20.	Results of 2 consecutively direct-AFB-smear negative and culture negative with 30-day intervals will indicate sputum conversion. Mostly, patients with sputum conversion will
Chest radiological examinations will be performed at month : 0, 3, 6, 12, and 18.	converse the positive to the negative results within the first 6-month of treatment duration.

Table 2. Patient monitoring during MDR-TB treatment and Assessment of sputum conversion [24]

8. Patient monitoring after completeness of the MDR-TB treatment [24]

For assessment of the MDR-TB relapse rate, direct AFB-smear examinations and cultures are
performed and assessed every 3 months in the first 6-month completeness of treatment and

then every 6 months for 18 months. Chest radiological examinations are preformed when indicated.

Cured	patient who treated with MDR-TB treatment regimen following the Thailand's 2012 National Tuberculosis Control Management (or NTP) Guidelines with consecutively 5- negative results of the 30 day-interval AFB smear examinations and cultures of the last 12 months of treatment duration
Treatment completed	patient with completeness of the MDR-TB treatment following the Thailand's 2012 NTP Guidelines but no consecutively AFB-smear examination and culture results during the last 12-month treatment duration
Died	patient with any cause of death during MDR-TB treatment following the Thailand's 2012 NTP Guidelines
Failed	patient treated with MDR-TB regimen following the Thailand's 2012 NTP Guidelines with 2 positive results of the 5 consecutive AFB-smear examinations and cultures during the last 12 months of treatment duration or patient with 1 positive-culture result of the last 3 consecutive cultures or patient with physician's decision to stop the MDR-TB treatment due to clinical unresponsiveness or various adverse-drug reactions
Default	patient with continuous interruption of the MDR-TB treatment following the Thailand's 2012 NTP Guidelines
Transfer out	partially MDR-TB treated patient with referring from (Transferring out) one setting to another setting with unknown treatment outcomes will be registered as " Transfer out "

Table 3. Classification of treatment outcomes [24]

9. MDR-TB management and treatment outcomes in Thailand between 2007-2009

The prevalence of laboratory-confirmed MDR-TB was 0.08%. Highest prevalence (0.21%) was found in the central part of Thailand. MDR-TB was mostly diagnosed and treated at the secondary care settings or general hospitals (31.5% and 31.14%), 24.3% and 25.08% of cases were diagnosed at the tertiary care settings and only 6.9% and 6.7% of the patients were diagnosed at the university hospitals, respectively [9]. The majority of the patients (63.82%) were registered as " after failure of the first-TB treatment " [9]. In Thailand, numbers of the secondary care settings or general hospitals are more than that of the tertiary care hospitals, this may reflex the above figures. Only 33.5% of cases were referred to the well-facilitated setting for directly observed treatment (DOT) [9]. Only 60.6% of MDR-TB cases were prescribed 4 oral second-line drugs and an injectable aminoglycoside drug [9] which recommended by the Thailand's 2012 National Tuberculosis Management Guidelines while the rests were prescribed various treatment regimens [24]. Only 57.5% of cases had completed treatment adherence [9]. Low DOT implementation can contribute to high default rates, high treatment failure rates, high death rates, and low cured rates. There was 24.2 % of patients with completeness of treatment, 29.1% cured, 20.5% default, 2.2% treatment failure, and 21.5% died [9]. Treatment failure and treatment default rates were higher among new case compared to the patients with previous TB treatment whereas higher death rates were found among the patients with previous TB treatment. This could be due to inadequately strict- and intensive-health education provision to the new cases and more severe disease at the time of diagnosis among the patients with previous TB treatment. Only 27.5% of cases with completed treatment were followed up more than 2 months [9].

A recent study in South Korea revealed that the treatment regimen was individualized based on the history of anti-TB drugs taken by the patient and the most DST result [69]. Three to seven anti-TB drugs were self-administered except injectable drugs during hospitalization [69]. Injectable drugs were prescribed for 6-7 months [69]. The total treatment duration was at least 18 months after sputum culture conversion [69]. If the medical treatment was expected to fail or had failed in patients with localized lung cavities, or bilateral lesions and anticipated adequate postoperative lung function, surgical resection was considered [69]. The treatment outcomes showed that 37.1% of patients had treatment success, and 4.5% of them died of all causes during the 3-4 years after treatment initiation [69]. The independent predictors of all-cause mortality were age, history of MDR-TB treatment, XDR-TB, and prothionamide resist-ance [69]. Currently, there is no DOTS programme implementation in South Korea [69] while Thailand has been implemented several years ago, but the treatment outcomes were better than that of Thailand [9, 69]. These different results of both projects should be intensively investigated and explained. Kliiman K et al. recently demonstrated that predictors of poor treatment outcomes in MDR-TB were previous TB treatment, ofloxacin resistance, positive-AFB smear, and HIV-infection/AIDS [70].

The criteria for capacity of establishment of the specialized MDR-TB centre that recommended by the Thailand' s 2012 NTP guidelines [24] are as the following : 1.authorized persons' recognition of the MDR-TB threats 2.good laboratory networks and good patient-referral system 3.good DOT system, and 4.consistently continuous care for MDR-TB patients.

10. XDR-TB treatment

A previous study in Peru by Mitnick CD et al. demonstrated that 48 (7.4%) of 651 tested-isolate patients had XDR-TB [71]. The results showed various individualized regimens prescribed for 47 patients with XDR-TB as the following : 1) 14.9% of the patients included ethambutol, 2) 34.0% included pyrazinamide, 3) 38.3% included streptomycin, 4) 19.1% included amikacin, 5) 53.2% included capreomycin, 6) 17.0% included kanamycin, 7) 21.3% included ciprofloxacin, 8) 12.8% included ofloxacin, 9) 42.6% included levofloxacin, 10) 2.1% included spafloxacin, 11) 72.3% included moxifloxacin, 12) 100% included cycloserine, 13) 66.0% included ethionamide, 14) 95.7% included para-aminosalicylic acid, 15) 100% included amoxicillin-clavulanate, 16) 44.7% included clarithromycin, 17) 97.9% included clofazimine, 18) 17.0% included rifabutin, 19) number of drugs in regimen (number without documented resistance or prior exposure for more than 1 month) : 19.1) 5.3 +/- 1.3 agents among all available agents, 19.2) 3.2 +/- 1.2

agents among 12 agents or classes for which routine DST was performed, 20) median duration of treatment with injectable agents : 15.4 months, and 21) median duration of treatment ranged 8.0- 24.9 months, median duration from treatment initiation to surgery : 11.6 months, and median duration of treatment for patients undergoing surgery : 31.2 months [70]. The median duration of follow-up was 19.4 months [71]. Treatment outcomes revealed that 60.4% of patients were cured or completed treatment [71]. This study is currently the up-to-date information of XDR-TB treatment. Positive AFB-smear, and urban residence could be predictors of poor treatment outcomes in XDR-TB [70]. For patients with mono/poly-resistant drug (s) TB, the recommended treatment regimens are shown in the Table 4 (13).

Mono/Poly-resistant Drug (s)	Regimen
Rifampicin mono-resistance	initial 2 months of isoniazid, pyrazinamide, and ethambutol, and followed by 10-16 months of isoniazid, ethambutol and a fluoroquinolone +/- initial 6 months of an injectable drug
Isoniazid mono-resistance	initial 2 months of rifampicin, pyrazinamide, and ethambutol, and followed by 4-7 months of rifampicin, and a fluoroquinolone (750-1,000 mg of levofloxacin or 400 mg of moxifloxacin substituted for isoniazid in the standard 6-month short-course regimen)
Rifampicin and pyrazinamide (+/- streptomycin) resistance	at least the initial 2-3 months of isoniazid, ethambutol, a fluoroquinolone, and an injectable drug (initial 6 months if extensive disease) for 18 months of total treatment duration
Rifampicin and ethambutol (+/- streptomycin) resistance	at least the initial 2-3 months of isoniazid, pyrazinamide, a fluoroquinolone, and an injectable drug (initial 6 months if extensive disease) for 18 months of total treatment duration
Isoniazid and pyrazinamide resistance	9-12 months of rifampicin, ethambutol,and a fluoroquinolon (longer if extensive disease)
Isoniazid and ethambutol resistance	9-12 months of rifampicin, pyrazinamide, and a fluoroquinolone (longer if extensive disease)
Isoniazid, pyrazinamide, and ethambutol (+/- streptomycin) resistance	at least the initial 2-3 months (6 months if extensive disease) of rifampicin, a fluoroquinolone, an oral second-line drug, an injectable drug for 18 months of total treatment duration

Table 4. Treatment of patients with mono-drug resistant and poly-drug resistant tuberculosis [13]

11. MDR/XDR-TB treatment-pipeline agents or compounds in clinical trials and related innovative researches

Currently, drugs in phase III clinical trials are moxifloxacin, gatifloxacin, and meropenem [72]. Heteronemin, nephalsterol, litosterol, and kahalalides are other interesting compounds which are in pre-clinical stage [72]. Okada M *et al.* conducted a study on granulysin and a new DNA vaccine against MDR/XDR-TB and revealed that agglutinating virus of Japan/Heat-Shock-Protein65DNA+Interleukin-12-12DNA vaccine provided strong therapeutic efficacy in killing MDR/XDR-TB bacilli in mice and monkey models [73]. A recent experiment using MDR-TB monkey models which received normal and genetically altered Bacilli Calmette Gue'rin (BCG) vaccines demonstrated that these 2 groups of monkeys survived well compared to the control group [74]. Another study in XDR-TB mice model showed ability of interleukin-7 to kill the bacilli [74].

12. Totally drug-resistant tuberculosis

Totally drug-resistant tuberculosis (TDR-TB or XXDR-TB) was recently defined as TB bacilli which resist to all first-line and the 6 second-line drugs (para-aminosalicylic acid, fluoroquinolones, aminoglycosides, thiamines, polypeptides, and cycloserine) [75]. Meanwhile, a recent report from the US-CDC listed 7 challenges that should be addressed before new terminology of TDR-TB should be considered for adopting [76], following are the challenges:

1. The definition should not hinge on resistance to all drugs tested, because the number of drugs tested varies widely between laboratories.

2. In vitro testing data suggest cross-resistance among different drugs within a class of drugs or closely related classes of drugs (e.g., polypeptides and aminoglycosides) is not 100%.

3. Research and reference laboratories in many countries do not test for resistance to the third-line drugs (linezolid, thioridazine, other phenothiazines, monobactams (meropenem, imipenem), macrolides, metronidazole and other imidazoles, clofazimine, and amoxicillin/clavulanic acid).

4. DST for several anti-TB drugs is not sufficiently reliable or reproducible; retesting the same isolate provides a different result in many cases.

5. There are several new anti-TB agents in development pipeline that will be prototypes for new classes of antimycobacterial drugs or add new chemical entities to existing class.

6. Avoiding the unintended implication that patients with TDR-TB should not or cannot be treated.

7. Global laboratory capacity for DST of *Mycobacterium tuberculosis* isolates remains limited [75]. Two cases of TDR-TB with controversies of terminology and treatment occurred in 2003 in Italy and firstly reported in 2007 [77]. Currently, in Thailand, patients with all anti-TB drug-resistance will be prescribed isoniazid alone for lifelong whereas no standardized treatment is recommended yet. During 21-22 March 2012, the WHO had convened a technical consultation to discuss the feasibility and implications of a definition to cover more advanced patterns of TB resistance than XDR-TB [78]. The WHO concluded that reports of severe patterns of anti-TB drug resistance (worse than XDR-TB alone) are increasing whereas a new definition of anti-TB drug resistance beyond XDR-TB is not recommended [78]. This undefined resistance patterns contributed to technical difficulties

with DST of several anti-TB agents, the lack of standardized DST methods for several present and new investigational drugs, and insufficient evidence to link such DST results to patients' treatment outcomes [78]. No DST methods for group 5 and new investigational agents currently exist [78]. Molecular DST for the second-line drugs cannot yet replace phenotypic methods [78]. Collaboration between the national TB control programme, Ministries of Public Health, and the pharmaceutical companies will be required to resolve the limitations of treatment options by the compassionate use of new anti-TB agents [78]. The WHO will be the lead in ensuring that better patient data provide a more robust information for future policy decision [78].

13. Conclusion

As countries are purchasing and using second-line drugs, the likelihood of misuse and developing of TB-resistant strains increases. Currently, WHO and its partners have reached the phase of expanding MDR-TB control as a component of a comprehensive TB control programme. Launching in 2002, the Global Fund to Fight AIDS, Tuberculosis and Malaria (GFATM) expected that requests for second-line drugs for MDR-TB management should go through the Green Light Committee to prevent their misuse. The number of Green Light Committee-approved MDR-TB control programme is increasing rapidly as a result of main streaming of MDR-TB management into general TB control efforts. Expanding projects and accelerating evidence gathering are essential to further develop international policies. The TB-endemic countries themselves and the ability of the technical agencies, as well as the donor community are the factors of future success to expand MDR-TB control programmes.

Author details

Attapon Cheepsattayakorn*

Address all correspondence to: attaponche@yahoo.com

10th Zonal Tuberculosis and Chest Disease Centre, Chiang Mai, 10th Office of Disease Prevention and Control, Chiang Mai, Department of Disease Control, Ministry of Public Health, Thailand, Thailand

References

[1] The WHO/IUATLD Global Project on Anti-tuberculosis Drug Resistance Surveillance. Anti-tuberculosis drug resistance in the world 1999-2002. Third Global Report. Communicable Diseases. Geneva : World Health Organization ; 2003.

[2]   The Bureau of Tuberculosis of Thailand' s Project on Anti-tuberculosis Drug Resistance
      Surveillance. Anti-tuberculosis drug resistance in Thailand 1997-1998. First Country
      Report. Nonthaburi, Thailand : Department of Disease Control, Ministry of Public
      Health; 1999.

[3]   The Bureau of Tuberculosis of Thailand ' s Project on Anti-tuberculosis Drug Resistance
      Surveillance. Anti-tuberculosis drug resistance in Thailand 2001-2002. Second Country
      Report. Nonthaburi, Thailand : Department of Disease Control, Ministry of Public
      Health; 2003.

[4]   The Bureau of Tuberculosis of Thailand ' s Project on Anti-tuberculosis Drug Resistance
      Surveillance. Anti-tuberculosis drug resistance in Thailand 2005-2006. Third Country
      Report. Nonthaburi, Thailand : Department of Disease Control, Ministry of Public
      Health; 2007.

[5]   Tuberculosis Annual Report-2008. Bangkok, Thailand : The Bureau of Tuberculosis of
      Thailand ; 2009.

[6]   Tuberculosis Annual Report-2003. Bangkok, Thailand : The Bureau of Tuberculosis of
      Thailand ; 2004.

[7]   Tuberculosis Annual Report-2011. Chiang Mai, Thailand : Tenth Zonal Tuberculosis
      and Chest Disease Centre, Tenth Office of Disease Prevention and Control, Chiang Mai,
      Thailand; 2012.

[8]   Tuberculosis Annual Report-2009. Chiang Mai, Thailand : Tenth Zonal Tuberculosis
      and Chest Disease Centre, Tenth Office of Disease Prevention and Control, Chiang Mai,
      Thailand; 2010.

[9]   The Bureau of Tuberculosis of Thailand ' s Research Project on Anti-tuberculosis Drug
      Resistance Surveillance. Situation of Multidrug-Resistant Tuberculosis in Thailand :
      Fiscal Year 2007-2009. Country Report. Nonthaburi, Thailand : Department of Disease
      Control, Ministry of Public Health; 2010.

[10] Scano F, Vitoria M, Burman W, Harries AD, Gilks CF, Havlir D. Management of HIV-
      infected patients with MDR- and XDR-TB in resource-limited settings. Int J Tuberc
      Lung Dis 2008; 12 (12) : 1370-1375.

[11] Jain A, Dixit P. Multidrug-resistant to extensively drug-resistant tuberculosis : what is
      next? J Biosci 2008 ; 33 (4) : 605-616.

[12] Gillespie SH. Evolution of drug resistance in *Mycobacterium tuberculosis* : clinical and
      molecular perspective. Antimicrob Agents Chemother 2002; 46 (2) : 267-274.

[13] Pinto L, Menzies D. Treatment of drug-resistant tuberculosis. Infect Drug Resist 2011;
      4: 129-135.

[14] Prasad R. Management of multidrug-resistant tuberculosis : practitioner' s view point.
      Indian J Tuberc 2007; 54 (1) : 3-11.

[15] Liu CH, Li HM, Li L, Hu YL, Wang Q, Yang N, *et al.* Anti-tuberculosis drug resistance patterns and trends in a tuberculosis referral hospital, 1997-2009. Epidemiol Infect 2011; 139 (12) : 1909-1918.

[16] Chakroborty A. Drug-resistant tuberculosis : an insurmountable epidemic ? Inflammopharmacology 2011; 19 (3) : 131-137.

[17] Arnadottir T. The Styblo model 20 years later : what holds true ? Int J Tuberc Lung Dis 2009; 13 (6) : 672-690.

[18] Gandhi NR, Andrews JR, Brust JC, Montreuil R, Weissman D, Heo M, *et al.* Risk factors for mortality among MDR- and XDR-TB patients in a high HIV prevalence setting. Int J Tuberc Lung Dis 2012; 16 (1) : 90-97.

[19] Marahatta SB. Multidrug-resistant tuberculosis burden and risk factors : an update. Kathmandu Univ Med J (KUMJ) 2010; 8 (29) : 116-125.

[20] Banerjee R, Schecter GF, Flood J, Porco TC. Extensively drug-resistant tuberculosis : new strains, new challenges. Expert Rev Anti Infect Ther 2008; 6 (5) : 713-724.

[21] Prasad R. Multidrug and extensively drug-resistant TB (M/XDR-TB) : problems and solutions. Indian J Tuberc 2010; 57 (4) : 180-191.

[22] Blomberg B. Antimicrobial resistance in developing countries. Tidsskr Nor Laegeforen 2008; 128 (21) : 2462-2466.

[23] Eurosurveillance editorial team. New WHO Europe Action Plan to fight MDR-TB. http//www.eurosurveillance.org/ViewArticle.aspx?ArticleId=199967   (accessed   4 August 2012).

[24] The Thailand' s 2012 National Tuberculosis Management Guidelines. Bangkok, Thailand : The Bureau of Tuberculosis of Thailand; 2012.

[25] Singh P, Katoch VM. Multidrug-resistant tuberculosis : current status and emerging tools for its management in India. J Commun Dis 2006; 38 (3) : 216-229.

[26] O' Grady J, Maeurer M, Mwaba P, Kapata N, Bates M, Hoelscher M, *et al.* New and improved diagnostics for detection of drug-resistant pulmonary tuberculosis. Curr Opin Pulm Med 2011; 17 (3) : 134-141.

[27] Nodieva A, Jansone I, Broka L, Pole I, Skenders G, Baumanis V. Recent nosocomial transmission and genotypes of multidrug-resistant *Mycobacterium tuberculosis*. Int J Tuberc Lung Dis 2010; 14 (4) : 427-433.

[28] Bodmer T, Strhle A. Diagnosing pulmonary tuberculosis with the Xpert MTB/RIF test. J Vis Exp 2012; 9 (62) : e3547. DOI : 10.3791/3547

[29] Syed J. The tuberculosis diagnostic pipeline. In : Clayden P, Chon L, Collins S, Harrington M, Jefferys R, Jimenez E, Morgan S, Swan T, Syed J, Wingfield C. (eds.) Treatment Action Group. HIV, tuberculosis, and viral hepatitis drugs, diagnosis, vaccines, immune-based therapies, and preventive technologies in development.

London : TAG; 2010. p107-124. http://www.treatmentactiongroup.org (accessed 31 August 2012).

[30] Mishra B, Rockey SM, Gupta S, Srinivasa H, Muralidharan S. Multidrug-resistant tuberculosis : the experience of an urban tertiary care hospital in South India using automated BACTEC 460 TB. Trop Doct 2012; 42 (1) : 35-37.

[31] Deun A Van, Martin A, Palomino JC. Diagnosis of drug-resistant tuberculosis : reliability and rapidity of detection. Int J Tuberc Lung Dis 2010; 14 (2) : 131-140.

[32] Bemer P, Palicova F, Ruesch-Gerdes S, Drugeon HB, Pfyffer GE. Multicenter evaluation of fully automated BACTEC mycobacteria growth indicator tube 960 system for susceptibility testing of *Mycobacterium tuberculosis*. J Clin Microbiol 2002; 40 (1) : 150-154.

[33] Dang TM, Nguyen TN, Wolbers M, Vo SK, Hoang TT, Nguyen HD, *et al.* Evaluation of microscopic observation drug susceptibility assay for diagnosis of multidrug-resistant tuberculosis in Vietnam. BMC Infect Dis 2012 Mar 1; 12 : 49.

[34] Guillerm M, Usdin M, Arkinstall J., editors. Tuberculosis diagnosis and drug sensitivity testing, an overview of the current diagnostic pipeline. Geneva : Me'decins Sans Frontie'res : Campaign for Access to Essential Medicines; 2006. http://www.access@geneva.msf.org and http://www.accessmed-msf.org (accessed 11 September 2012).

[35] Bonnet M, Gagnidze L, Varaine F, Ramsay A, Githui W, Guerin PJ. Evaluation of FASTPlaqueTB™ to diagnose smear-negative tuberculosis in a peripheral clinic in Kenya. Int J Tuberc Lung Dis 2009; 13 (9) : 1112-1118.

[36] Piuri M, Jacobs WR Jr, Hatfull GF. Fluoromycobacteriophages for rapid, specific, and sensitive antibiotic susceptibility testing of *Mycobacterium tuberculosis*. PLoS ONE 2009; 4(3): e4870. DOI: 10.1371/journal.pone.0004870

[37] Rondo'n L, Piuri M, Jacobs WR Jr, Waard Jde, Hatfull GF, Takiff HE. Evaluation of fluoromycobacteriophages for detecting drug resistance in *Mycobacterium tuberculosis*. J Clin Microbiol 2011; 49 (5) : 1838-1842.

[38] Musa HR, Ambroggi M, Souto A, Aengeby KAK. Drug susceptibility testing of *Mycobacterium tuberculosis* by a nitrate reductase assay applied directly on microscopy-positive sputum samples. J Clin Microbiol 2005; 43 (7) : 3159-3161.

[39] Martin A, Paasch F, Von Groll A, Fissette K, Almeida P, Varaine F, *et al.* Thin-layer agar for detection of resistance to rifampicin, ofloxacin and kanamycin in *Mycobacterium tuberculosis* isolates. Int J Tuberc Lung Dis 2009; 13 (10) : 1301-1304.

[40] Minion J, Leung E, Menzies, Pai M. Microscopic-observation drug susceptibility and thin layer agar assays for the detection of drug resistant tuberculosis : a systematic review and meta-analysis. Lancet Infect Dis 2010; 10 (10) : 688-698.

[41] Martin A, Portaels F, Palomino JC. Colorimetric redox-indicator methods for the rapid detection of multidrug resistance in *Mycobacterium tuberculosis* : a systematic review and meta-analysis. J Antimicrob Chemother 2007; 59 (2) : 175-183.

[42] Martin A, Paasch F, Docx S, Fissette K, Imperiale B, Ribo'n W, *et al.* Multicenter laboratory validation of the colorimetric-redox indicator (CRI) assay for the rapid detection of extensively drug-resistant (XDR) *Mycobacterium tuberculosis.* J Antimicrob Chemother 2011; 66 (4) : 827-833.

[43] Rossau R, Traore H, Beenhouwer Hde, Mijs W, Jannes G, Rijk Pde, *et al.* Evaluation of the INNO-LiPA Rif.TB assay, a reverse hybridization assay for the simultaneous detection of *Mycobacterium tuberculosis* complex and its resistance to rifampicin. Antimicrob Agents Chemother 1997; 41 (10) : 2093-2098.

[44] Viveiros M, Leandro C, Rodrigues L, Almeida J, Bettencourt R, Couto I, *et al.* Direct application of the INNO-LiPA Rif.TB line-probe assay for rapid identification of *Mycobacterium tuberculosis* complex strains and detection of rifampicin resistance in 360 smear-positive respiratory specimens from an area of high incidence of multidrug-resistant tuberculosis. J Clin Microbiol 2005; 43 (9) : 4880-4884.

[45] Abebe G, Paasch F, Apers L, Rigouts L, Colebunders R. Tuberculosis-drug resistance testing by molecular methods : opportunities and challenges in resource-limited settings. J Microbiol Methods 2011; 84 (2) : 155-160.

[46] O'Grady J, Bates M, Chilukutu L, Mzyece J, Cheelo B, Chilufya M, *et al.* Evaluation of the Xpert MTB/RIF assay at a tertiary care referral hospital in a setting where tuberculosis and HIV infection are highly endemic. Clin Infect Dis 2012 Aug 23. [Epub ahead of print].

[47] Rachow A, Zumla A, Heinrich N, Rojas-Ponce G, Mtafya B, Reither K, *et al.* Rapid and accurate detection of *Mycobacterium tuberculosis* in sputum samples by Cepheid Xpert MTB/RIF assay-a clinical validation study. PLoS ONE 2011; 6 (6) : e20458. DOI : 10.1371/journal.pone.0020458

[48] Shimizu Y, Dobashi K, Yoshikawa Y, Yabe S, Higuchi S, Koike Y, *et al.* Five-antituberculosis drug-resistance genes detection using array system. J Clin Biochem Nutr 2008; 42 (3) : 228-234.

[49] Wilson ML. Recent advances in the laboratory detection of *Mycobacterium tuberculosis* complex and drug resistance. Clin Infect Dis 2011; 52 (11) : 1350-1355.

[50] Cha J, Lee HY, Lee KS, Koh WJ, Kwon OJ, Yi CA, *et al.* Radiological findings of extensively drug-resistant pulmonary tuberculosis in non-AIDS adults : comparisons with findings of multidrug-resistant and drug-sensitive tuberculosis. Korean J Radiol 2009; 10 (3) : 207-216.

[51] Lee ES, Park CM, Goo JM, Yim JJ, Kim HR, Lee IS, *et al.* Computed tomography features of extensively drug-resistant pulmonary tuberculosis in non-HIV-infected patients. J Comput Assist Tomogr 2010; 34 (4) : 559-563.

[52] Sneag DB, Schaaf HS, Cotton MF, Zar HJ. Failure of chemoprophylaxis with standard antituberculosis agents in child contacts of multidrug-resistant tuberculosis cases. Pediatr Infect Dis J 2007; 26 (12) : 1142-1146.

[53] Ahuja SD, Ashkin D, Avendano M, Banerjee R, Bauer M, Bayona JN, et al. Multidrug-resistant pulmonary tuberculosis treatment regimens and patient outcomes : an individual patient data meta-analysis of 9,153 patients. PLoS Med 2012; 9 (8) : e1001300. DOI : 10.1371/journal.pmed.1001300

[54] Falzon D, Jaramillo E, Schünemenn HJ, Arentz M, Bauer M, Bayona J , et al. WHO guidelines for the programmatic management of drug-resistant tuberculosis. Eur Respir J 2011; 38 (3) : 516-528.

[55] Nathanson E, Weezenbeek L-van, Rich ML, Gupta R, Bayona J, Blöndal K, et al. Multidrug-resistant tuberculosis management in resource-limited settings. Emerg Infect Dis 2006; 12 (9) : 1389-1397.

[56] Cheepsattayakorn A, Cheepsattayakorn R. The outcome of tuberculosis control in special high-risk populations in northern Thailand : an observational study. Journal of Health Systems Research 2009; 3 (4) : 558-566.

[57] Joseph P, Desai VBR, Fredrick JS, Ramachandran R, Raman B, Wares F, et al. Outcome of standardized treatment for patients with MDR-TB from Tamil Nadu, India. Indian J Med Res 2011; 133 (5) : 529-534.

[58] Heller T, Lessells RJ, Wallrauch CG, Bärnighausen T, Cooke GS, Mhlongo L, et al. Community-based treatment for multidrug-resistant tuberculosis in rural KwaZulu-Natal, South Africa. Int J Tuberc Lung Dis 2010; 14 (4) : 420-426.

[59] Kurbatova EV, Gammino VM, Bayona J, Becerra MC, Danilovitz M, Falzon D, et al. Predictors of sputum culture conversion among patients treated for multidrug-resistant tuberculosis. Int J Tuberc Lung Dis 2012; 16 (10) : 1335-1343.

[60] Dheda K, Shean K, Zumla A, Badri M, Streicher EM, Page-Shipp L, et al. Early treatment outcomes and HIV status of patients with extensively drug-resistant tuberculosis in South Africa : a retrospective cohort study. Lancet 2010; 375 (9728) : 1798-1807.

[61] Well CD. Global impact of multidrug-resistant pulmonary tuberculosis among HIV-infected and other immunocompromised hosts : epidemiology, diagnosis, and strategies for management. Curr Infect Dis Rep 2010; 12 (3) : 192-197.

[62] Shenoi SV, Brooks RP, Barbour R, Altice F, Zelterman D, Moll AP, et al. Survival from XDR-TB is associated with modifiable clinical characteristics in rural South Africa. PLoS ONE 2012;7(3):e31786. DOI : 10.1371/journal.pone.0031786

[63] LoBue P. Extensively drug-resistant tuberculosis. Curr Opin Infect Dis 2009; 22 (2) : 167-173.

[64] Monedero I, Caminero JA. MDR-/XDR-TB management : what it was, current standards and what is ahead. Expert Rev Respir Med 2009; 3 (2) : 133-145.

[65] Monedero I, Caminero JA. Management of multidrug-resistant tuberculosis : an update. Ther Adv Respir Dis 2010; 4 (2) : 117-127.

[66] Schaaf HS, Marais BJ. Management of multidrug-resistant tuberculosis in children : a survival guide for paediatricians. Paediatr Respir Rev 2011; 12 (1) : 31-38.

[67] Mellado Peña MJ, Baquero-Artigao F, Moreno-Perez D; Grupo de Trabajo de Tuberculosis de la Sociedad Española de Infecologia Pedia'trica. Recommendations of the Spanish Society for Pediatric Infectious Diseases (SEIP) on the management of drug-resistant tuberculosis. An Pediatr (Barc) 2009; 71 (5) : 447-458.

[68] Ozkutuk N, Surucuoglu S, Gazi H, Coskun M, Ozkutuk A, Ozbakkaloglu B. Second-line drug susceptibilities of multidrug-resistant *Mycobacterium tuberculosis* isolates in Aegean region-Turkey. Turk J Med Sci 2008; 38 (3) : 245-250.

[69] Jeon DS, Shin DO, Park SK, Seo JE, Seo HS, Cho YS, *et al.* Treatment outcome and mortality among patients with multidrug-resistant tuberculosis in tuberculosis hospitals of the public sector. J Korean Med Sci 2011; 26 (1) : 33-41.

[70] Kliiman K, Altraja A. Predictors of poor treatment outcome in multi- and extensively drug-resistant pulmonary TB. Eur Respir J 2009; 33 (5) : 1085-1094.

[71] Mitnick CD, Shin SS, Seung KJ, Rich ML, Atwood SS, Furin JJ, *et al.* Comprehensive treatment of extensively drug-resistant tuberculosis. N Engl J Med 2008; 359 (6) : 563-574.

[72] Cheepsattayakorn A, Cheepsattayakorn R. Novel compounds and drugs and recent patents in treating multidrug-resistant and extensively drug-resistant tuberculosis. Recent Pat Antiinfect Drug Discov 2012; 7 (2) : 141-156.

[73] Okada M, Kita Y, Nakajima T, Kanamura N, Hashimoto S, Nagasawa T, *et al.* Novel therapeutic vaccine : granulysin and new DNA vaccine against tuberculosis. Human vaccines 2011; 7 Supplement : 60-67.

[74] Institute of Medicine (US) Forum on Drug Discovery, Development, and Translation; Russian Academy of Medical Science. The New Profile of Drug-Resistant Tuberculosis in Russia : A Global and Local Perspective : Summary of a joint Workshop. Washington (DC) : National Academies Press (US); 2011. 6, Treatment of Drug-Resistant TB. http:// www.ncbi.nlm.nih.gov/book/NBK62451/ (accessed 1 October 2012).

[75] Caminero JA. Treatment of tuberculosis according to the different pattern of resistance. Med Clin (Barc) 2010; 134 (4) : 173-181.

[76] Cegielski P, Nunn P, Kurbatova EV, Weyer K, Dalton TL, Wares DF, *et al.* Challenges and controversies in defining totally drug-resistant tuberculosis. Emerg Infect Dis. http://dx.doi.org/10.3201/eid1811.120256,   http://dx.doi.org/10.3201/eid1811.120256, http:///www..cdc.gov/Other/disclaimer.html, and http://www.cdc.gov/eid/article/ 18/11/12-0256_article.htm (accessed 1 October 2012).

[77] Reichman L. Information about tuberculosis. http://www.tbfacts.org/xdr-tb.html (accessed 1 October 2012).

[78] World Health Organization : Totally Drug-Resistant TB : a WHO consultation on the diagnostic definition and treatment options. http://www.who.int/.../tb/.../ Report_Meeting_totallydrugresistant... (accessed 1 October 2012).

Chapter 13

Epidemiology of
Multidrug Resistant Tuberculosis (MDR-TB)

Dhammika Nayoma Magana-Arachchi

Additional information is available at the end of the chapter

1. Introduction

An understanding of the epidemiology of multidrug resistant tuberculosis (MDR-TB) and the extensively drug-resistant tuberculosis (XDR-TB) is critical for effective control of the global burden of tuberculosis (TB) which is caused by the organisms belonging to the *Mycobacterium tuberculosis* complex. Epidemiology of MDR-TB and XDR-TB will be reviewed here.

The history of tuberculosis treatment has observed sequential development of resistance to anti-tuberculosis drugs over the decades. Para amino salicylic acid (PAS) and isoniazid (INH) were introduced to reduce the development of streptomycin (SM) resistance, which heralded the era of combination treatment for tuberculosis [1]. Within 20 years, resistance to both INH and SM was already a challenge in the use of INH, SM and PAS as the standard anti-tuberculosis regimen. With the discovery of rifampicin (RMP) in 1966 [2] and the expansion of its use between 1970 and 1990, patients who were already carriers of isoniazid (INH) resistant *Mycobacterium tuberculosis* strains became resistant to RMP. This was the start of a progressively growing problem, multi drug resistant tuberculosis (MDR-TB), which has reached epidemic proportions in some countries. In the last two decades, with the misuse of other drugs with anti-tuberculosis action, in particular the fluoroquinolones (FQs), the most effective among the second-line drugs, resistance has dramatically increased to extensively drug-resistant TB (XDR-TB) which is defined as resistance to at least RMP and INH (the definition of multidrug-resistant tuberculosis (MDR-TB)), in addition to any fluoroquinolone, and at least one of the three injectable anti-tuberculosis (TB) drugs capreomycin, kanamycin and amikacin [3].

1.1. Epidemiology

John Last has defined epidemiology as "The study of the distribution and determinants of health-related states or events in specified populations, and the application of this study to the control of health problems" [4]. Epidemiologists are concerned not only with death, illness and disability, but also with more positive health states and, most importantly, with the means to improve health [5]. Epidemiological studies are classified as either observational or experimental. Various methods can be used to carry out epidemiological investigations: surveillance and descriptive studies are used to study distribution while analytical studies are used to study determinants.

The two mostly common terms used in epidemiology are the 'prevalence' and the 'incidence'. The incidence of disease represents the rate of occurrence of new cases arising in a given period in a specified population, while prevalence is the frequency of existing cases in a defined population at a given point in time [5]. These are fundamentally different ways of measuring occurrence, and the relation between incidence and prevalence varies among diseases [5]. [For a comprehensive study on epidemiology, please refer the World Health Organization (WHO) manual on Basic Epidemiology].

1.2. Epidemiology of tuberculosis

Despite the availability of highly efficacious treatment for decades, TB remains a major global health problem. In 1993, WHO declared TB a global public health emergency, at a time when an estimated 7–8 million cases and 1.3–1.6 million deaths occurred each year. In 2010, there were an estimated 8.5–9.2 million cases and 1.2–1.5 million deaths from TB [6]. According to the newest report, has observed a gradual decline in the absolute number of TB cases since 2006 and also in the incidence rates of TB since 2002 [6].

2. Global epidemiology of MDR-TB

2.1. Global epidemiology of MDR-TB (global tuberculosis control: WHO report 2011)

Globally, around 50 000 cases of MDR-TB were notified to WHO in 2010, mostly by European countries and South Africa. This represented 18% of the 290 000 (range, 210 000–380 000) cases of MDR-TB estimated to exist among patients with pulmonary TB who were notified in 2010. The proportion of TB patients estimated to have MDR-TB that were actually diagnosed was under 10% in all of the 27 high MDR-TB countries outside the European Region, with the notable exception of South Africa where 81% of estimated cases were diagnosed. In, 15 high MDR-TB burden countries in the European Region, the proportion of estimated cases that were diagnosed ranged from 24% (in Tajikistan) to over 90% of cases (in Belarus and Kazakhstan); no data were reported from Lithuania. In Russian Federation, which ranks third in terms of estimated numbers of cases of MDR-TB at the global level, the proportion of estimated cases that were diagnosed was 44% in 2010. The numbers of patients diagnosed with MDR-TB and started on treatment with recommended second-line drug regimens in the high MDR-TB burden countries in 2010, at just under 40 000, was less than the number of cases notified [6]

2.2. Regimen surveys and definitions of patients registration groups for treatment of tuberculosis

'Regimen surveys' measure first-line and/or second-line drug resistance among a group of selected patients that cannot be considered representative of a patient population [7]. These surveys help to determine the predominant patterns of drug resistance, and are useful in providing guidance on appropriate regimens for MDR-TB treatment for particular patient groups. These include return cases after treatment failure, chronic cases and symptomatic contacts of MDR-TB cases. According to WHO, Regimen surveys should be conducted in the process of developing MDR-TB treatment programmes, or within selected centres or diagnostic units that regularly address high-risk cases.

The fourth edition of WHO *Guidelines for treatment of tuberculosis* defines patient registration groups by history of previous treatment [8]. [For a comprehensive study on definitions, please refer the document WHO/HTM/TB/2009.420].

2.2.1. New case

For the purpose of surveillance, a 'new case' is defined as a newly registered episode of TB in a patient who, in response to direct questioning denies having had any prior anti-tuberculosis treatment (for up to one month), and in countries where adequate documentation is available, for whom there is no evidence of such history. Determining the proportion of drug resistance among new cases is vital in the assessment of recent transmission.

2.2.2. Previously treated case

For the purpose of surveillance, a 'previously treated case' is defined as a newly registered episode of TB in a patient who, in response to direct questioning admits having been treated for TB for one month or more, or, in countries where adequate documentation is available, there is evidence of such history.

2.2.3. Primary resistance

Patients with TB resistant to one or more anti-tuberculosis drugs, but who have never been previously treated for TB, are said to have "primary resistance" (or "initial resistance") due to transmission of a drug-resistant strain.

2.2.4. Acquired resistance

Patients diagnosed with TB who start anti-tuberculosis treatment and subsequently acquire resistance to one or more of the drugs used during the treatment, are said to have developed "acquired resistance". In the past, resistance among previously treated cases (defined as cases with ≥ one month history of treatment) was used as a proxy for acquired resistance; however, this patient category is now known to also be comprised of patients who have been re-infected with a resistant strain, and patients who were primarily infected with a resistant strain and subsequently failed therapy or relapsed.

2.2.5. Cured

A patient who has completed a course of anti-TB treatment according to programme protocol and has at least five consecutive negative cultures from samples collected at least 30 days apart in the final 12 months of treatment. If only one positive culture is reported during that time, and there is no concomitant clinical evidence of deterioration, a patient may still be considered cured, provided that this positive culture is followed by a minimum of three consecutive negative cultures taken at least 30 days apart.

2.2.6. Failed

Anti-TB treatment will be considered to have failed if two or more of the five cultures recorded in the final 12 months of therapy are positive, or if any one of the final three cultures is positive. Treatment will also be considered to have failed if a clinical decision has been made to terminate treatment early because of poor clinical or radiological response or adverse events. These latter failures can be indicated separately in order to do sub-analysis.

3. Surveillance studies for the assessment of resistance rates and the detection of MDR-TB

MDR-TB poses a therapeutic challenge and is associated with increased mortality. Surveillance studies for the assessment of resistance rates and the detection of MDRTB are therefore crucial in order to optimize empiric drug therapy and to prevent the dissemination of resistant strains in a community [9]. The extent of the problem of MDR-TB has been examined by the WHO in cross-sectional surveys of drug resistance in either clinical series or whole-country cohorts [10]. Cross-sectional surveys almost certainly underestimate the burden and number of cases of MDR-TB because they do not take into account the numerical burden of TB in the high-burden countries [11]. When the exercise is repeated with a mathematical modeling design using drug-resistance estimates and the number of cases of TB, a more accurate picture of the global MDR-TB burden is claimed [12].

3.1. Global project of drug resistance surveillance

The WHO and the IUATLD (International Union against Tuberculosis and Lung Disease) have established a global project of drug resistance surveillance that is based on standard epidemiological methods and quality control through an extensive network of reference laboratories. The Global Project has served as a common platform for country, regional and global level evaluation of the magnitude and trends in anti-tuberculosis drug resistance quantified the growing global burden of MDR-TB and started to document the spread of XDR-TB. Since its launch in 1994, the Global Project has collected and analyzed data on drug resistance from surveys of sampled patients and from national surveillance systems from an ever increasing number of settings around the world [7].

The review of Cohn et al, 1997 represented a comprehensive description of worldwide drug resistance surveys performed during the 1990s. According to the study, resistance to multiple drugs varied by geographic region and was more common when resistance was acquired rather than primary. The rate of multidrug resistance (and occasionally other drugs) was low in most surveys of primary resistance, ranging from 0 to 10.8% (median rate, 0.5%); however, for acquired resistance, the rate of multidrug resistance ranged from 0 to 48.0% (median rate, 12.2%). For surveys that did not distinguish between primary and acquired resistance, the range was 0.5% to 14.3% (median rate, 2.3%). In terms of antituberculous drug resistance, they found a great deal of variability between different countries, and within some countries, differences between regions or cities [13].

The review of Caminero et al of 2010 [14], broadly discuss the epidemiological data of the global report, issued in 2008. The report included drug susceptibility data from 90 726 patients in 83 countries and territories from year 2002 to 2007. The median prevalence of resistance in new cases of TB was 11.1% for any drug and 1.6% for MDR-TB. The prevalence of MDR-TB in new TB cases ranged from 0% in eight countries to 22.3% in Baku, Azerbaijan, and 19.4% in the Republic of Moldova. Of the 20 settings with the highest proportion of MDR-TB in new cases, 14 were located in countries of the former Soviet Union (between 6.8% and 22.3% in nine countries, including Moldovia and Azerbaijan) and four in China (7% in two provinces in China) [15, 16], A trend analysis of the 2008 report shows that between 1994 and 2007 the prevalence of MDR-TB in new cases (initial resistance) increased substantially in South Korea and two Russian Oblasts, Tomsk and Orel. By contrast, the prevalence remained stable in Estonia and Latvia, both of which have high rates of initial MDR-TB. The prevalence of MDR-TB in all TB cases decreased in Hong Kong and the United States [14].

Of 37 countries and territories that reported representative data on XDR-TB, five countries, all from the former Soviet Union, each reported 25 or more cases of XDR-TB, with MDR-TB prevalence ranging from 6.6% to 23.7% [15, 16], data from Eastern Mediterranean countries showed that the prevalence of initial MDR-TB was higher than previously estimated, with the exception of Morocco and Lebanon, with rates of respectively 0.5% and 1.1%. Initial MDR-TB rates in Jordan and Yemen were respectively 5.4% and 2.9%. The Americas, Central Europe and Africa reported the lowest rates of initial MDR-TB, with the notable exceptions of Peru, Rwanda and Guatemala, which reported rates of respectively 5.3%, 3.9% and 3.0%. [15, 16]. Data on previously treated cases from the WHO/ Union 2008 report were available for 66 countries and two regions of China [15]. Drug susceptibility testing (DST) results were available for 12 977 patients. Resistance to at least one anti-tuberculosis drug ranged from 0% in three European countries to 85.9% in Tashkent, Uzbekistan. The highest proportions of MDR-TB were reported in Tashkent (60.0%) and Baku, Azerbaijan (55.8%). data from Gujarat State, India, providing the first reliable descriptions of previously treated cases in India, showed 17.2% MDR-TB in this group [15].

The 2008 WHO/Union report also included a global estimation of the MDR-TB problem [14]. Based on drug resistance data from 114 countries and two regions of China reporting to this project, combined with nine other epidemiological factors, the proportion of MDR-TB among new, previously treated and combined cases was estimated for countries with no survey information available. The estimated proportion of MDR-TB for all countries was then applied to incident TB cases (also based on indirect estimates). It was calculated that 4 89 139 (95% confidence limits [95%CL] 455 093–614 215) cases emerged in 2006, and that the global proportion of MDR-TB among all cases was 4.8% (95%CL 4.6–6.0). India, China and the Russian Federation were estimated to have the highest number of MDR-TB cases: India and China have approximately 50% of the global burden and the Russian Federation a further 7%. Twenty seven countries accounted for 86% of the world's MDRTB burden [14].

Caminero et al, divided the world into four large regions according to the influence of the three factors i.e., past and present management of TB and transmission of MDR-TB.

1. Countries with an epidemic: high prevalence and incidence of MDR-TB.

2. Countries with high MDR-TB prevalence but low or decreasing incidence.

3. Countries with low prevalence and incidence of MDR-TB and

4. Countries with low prevalence but an increasing incidence of MDR-TB.

The fourth edition of WHO *Guidelines for surveillance of drug resistance in tuberculosis* is an updated version of earlier editions published in 1994, 1997 and 2003. These guidelines incorporate the 2007 WHO *Interim recommendations for the surveillance of drug resistance in tuberculosis* and the conclusions of an Expert Committee Meeting on Anti-Tuberculosis Drug Resistance Surveys held in Geneva in September 2008. In addition experience gained from 15 years of the Global Project on Anti-Tuberculosis Drug Resistance Surveillance is also included [7].

Given below are some of the updates and clarifications in surveillance methodology that have been incorporated into the 4th edition:

1. At a minimum, surveillance should evaluate susceptibility to the following drugs:

a. Isoniazid and rifampicin;

b. If resistance is detected to rifampicin, then susceptibility to the fluoroquinolones and second- line injectable agents most often used in the setting have be tested. Testing for susceptibility to the first-line drug ethambutol should also be considered.

2. Statistical and epidemiological methodology is a fundamental aspect of designing surveys that sample patients, and appropriate technical assistance should be received in the early stages of planning. In particular, for surveys that use cluster-based sampling methods, results should be adjusted to correct for biases introduced by these sampling techniques. Missing values should also be accounted for, e.g. using multiple imputation techniques when possible.

3. MDR-TB management is a component of the Stop TB Strategy and WHO Member States have committed themselves to achieve universal access to diagnosis and treatment by 2015. Therefore, all drug resistance surveillance activities should be linked to patient treatment and care. Planning a comprehensive treatment programme for patients identified during a survey as having drug-resistant TB should run in parallel to planning the survey itself.

3.2. MDR-TB and immigration

Gilad et al [9] assessed the incidence of TB in Southern Israel in the period between 1992 and 1997, and studied the prevalence of resistance to anti-TB drugs and its distribution among the various subpopulations inhabiting that region, with the intention of tailoring the empirical anti-TB treatment guidelines to those subpopulations. This study described the unique epidemiology of drug-resistant TB in Southern Israel, a region inhabited by both native and immigrant populations. Significant differences in age, gender, and resistance rates were found among the four distinct subpopulations inhabiting the Negev region. They attributed the observed differences to immigration from countries of high prevalence of drug-resistant TB. According to an earlier 10-year survey (1978- 1987) of TB in the Negev, Ethiopian immigrants and Bedouin Arabs comprised 76% of TB cases and 33% of them were extrapulmonary TB [17]. However the study of Gilad et al [9], recorded only 20% of isolates as extrapulmonary, and Ethiopian immigrants and Bedouin Arabs comprised only 40% of the cases. These differences demonstrate how dynamic this disease might be, tremendously influenced by immigration, and demonstrate the importance of continued surveillance in such a setup [9].

A worldwide survey of drug resistance rates by the WHO [18] demonstrated high rates of resistance among isolates in the former Soviet Union, with the highest rates detected in Latvia. The Resistance rates observed rom the study for the immigrants from the former Soviet Union (IFSU) were much higher than those encountered in the Russian republic for every drug or drug combination [9]. These rates were very similar to those found in Latvia, and were even higher overall (50% and 41.5%, respectively). In this current era, import of infectious diseases across international borders occurs much readily [9]. The studies done in Germany and Canada also had reported an increased incidence of multidrug resistance due to the immigration [19-21].

These studies have shown the impact of immigration on the incidence and distribution of drug-resistant TB in a particular country and the importance of continuous surveillance and immediate therapeutic decisions to prevent the dissemination of such resistant strains to their general populations [9].

3.3. HIV and MDR-TB

The epidemiological impact of HIV on the epidemic of drug-resistant TB is not known and may depend on several factors. HIV-positive TB cases are more likely to be smear negative. In addition, delayed diagnosis of drug resistance and unavailability of treatment (particularly in previous years) have led to high death rates in people living with HIV. Both of these factors (smear negativity and short duration of disease due to mortality) may suggest a lower rate of general transmission. However, HIV-positive cases progress more rapidly to disease and in settings where MDR-TB is prevalent (either in the general population or in the local population such as a hospital or a district), this may lead to rapid development of a pool of drug-resistant TB patients or an outbreak [7].

According to Cohn et al, 1997 [13], though the association of MDR-TB with AIDS has been well documented during outbreaks [22-24], the role of HIV infection as a risk factor for the development of drug-resistant TB in other settings was not clear [25]. In Kenya, Malawi, Tanzania, COte d'Ivoire, and France, drug resistance was not associated with HIV infection [26-30]. In contrast, in a survey of eight metropolitan areas of the United States, HIV infection was associated with resistance to antituberculous drugs, both within and outside the New York City area [31]. The acquired MDR-TB also occurs in largely immunocompetent hosts, which was seen in India, Korea, Nepal, and Bolivia [32-35].

The studies by Borrell and Gagneux [36] pointed out that, from a scientific point of view, the actual evidence for primary transmission of MDR -TB in HIV-negative individuals that has been confirmed by molecular methods is very limited, and that more studies including molecular data are needed to know the true extent of primary MDR-TB & XDR –TB in a general population.

3.4. Inadequate treatment and development of MDR and XDR-TB

Multidrug-resistant tuberculosis (MDR-TB) is a major challenge for TB control worldwide. Inadequate treatment of MDR-TB inevitably results in high mortality and the development of XDR-TB [37]. The study of Jeon et al, 2011 [38], shows how inadequate treatment has contributed to the high prevalence of MDR and XDR-TB in Korea. According to Jeon et al, the three TB referral hospitals in the public sector are responsible for the management of MDR-TB in the public sector of Korea. This study showed poor outcome for patients with MDR-TB at the 3 TB hospitals in Korea: low treatment success rate (37.1%), high default rate (37.1%), and high all-cause mortality rate (31.2 %) during the 3-4 yr after treatment initiation. Since the National Tuberculosis Program (NTP) of Korea has focused on new cases, there have been limited nationwide data about the incidence and prevalence of MDR-TB and its treatment outcomes. Treatment success rate of their study was the lowest ever reported among MDR-TB cohorts in Korea [38].

4. Molecular epidemiology of MDR-TB

4.1. Molecular epidemiology

Many different definitions of molecular epidemiology have been published and all mention the use of molecular tools, but not all explicitly mention epidemiology. Molecular epidemiology is not just molecular taxonomy, phylogeny, or population genetics but the application of these techniques to epidemiologic problems [39]. Epidemiology attempts to identify factors that determine disease distribution in time and place, as well as factors that determine disease transmission, manifestation, and progression. Further, epidemiology is always motivated by an opportunity or possibility for intervention and prevention [39]. What distinguishes molecular epidemiology is both the "molecular," the use of the techniques of molecular biology to characterize nucleic acid- or amino acid-based content, and the "epidemiology," the study of the distribution and determinants of disease occurrence in human populations [39].

Molecular epidemiology makes use of the genetic diversity within strains of infectious organisms to track the transmission of these organisms in human populations and to evaluate the host and parasite -specific risk factors for disease spread.

Therefore molecular epidemiologic techniques can be incorporated into almost any epidemiologic assessment to improve exposure and outcome measures

4.2. Molecular epidemiology of TB

The molecular epidemiologic approach to studying tuberculosis epidemiology has identified several new observations that could not have been obtained by conventional epidemiologic or laboratory approaches [39]. Mycobacterial strain typing by means of molecular methods has become an important instrument for tuberculosis surveillance, control and prevention [40]. Among DNA fingerprinting methods which restriction fragment length polymorphism (RFLP) typing is the most common method used has permitted novel investigations of the epidemiology and pathogenesis of tuberculosis. The use of IS6110, an insertion sequence which is present in *Mycobacterium tuberculosis*, is generally considered to be the gold standard for tuberculosis molecular epidemiology studies [41], but other molecular typing techniques could be used as adjuncts in selected circumstances [42].

Spoligotyping is a technique based on the polymorphism of the direct repeat (DR) locus present in *M. tuberculosis* DNA. The DR sequences are composed of multiple 36bp copies, interspersed by short non repetitive sequences [43]. The direct-repeat locus in *M. tuberculosis* contains 10 to 50 copies of a 36-bp direct repeat, which are separated from one another by spacers that have different sequences. However, the spacer sequences between any two specific direct repeats are conserved among strains. Because strains differ in terms of the presence or absence of specific spacers, the pattern of spacers in a strain can be used for genotyping (spacer oligonucleotide typing, or "spoligotyping"). Spoligotyping has two advantages over IS6110-based genotyping. As small amounts of DNA are required, it can be performed on clinical samples or on strains of *M. tuberculosis* shortly after their inoculation into liquid culture. In addition the results of spoligotyping, which are expressed as positive or negative for each spacer, can be expressed in a digital format. However, spoligotyping has less power to discriminate among *M. tuberculosis* strains than does IS6110-based genotyping.

Mycobacterial interspersed repeat units (MIRU) genotyping categorizes the number and size of the repeats in each of 12 independent MIRUs, with the use of a polymerase-chain-reaction (PCR) assay, followed by gel electrophoresis to categorize the number and size of repeats in 12 independent loci, each of which has a unique repeated sequence. Two to eight alleles are at each of the 12 loci, yielding approximately 20 million possible combinations of alleles. The discriminatory power of MIRU genotyping is almost as great as that of IS6110-based genotyping. Unlike IS6110-based genotyping, MIRU analysis can be automated and can thus be used to evaluate large numbers of strains, yielding intrinsically digital results that can be easily catalogued on a computer data base.

The PGRS, the DR and the GTG repeated sequences have mainly been used for sub typing strains for which differentiation by IS6110 finger printing appeared insufficient. This is useful when *M. tuberculosis* strains contain no or lesser than six copies of IS*6110*. According to a recorded study in Sri Lanka, 68% of the isolates had less than five copies which were similar to that of other countries in the Asian region, such as India, Malaysia, Oman and Hong Kong [44].

The study by Ghebremichael et al [45] determined the transmission pattern of TB strains in Sweden. By MIRU-VNTR 31 (45%) of the 69 patients with Beijing strains were found in altogether 7 clusters (2–11 per cluster), yielding 45 different patterns. Thus the MIRU-VNTR typing, with fewer and larger clusters, was less discriminatory than IS*6110* RFLP. The two strains where a possible epidemiological linkage was established differed in one allele and thus did not cluster in MIRU-VNTR. All strains that clustered by MIRU-VNTR were identical also by RD deletions, mutT gene polymorphism and Rv3135 gene analysis, but not by spoligotyping and IS1547. Four of the IS*6110* RFLP clusters contained isolates that differed by MIRU-VNTR. The combination of MIRUVNTR with RFLP resulted in the disappearance of two clusters, and a reduction of the number of isolates in two clusters, compared to the clustering observed with IS*6110* RFLP clustering alone. In this study they found that patients with DR Beijing strains have been diagnosed for more than a decade in Sweden. The majority of the patients were foreign born, and their country of origin reflects areas where the Beijing genotype is prevalent [45].

4.3. Molecular epidemiology of MDR-TB

A study by Calver et al [46], investigated an outbreak of tuberculosis using a molecular epidemiologic approach and clinical and epidemiologic data to identify inadequacies in the implemented DOTS-plus strategy that lead to the emergence of pre–XDR TB and XDR TB in South Africa. They genotyped the drug-resistant *M. tuberculosis* isolates using molecular techniques including insertion sequence (IS) *6110* RFLP, spoligotyping and MIRU typing (12-loci format). Genotyping results indicated an on-going transmission of drug-resistant TB, and contact tracing among case-patients in the largest cluster demonstrated multiple possible points of contact. Phylogenetic analysis demonstrated stepwise evolution of drug resistance, despite stringent treatment adherence. These findings suggested that existing TB control measures in South Africa were inadequate to control the spread of drug-resistant TB in their HIV co-infected population. Diagnosis delay and inappropriate therapy facilitated disease transmission and drug resistance.

Hsu et al, 2010 [47], investigated the transmission and predominant genotypes of MDR- TB in Eastern Taiwan using both spoligotyping and MIRU-VNTR. Of the tested MDR isolates of 73 (94%) Spoligotyping, identified the Beijing strain as the predominant genotype (n = 48, 66%), followed by Haarlem H3 (n = 15, 21%), T1 (n = 3, 4%) and East-African Indian 2 MANILLA (n = 1, 1%). Six (8%) isolates did not match any spoligotype in the SpolDB4 database. Using MIRU-VNTR typing, they observed a unique pattern in 27 isolates, and 46 had clustered pattern strains (10 clusters). According to them by MIRU-VNTR they observed an isolate in cluster 9, however from spoligotyping, it had a unique pattern and therefore they did not considered it as a clustered pattern strain. By considering both spoliotyping and MIRU-VNTR into account, 28 (38.4%) isolates were judged to have a unique pattern and 45 (61.6%) were clustered pattern strains (classifying into 10 clusters). Assuming that there was one source case in each cluster and the rest in the cluster were due to transmission, Hsu et al, concluded that 47.9% ([45 − 10]/ 73) of the patients had MDR-TB due to recent transmission [47].

To better understand the epidemiology of MDRTB, the New York City Tuberculosis Control Program began DNA genotyping of MDRTB strains from new cases in 1995 [48]. The objectives of the study were to provide descriptive molecular epidemiology of MDRTB cases in the city during 1995–1997 and to identify predominant MDR strains present during the three years, as well as the extent and risk factors for clustering among the tested cases. Genotyping results were available for 234 patients; 153 (65.4%) were clustered, 126 (82.3%) of them in eight clusters of >4 patients. Epidemiologic links were identified for 30 (12.8%) patients; most had been exposed to patients diagnosed before the study period. From the analysis, the largest cluster observed was from the "W" strain (59 patients) representing almost 25% of the 241 MDRTB patients during the 3 years. This strain caused a well-documented multi-institutional outbreak in New York City from 1990 through 1993 [49-53]. Strain "W1", which was isolated in seven patients, is a variant of the W strain. It had an additional IS6110 copy and was a part of the W strain outbreak [52, 53]. Forty percent (12 of 30) of the epidemiologic links in this cohort were to patients with these two strains. According to Munsiff et al [48] these strains were likely transmitted in the early 1990s when MDRTB outbreaks and tuberculosis transmission were widespread in New York.

To analyze the molecular epidemiology of M. tuberculosis strains at a hospital in Buenos Aires, Argentina, and mutations related to MDR and XDR-TB, Gonzalo et al [54], conducted a prospective case –control study. Spoligotyping identified predominance of the Haarlem family among the MDR TB cases (family responsible for the 1990s [55] outbreak) as well as the LAM and T families. A similar strain family distribution was reported for the French Departments of the Americas [56] and Turkey [57]. The Beijing family was seldom encountered in these areas, which is in line with recent observations in 7 countries in South America, including Argentina [58]. According to them [54] the MDR TB Haarlem2 strain appears to be more successful than other circulating MDR- TB strains and also than its susceptible counterpart (of 25 Haarlem2 strains, 20 were MDR TB).

By genotyping all isolates and combining with the mutational results, Perdigão et al [59] were able to assess the isolates' genetic relatedness and determine possible transmission events. According to their study strains belonging to family Lisboa, characterized several years ago, were responsible for the majority of the MDR-TB. Even more alarming was the high prevalence of extensive drug-resistant tuberculosis (XDR-TB) among the MDR-TB isolates, which was found to be 53%.

4.4. Transmission of MDR-TB and XDR-TB

Mathematical models predict that the future of the multidrug-resistant (MDR) and extensively drug-resistant (XDR) tuberculosis (TB) epidemic will depend to a large extent on the trans- mission efficiency or relative fitness of drug-resistant Mycobacterium tuberculosis compared to drug-susceptible strains. Molecular epidemiological studies comparing the spread of drug-resistant to that of drug-susceptible strains have yielded conflicting results: MDR strains can be up to 10 times more or 10 times less transmissible than pan-susceptible strains [36].

Experimental work performed with model organisms has highlighted a level of complexity in the biology of bacterial drug resistance that is generally not considered during standard epidemiological studies of TB transmission. However, much more work is needed to understand the detailed molecular mechanisms and evolutionary forces that drive drug resistance in this pathogen. Such increased knowledge will allow for better epidemiological predictions and assist in the development of new tools and strategies to fight drug resistant TB [36].

In infectious disease epidemiology, the relevant measure that reflects the reproductive fitness of a pathogen is the number of secondary cases generated; this measure is also known as the basic reproductive rate, R_0 [60]. In addition to the absolute number of secondary cases (i.e., absolute fitness), an often more useful measure is that of 'relative fitness', where the success of a particular pathogen variant is compared to the success of another. For example, the fitness of a drug-resistant bacterial strain can be expressed relative to the fitness of a drug-susceptible strain. In addition to epidemiological measures of relative fitness, differences in relative fitness can be measured experimentally [36].

The results of experimental studies performed with strains resistant to INH, SM or RMP suggested that, in clinical settings, there was a strong selection pressure for drug resistance-conferring mutations that cause minimal fitness defects [61]. Although these findings support the notion that virulence and competitive fitness assays can be predictive of the epidemiology of drug-resistant TB, they do not capture the overall complexity of the life cycle of *M. tuberculosis* [36]. Although several mechanisms of compensatory evolution have been described in other bacteria [62] little work has been done on this topic in *M. tuberculosis*.

Various molecular tools have been developed to genotype *M. tuberculosis* strains [63]. These tools have been applied to molecular epidemiological investigation of TB transmission for many years. According to the standard concept, patient isolates sharing a particular genotype or DNA 'fingerprint' can be considered epidemiologically linked and represent cases of active TB transmission (i.e., they are clustered TB cases), whereas strains with distinct or 'unique' DNA patterns are thought to reflect reactivation of latent infections. They compared molecular epidemiological fitness estimates from two previous reviews and more recent studies [60, 64]. Overall, the relative fitness estimates for MDR-TB vary dramatically, ranging from an almost 10-fold increased fitness compared to fully drug-susceptible strains found in a study from Russia [65] to about 10-fold lower fitness in Mexico [66] other studies have reported that MDR strains do not cause any secondary cases at all [67]. The reasons for this high variability in relative fitness of MDR strains have likely to do with the differences in study design and setting, differences in sample size and different methodologies and also to the variation in the quality of the TB control programmes [36]. According to Borrell and Gagneux, in addition to methodological, socio-economic and environmental factors, the variation in MDR fitness also reflects biological heterogeneity. Current epidemiological evidence for transmission of MDR- and XDR-TB, particularly compared to pan-susceptible TB, is very inconclusive. This can be partially explained by the fact that *M. tuberculosis* is more genetically diverse than is often appreciated [68] and because drug-resistant strains can exhibit heterogeneous fitness compared to drug-susceptible strains [36].

5. Conclusion

An understanding of the epidemiology of multidrug resistant tuberculosis (MDR-TB) and the extensively drug-resistant tuberculosis (XDR-TB) is critical for effective control of the global burden of tuberculosis (TB). For a comprehensive study on epidemiology of multidrug resistant tuberculosis (MDR-TB), please refer the reviews in the reference list.

6. Future studies

Future Studies on Epidemiology

In all epidemiological studies it is essential to have a clear definition of a case of the disease being investigated by delineating the symptoms, signs or other characteristics indicating that a person has the disease. A clear definition of an exposed person is also necessary. This definition must include all the characteristics that identify a person as being exposed to the factor in question. In the absence of clear definitions of disease and exposure, it is very difficult to interpret the data from an epidemiological study.

Future Studies on Transmission of TB

Future epidemiological studies on the transmission of drug-resistant TB should incorporate more comprehensive strain data, including specific drug resistance-conferring mutations and information on the strain genetic background. These variables, as well as their interaction, could play an important role in the transmission success of particular drug-resistant variants.

Future Studies on HIV/TB

The investigators who conduct the studies on HIV/ TB need to consider other possible risk factors for drug resistance such as demographics; prior therapy, socioeconomic status, and quality of TB control programs, etc.

Acknowledgements

The research works on TB were supported by the grants, RG/2006/HS/07 NSF and 07-47 of NRC and by IFS, Sri Lanka. I am expressing my sincere gratitude to Professor Jennifer Perera and Dr. N.V. Chandrasekaran for their valuable guidance and Dr. D. Medagedara and Professor V. Thevanesam for their support in tuberculosis research and to Ms. R. P. Wanigatunge for technical support in preparation of manuscript.

Author details

Dhammika Nayoma Magana-Arachchi

Address all correspondence to: nayomam@yahoo.com

Cell Biology, Institute of Fundamental Studies, Kandy, Sri Lanka

References

[1] Chiang CY. State of the Art Series on Drug-resistant Tuberculosis: It's Time to Protect Fluoroquinolones. International Journal of Tuberculosis and Lung Disease 2009;13(11) 1319.

[2] Maggi N, Pasqualucci CR, Ballotta R, Sensi P. Rifampicin: A New Orally Active Rifamycin. Chemotherapia 1966;11: 285–292.

[3] Migliori GB, Besozzi G, Girardi E, Kliiman K, Lange C, Toungoussova OS, Ferrara G, Cirillo DM, Gori A, Matteelli A, Spanevello A, Codecasa LR, Raviglione MC, SMIRA/TBNET Study Group. Clinical and Operational Value of the Extensively Drug-Resistant Tuberculosis Definition. European Respiratory Journal 2007;30 623–626.

[4] Jamison DT, Breman JG, Measham AR, Alleyne G, Claeson M, Evans DB, et al., editors. Disease Control Priorities in Developing Countries. New York: Oxford University Press; 2006.

[5] Bonita R, Beaglehole R, Kjellström T. Basic Epidemiology. 2nd Edition. World Health Organization. 2006.

[6] Towards Universal Access to Diagnosis and Treatment of Multidrug-Resistant and Extensively Drug-resistant Tuberculosis. by 2015: WHO Progress Report 2011. WHO/HTM/TB/2011.3

[7] Guidelines for Surveillance of Drug Resistance in Tuberculosis – 4th ed. Geneva, World Health Organization, 2009 (WHO/HTM/TB / 2009.422.)

[8] Guidelines for Treatment of Tuberculosis. Fourth Edition. Geneva, World Health Organization, 2009, (document WHO/HTM/TB /2009.420).

[9] Gilad J, Borer A, Riesenberg K, Peled N, Schlaeffer F. Epidemiology and Ethnic Distribution of Multidrug-Resistant Tuberculosis in Southern Israel 1992–1997* The Impact of Immigration. Clinical Investigations CHEST 2000;117 738–743.

[10] Espinal MA, Laszlo A, Simonsen L et al. Global Trends in the Resistance to Antituberculosis Drugs. New England Journal of Medicine 2001;344 1294–1303.

[11] Ormerod. LP. Multidrug-resistant Tuberculosis (MDR-TB): Epidemiology, Prevention and Treatment. British Medical Bulletin 2005;73 and 74 17–24. DOI: 10.1093/bmb / ldh047

[12] Dye C, Espinal MA, Watt CJ et al. Worldwide Incidence of Multidrug-resistant Tuberculosis. Journal of Infectious Diseases 2002;185 1197–2002.

[13] Cohn DL, Bustreo F, Raviglione MC. Drug-Resistant Tuberculosis: Review of the Worldwide Situation and the WHO/IUATLD Global Surveillance Project. Clinical Infectious Diseases 1997;24 (Suppl 1) S121-30.

[14] Caminero JA. Multidrug-Resistant Tuberculosis: Epidemiology, Risk Factors and Case Finding. International Journal of Tuberculosis and Lung Disease 2010;14(4) 382–390.

[15] World Health Organization. The WHO/IUATLD Global Project on Anti-Tuberculosis Drug Resistance Surveillance. Antituberculosis Drug Resistance in the World. Report no. 4. WHO/ HTM/TB/2008.394. Geneva, Switzerland: WHO, 2008: pp 1– 120.

[16] Wright A, Zignol M, Van Deun A, Falzon D, Gerdes SR, Feldman K, Hoffner S, Drobniewski F, Barrera L, van Soolingen D, Boulabhal F, Paramasivan CN, Kam KM, Mitarai S, Nunn P, Raviglione M. Epidemiology of Antituberculosis Drug Resistance 2002–07: An Update Analysis of the Global Project on Anti-Tuberculosis Drug Resistance Surveillance. Lancet 2009;373 1861–1873.

[17] Dolberg OT, Alkan M, Schlaeffer F. Tuberculosis in Israel: A 10-year Survey of an Immigrant Population. Israel Journal of Medical Sciences 1991;27 386–389.

[18] Pablos-Mendez A, Raviglione MC, Laszlo A, et al. Global Surveillance for Antituberculosis-drug Resistance 1994–1997. New England Journal of Medicine 1998;338 1641–1649.

[19] Niemann S, Rusch-Gerdes S, Richter E. IS6110 Fingerprinting of Drug-Resistant Mycobacterium tuberculosis Strains Isolated in Germany during 1995. Journal of Clinical Microbiology 1997;35 3015–3020.

[20] Cowie RL, Sharpe JW. Tuberculosis among Immigrants: Interval from Arrival in Canada to Diagnosis; A 5-year Study in Southern Alberta. Canadian Medical Association Journal 1998;158 611– 612.

[21] Mans BJ, Fanning EA, Cowie RL. Antituberculosis Drug Resistance in Immigrants to Alberta, Canada, with Tuberculosis, 1982–1994. International Journal of Tuberculosis and Lung Disease 1997;1 225–230.

[22] Fischl MA, Uttamchandani RB, Daikos GL, et al. An Outbreak of Tuberculosis Caused by Multiple-drug-resistant Tubercle Bacilli among Patients with HIV Infection. Annals of Internal Medicine 1992;117 177-83.

[23] Dooley SW, Jarvis WR, Martone WJ, Snider DE Jr. Multidrug-resistant Tuberculosis [Editorial]. Annals of Internal Medicine 1992;117 257-259.

[24] Small PM, Shafer RW, Hopewell PC, et al. Exogenous Reinfection with Multidrug-resistant *Mycobacterium tuberculosis* in Patients with Advanced HIV Infection. New England Journal of Medicine 1993;328 1137-44.

[25] Nunn P, Felten M. Surveillance of Resistance to Antituberculosis Drugs in Developing Countries. Tubercle and Lung Disease 1994;75 163-167.

[26] Githui W, Nunn P, Juma E, et al. Cohort Study of HIV-positive and HIV-negative Tuberculosis, Nairobi, Kenya: Comparison of Bacteriological Results. Tubercle and Lung Disease 1992;73 203-209.

[27] Glynn JR, Jenkins PA, Fine PEM, et al. Patterns of Initial and Acquired Antituberculosis Drug Resistance in Karonga District, Malawi. Lancet 1995;345 907-910.

[28] Dupon M, Texier-Maugein J, Leroy V, Sentilhes A, Pellegrin JL, Morlat P, Ragnaud JM, Chêne G, Dabis F. Tuberculosis and HIV Infection: A Cohort Study of Incidence and Susceptibility to Antituberculous Drugs, Bordeaux, 1985-1993. Groupe d'Epidémiologie Clinique du SIDA en Aquitaine. AIDS 1995;9 577-583.

[29] Braun MM, Kilburn JO, Smithwick RW, Coulibaly IM, Coulibaly D, Silcox VA, Gnaore E, Adjorlolo G, De Cock KM. HIV Infection and Primary Resistance to Antituberculosis Drugs in Abidjan, COte d'Ivoire. AIDS 1992;6 1327-1330.

[30] Chum HJ, O'Brien RJ, Chonde TM, Graf P, Rieder HL. An Epidemiological Study of Tuberculosis and HIV Infection in Tanzania, 1991-1993. AIDS 1996;10 299-309.

[31] Gordin FM, Nelson ET, Matts JP, Cohn DL, Ernst J, Benator D, Besch CL, Crane LR, Sampson JH, Bragg PS, El-Sadr W. The Impact of Human Immunodeficiency Virus Infection on Drug Resistant Tuberculosis. American Journal of Respiratory and Critical Care Medicine 1996;154(5) 1478-1483.

[32] Trivedi SS, Desai SG. Primary Antituberculosis Drug Resistance and Acquired Rifampicin Resistance in Gujarat, India. Tubercle 1988;69 37-42.

[33] Kim SJ, Hong YP. Drug Resistance of *Mycobacterium tuberculosis* in Korea. Tubercle and Lung Disease 1992;73 219-224.

[34] Takahashi M, Maskay NL. Drug Resistance of *M. tuberculosis* and Comparison of Drug Sensitivity Test in Nepal. Kekkaku 1993;68 91-97.

[35] De Caballero RS. Estudio de resistencia del *Mycobacterium tuberculosis* a la uimioterapia especifica en 1008 casos. Anuario Ateneo Medicina 1989-1990; 12-14.

[36] Borrell S, Gagneux S. Infectiousness, Reproductive Fitness and Evolution of Drug-Resistant *Mycobacterium Tuberculosis*. International Journal of Tuberculosis and Lung Disease 2009;13(12) 1456–1466.

[37] Jassal M, Bishai WR. Extensively Drug-resistant Tuberculosis. Lancet Infectious Diseases 2009;9 19-30

[38] Jeon DS, Shin DO, Park SK, Seo JE, Seo HS, Cho YS, Lee JY, Kim DY, Kong SJ, Kim YS, Shim TS. Treatment Outcome and Mortality among Patients with Multidrug-resistant

Tuberculosis in Tuberculosis Hospitals of the Public Sector. Infectious Diseases, Microbiology and Parasitology. Journal of Korean Medical Science 2011;26 33-41.

[39] Foxman B, Riley L. Molecular Epidemiology: Focus on Infection. American Journal of Epidemiology 2001;153 1135–1141.

[40] van Soolingen D. Utility of Molecular Epidemiology of Tuberculosis. European Respiratory Journal 1998;11 795-797.

[41] van Embden JDA, Cave MD, Crawford JT, Dale JW, Eisenach KD, Gicquel B, Hermans P, Martin C, Mcadam R, Shinnick TM, Small PM. Strain Identification of *Mycobacterium tuberculosis* by DNA Fingerprinting: Recommendation for a Standardized Methodology. Journal of Clinical Microbiology 1993;31(2) 406-409.

[42] Cohn DL, O'Brien RJ. The Use of Restriction Fragment Length Polymorphism (RFLP) Analysis for Epidemiological Studies of Tuberculosis in Developing Countries. International Journal of Tuberculosis and Lung Disease 1998;2(1) 16-26.

[43] Kamerbeek J, Schouls L, Kolk A, van Agterveld M, van Soolingen D, Kuijper S, Bunschoten A, Molhuizen H, Shaw R, Goyal M, van Embden J. Simultaneous Detection and Strain Differentiation of *M. tuberculosis* for Diagnosis and Epidemiology. Journal of Clinical Microbiology 1997;35(4) 907-914.

[44] Magana Arachchi DN, Perera AJ, Senaratne V, Chandrasekaran NV. Pattern of Drug Resistance and RFLP Analysis on *Mycobacterium tuberculosis* Strains Isolated from Recurrent Tuberculosis Patients. Southeast Asian Journal of Tropical Medicine and Public Health 2010;41(3) 583-589.

[45] Ghebremichael S, Groenheit R, Pennhag A, Koivula T, Andersson E, Bruchfeld J, Hoffner S, Romanus V, Källenius G. Drug Resistant *Mycobacterium tuberculosis* of the Beijing Genotype Does Not Spread in Sweden. PLoS ONE 2010;5(5) e10893. doi:10.1371/journal.pone.0010893

[46] Calver AD, Falmer AA, Murray M, Strauss OJ, Streicher EM, Hanekom M, Liversage T, Masibi M, van Helden PD, Warren RM, and Victor TC. Emergence of Increased Resistance and Extensively Drug-Resistant Tuberculosis Despite Treatment Adherence, South Africa. Emerging Infectious Diseases 16(2);2010 264-271.

[47] Hsu AH, Lin CB, Lee YS, Chiang CY, Chen LK, Tsai YS, Lee JJ. Molecular Epidemiology of Multidrug-resistant *Mycobacterium tuberculosis* in Eastern Taiwan. International Journal of Tuberculosis and Lung Disease 2010;14(6) 924–926.

[48] Munsiff SS, Bassoff T, Nivin B, Li J, Sharma A, Bifani P, Mathema B, Driscoll J, Kreiswirth BN. Molecular Epidemiology of Multidrug-Resistant Tuberculosis, New York City, 1995–1997. Emerging Infectious Diseases 2002;8(11) 1230-1238.

[49] Centers for Disease Control and Prevention. Nosocomial Transmission of Multidrug-resistant Tuberculosis among HIV-infected Persons—Florida and New York, 1988-1991. MMWR Morb Mortal Wkly Rep, 1991;40 589–91.

[50] Valway SE, Richards SB, Kovacovich J, Greifinger RB, Crawford JT, Dooley SW. Outbreak of Multidrug-resistant Tuberculosis in a New York State Prison. American Journal of Epidemiology 1994;140 113–122.

[51] Coronado VG, Beck-Sague CM, Hutton MD, Davis BJ, Nicholas P, Villareal C, et al. Transmission of Multidrug-resistant *Mycobacterium tuberculosis* among Persons with Human Immunodeficiency Virus Infection in an Urban Hospital: Epidemiological and Restriction Fragment Length Polymorphism Analysis. Journal of Infectious Diseases 1993;168 1052– 1055.

[52] Frieden TR, Sherman LF, Maw KL, Fujiwara PI, Crawford JT, Nivin B, et al. A Multi-institutional Outbreak of Highly Drug Resistant Tuberculosis. Journal of the American Medical Association 1996;276 1229–1235.

[53] Nivin B, Nicholas P, Gayer M, Frieden TR, Fujiwara P. A Continuing Outbreak of Multidrug-resistant Tuberculosis, with Transmission in a Hospital Nursery. Clinical Infectious Diseases 1998;26 303–307.

[54] Gonzalo X, Ambroggi M, Cordova E, Brown T, Poggi S, Drobniewski F. Molecular Epidemiology of Mycobacterium tuberculosis, Buenos Aires, Argentina. Emerging Infectious Diseases [Serial on the Internet]. 2011 Mar [2012 September] http://dx.doi.org/10.3201 /eid1703100394

[55] Ritacco V, Di Lonardo M, Reniero A, Ambroggi M, Barrera L, Dambrosi A, Lopez B, Isola N, de Kantor IN. Nosocomial Spread of Human Immunodeficiency Virus–related Multidrug-resistant Tuberculosis in Buenos Aires. Journal of Infectious Diseases. 1997;176 637–642.

[56] Brudey K, Filliol I, Ferdinand S, Guernier V, Duval P, Maubert B, Sola C, Rastogi N. Long-term Population-based Genotyping Study of *Mycobacterium tuberculosis* Complex Isolates in the French Departments of the Americas. Journal of Clinical Microbiology 2006;44 183–191.

[57] Durmaz R, Zozio T, Gunal S, Yaman A, Cavusoglu C, Guney C, Sola C, Rastogi N. Genetic Diversity and Major Spoligotype Families of Drug-resistant *Mycobacterium tuberculosis* Clinical Isolates from Different Regions in Turkey. Infection, Genetics and Evolution 2007;7 513–519.

[58] Ritacco V, López B, Cafrune PI, Ferrazoli L, Suffys PN, Candia N, Vásquez L, Realpe T, Fernández J, Lima KV, Zurita J, Robledo J, Rossetti ML, Kritski AL, Telles MA, Palomino JC, Heersma H, van Soolingen D, Kremer K, Barrera L. *Mycobacterium tuberculosis* Strains of the Beijing Genotype are Rarely Observed in Tuberculosis Patients in South America. Memórias do Instituto Oswaldo Cruz 2008;103 489–492.

[59] Perdigão J, Macedo R, João I, Fernandes E, Brum L, Portugal I. Multidrug-resistant Tuberculosis in Lisbon, Portugal: A Molecular Epidemiological Perspective. Microbial Drug Resistance 2008;14(2) 133-143.

[60] Dye C, Williams BG, Espinal MA, Raviglione MC. Erasing the World's Slow Stain: Strategies to Beat Multidrug-resistant Tuberculosis. Science 2002;295 2042–2046.

[61] Bottger EC, Springer B. Tuberculosis: Drug Resistance, Fitness and Strategies for Global Control. European Journal of Pediatrics 2008;167 141– 148.

[62] Maisnier-Patin S, Andersson DI. Adaptation to the Deleterious Effects of Antimicrobial Drug Resistance Mutations by Compensatory Evolution. Research in Microbiology 2004;155 360–369.

[63] Mathema B, Kurepina NE, Bifani PJ, Kreiswirth BN. Molecular Epidemiology of Tuberculosis: Current Insights. Clinical Microbiology Reviews 2006;19 658–685.

[64] Cohen T, Sommers B, Murray M. The Effect of Drug Resistance on the Fitness of *Mycobacterium tuberculosis*. Lancet Infectious Diseases 2003;3 13–21.

[65] Toungoussova OS, Sandven P, Mariandyshev AO, Nizovtseva, NI, Bjune G, Caugant DA. Spread of Drug-resistant *Mycobacterium tuberculosis* Strains of the Beijing Genotype in the Archangel Oblast, Russia. Journal of Clinical Microbiology 2002;40 1930– 1937.

[66] Garcia-Garcia ML, Ponce de Leon A, Jimenez-Corona ME, et al. Clinical Consequences and Transmissibility of Drug-resistant Tuberculosis in Southern Mexico. Archives of Internal Medicine 2000;160 630–636.

[67] Burgos M, DeRiemer K, Small PM, Hopewell PC, Daley CL. Effect of Drug Resistance on the Generation of Secondary Cases of Tuberculosis. Journal of Infectious Diseases 2003;188 1878–1884

[68] Hershberg R, Lipatov M, Small PM, Sheffer H, Niemann S, Homolka S, Roach JC, Kremer K, Petrov DA, Feldman MW, Gagneux S. High Functional Diversity in *Mycobacterium tuberculosis* Driven by Genetic Drift and Human Demography. PLoS Biology 2008;6(12): e311.

Permissions

The contributors of this book come from diverse backgrounds, making this book a truly international effort. This book will bring forth new frontiers with its revolutionizing research information and detailed analysis of the nascent developments around the world.

We would like to thank Dr. Bassam H. Mahboub and Dr. Mayank G. Vats, for lending their expertise to make the book truly unique. They have played a crucial role in the development of this book. Without their invaluable contribution this book wouldn't have been possible. They have made vital efforts to compile up to date information on the varied aspects of this subject to make this book a valuable addition to the collection of many professionals and students.

This book was conceptualized with the vision of imparting up-to-date information and advanced data in this field. To ensure the same, a matchless editorial board was set up. Every individual on the board went through rigorous rounds of assessment to prove their worth. After which they invested a large part of their time researching and compiling the most relevant data for our readers. Conferences and sessions were held from time to time between the editorial board and the contributing authors to present the data in the most comprehensible form. The editorial team has worked tirelessly to provide valuable and valid information to help people across the globe.

Every chapter published in this book has been scrutinized by our experts. Their significance has been extensively debated. The topics covered herein carry significant findings which will fuel the growth of the discipline. They may even be implemented as practical applications or may be referred to as a beginning point for another development. Chapters in this book were first published by InTech; hereby published with permission under the Creative Commons Attribution License or equivalent.

The editorial board has been involved in producing this book since its inception. They have spent rigorous hours researching and exploring the diverse topics which have resulted in the successful publishing of this book. They have passed on their knowledge of decades through this book. To expedite this challenging task, the publisher supported the team at every step. A small team of assistant editors was also appointed to further simplify the editing procedure and attain best results for the readers.

Our editorial team has been hand-picked from every corner of the world. Their multi-ethnicity adds dynamic inputs to the discussions which result in innovative outcomes. These outcomes are then further discussed with the researchers and contributors who give their valuable feedback and opinion regarding the same. The feedback is then collaborated with the researches and they are edited in a comprehensive manner to aid the understanding of the subject.

Apart from the editorial board, the designing team has also invested a significant amount of their time in understanding the subject and creating the most relevant covers. They scrutinized every image to scout for the most suitable representation of the subject and create an appropriate cover for the book.

The publishing team has been involved in this book since its early stages. They were actively engaged in every process, be it collecting the data, connecting with the contributors or procuring relevant information. The team has been an ardent support to the editorial, designing and production team. Their endless efforts to recruit the best for this project, has resulted in the accomplishment of this book. They are a veteran in the field of academics and their pool of knowledge is as vast as their experience in printing. Their expertise and guidance has proved useful at every step. Their uncompromising quality standards have made this book an exceptional effort. Their encouragement from time to time has been an inspiration for everyone.

The publisher and the editorial board hope that this book will prove to be a valuable piece of knowledge for researchers, students, practitioners and scholars across the globe.

List of Contributors

Beatrice Saviola
Basic Medical Sciences, College of Osteopathic Medicine, Western University of Health Sciences, Pomona CA, USA

Armando Acosta, Yamile Lopez, Maria Elena Sarmiento and Nadine Alvarez
Instituto Finlay, La Habana, Cuba

Norazmi Mohd Nor
School of Health Sciences and Institute for Research in Molecular Medicine, Universiti Sains Malaysia, Kubang Kerian, Malaysia

Rogelio Hernández Pando
Experimental Pathology Section, National Institute of Medical Sciences and Nutrition, Mexico City, Mexico

Aharona Glatman-Freedman
New York Medical College, Valhalla, New York, USA

Zeev Theodor Handzel
Pediatric Research Laboratory, Pediatric Division, Kaplan Medical Center, Associated with the Hadassah and Hebrew University-Jerusalem, Rehovot, Israel

Mahavir Singh
LIONEX Diagnostics and Therapeutics GmbH, Braunschweig, Germany
Department of Genome Analytics, Helmholtz Centre for Infection Research, Braunschweig, Germany

Matthias Stehr and Ayssar A. Elamin
LIONEX Diagnostics and Therapeutics GmbH, Braunschweig, Germany

Ruiru Shi
Sino-US Tuberculosis Research Center and Clinical Laboratory Department of Henan Provincial Chest Hospital, Zhengzhou, Henan, China

Isamu Sugawara
Center of Tuberculosis Diagnosis and Treatment, Shanghai Pulmonary Hospital, Tongji, University School of Medicine, Shanghai, China

Raquel Lima de Figueiredo Teixeira, Márcia Quinhones Pires Lopes, Philip Noel Suffys and Adalberto Rezende Santos
Laboratory of Molecular Biology Applied to Mycobacteria – Oswaldo Cruz Institute – Fiocruz, Rio de Janeiro, Brazil

Márcia Quinhones Pires Lopes, Rafael Santos Pinto, Lizânia Borges Spinassé, Raquel Lima de Figueiredo Teixeira, Philip Noel Suffys and Adalberto Rezende Santos
Laboratory of Molecular Biology Applied to Mycobacteria – Oswaldo Cruz Institute – Fiocruz, Av. Brasil, Rio de Janeiro, RJ, Brazil

Antonio Basilio de Miranda
Laboratory of Computational and Systems Biology – Oswaldo Cruz Institute – Fiocruz, Rio de Janeiro, Brazil

Fernanda Carvalho Queiroz Mello and José Roberto Lapa e Silva
Medical School - Hospital Complex HUCFF-IDT - Federal University of Rio de Janeiro (UFRJ), Rio de Janeiro, Brazil

Hum Nath Jnawali and Sungweon Ryoo
Korean Institute of Tuberculosis, Osong Saengmyeong, Cheongwon-gun, Chungcheong-bukdo, Republic of Korea

Gunes Senol
Infectious Diseases and Clinical Microbiology, Izmir Chest Diseases and Chest Surgery Training Hospital, Izmir, Turkey

Mochammad Hatta and A. R. Sultan
Departments of Medical Microbiology, Molecular Biology and Immunology Laboratory, Faculty of Medicine, Hasanuddin University, Makassar, Indonesia

Zakaria Hmama
Division of Infectious diseases, Department of Medicine, University of British Columbia, BC, Canada

Attapon Cheepsattayakorn
10th Zonal Tuberculosis and Chest Disease Centre, Chiang Mai, 10th Office of Disease Prevention and Control, Chiang Mai, Department of Disease Control, Ministry of Public Health, Thailand

Dhammika Nayoma Magana-Arachchi
Cell Biology, Institute of Fundamental Studies, Kandy, Sri Lanka

Printed in the USA
CPSIA information can be obtained
at www.ICGtesting.com
JSHW011443221024
72173JS00004B/923